Issues in Hospital Administration

The Milbank Readers
John B. McKinlay, general editor

Issues in Hospital Administration

Milbank Reader 9

edited by John B. McKinlay

The MIT Press
Cambridge, Massachusetts
London, England

© 1982 by
The Massachusetts Institute of Technology

Printed and bound in the United States of America

Library of Congress Cataloging in Publication Data

Main entry under title:
Issues in hospital administration.

(The Milbank reader series : 9)
Bibliography: p.
Includes index.
1. Hospitals—Administration—Addresses, essays, lectures.
2. Hospitals—United States—Administration—Addresses, essays,
lectures. I. McKinlay, John B. II. Series. [DNLM: 1. Hospital
administration—Collected works. WX 150 I86]
RA971.I85   362.1′1′06   81–12384
ISBN 0–262–63085–0 (pbk.) AACR2
     0–262–13184–6 (hard)

Contents

Foreword

During 1973–74, the Milbank Memorial Fund, in conjunction with Prodist (New York), produced four edited volumes that drew together and organized published papers from the well-known and respected *Milbank Memorial Fund Quarterly*. In producing these four initial resource books (*Research Methods in Health Care, Politics and Law in Health Care Policy, Economic Aspects of Health Care*, and *Organizational Issues in the Delivery of Health Services*), the Fund had attempted to respond to heavy and continuing requests for accessibility and economy of the Milbank papers. The success of the four books exceeded even the most optimistic expectations, and all are now, unfortunately, out of print. They were adopted as course texts by many different health-related disciplines, were used widely throughout North America and abroad, were acquired by many university and professional libraries and were favorably reviewed in internationally respected professional journals.

The foreword to the earlier series noted that we always "planned to keep this series active and responsive to changing needs. Suggestions for future volumes will be welcome." Since their release, there have been numerous inquiries, requests, and suggestions for further volumes dealing with new and emerging issues concerning health care and social policy. The titles included in this second wave of edited volumes attempt to respond again to this widespread enthusiasm and need.

A venture of this nature has several obvious limitations. First of all, the universe from which the contributions were selected was limited to the *Milbank Memorial Fund Quarterly/Health and Society* and to several books produced by the Fund as a result of round-table meetings on particular health-care issues. However, more than enough rich material by eminent scholars was available for at least the present volumes. For the editor, a major problem was to decide which of several excellent papers had to be omitted (for reasons of economy, coverage, datedness, etc.) rather than what was available for inclusion in each volume. It should be emphasized that all of the authors represented here have progressed in their thinking and have advanced their work in other journals and books since original publication of the papers. Some have altered their theoretical orientation and some even their substantive interests. Wherever possible the editor has selected contributions published since the early 1970s. Indeed, most of the articles were first published within the last three or four years. Articles that were widely recognized as classic statements were selected from earlier years. Finally, several contributions dealt with a breadth of issues and were of sufficient quality to warrant their inclusion in more than one volume. Since each volume is likely to appeal to somewhat different readerships, this duplication was not considered problematic but rather enhanced the treatment of some health-care issues and the value of each volume.

It is hoped that this new series will help teachers, researchers, policymakers, public administrators, and especially students to overcome an ever-increasing problem: namely, how to gain easy and economical access to the rich resources contained in recent Milbank Memorial Fund publications.

Introduction

The fifteen papers in this volume focus on some of the most important issues presently facing hospital administrators. The first section, on general issues, begins with a careful study of seventeen hospitals by W. Richard Scott and his colleagues. They relate certain hospital characteristics to measures of services, outcomes, and costs. These authors believe that their general research approach, which combines measures of organizational structure, processes, and outcomes into a single design and which attempts to adjust process and outcome measures for differences in the types of clients served, is a promising direction for future research. They caution however against making any generalizations based on their small sample of hospitals. Edward Morse and his colleagues employ survey data from 338 government, nonfederal, and voluntary general service hospitals to examine the impact of several dimensions of organizational structure on indicators of hospital efficiency and level of adoption of new medical technology. They focus particularly on the degree to which resource allocation decision making is centralized as well as on levels of visibility of medical and economic consequences. It appears that, in terms of efficiency, organizational structure is an important factor in determining whether gains in effectiveness outweigh expenses associated with the adoption of new medical technology. The third paper by Ralph Berry is also based on empirical research and attempts a detailed analysis to identify and measure the effects of factors that significantly influence the cost and efficiency of the short-term general hospital system in the United States. His analysis involves data on approximately 6,000 hospitals for the years 1965, 1966, and 1967 and employs a model that expresses hospital cost as a function of the level of output, the quality of services provided, the scope of services provided, factor prices and relative efficiency. His analysis does provide insight into the factors affecting hospital cost: hospital services are produced subject to economics of scale but the absolute magnitudes are rather insignificant; on the basis of the limited data available, he concludes that quality does affect costs; medical education is a significant factor affecting hospital costs;

and product mix also has a significant impact on costs. In a study of five typical hospitals and a specialized treatment center, Christopher Zook and his colleagues found that more than half of all patients, and 60 percent of all costs, were attributable to repeated admissions for the same disease. The fiscal and clinical nature of repeated hospitalizations suggests changes for national health care policy. These will require more sensitive identification of patients "at risk" to "medical recidivism," and insurance mechanisms that relate more rationally and equitably to long-term needs. Lois Myers and Steven Schroeder are concerned with the serious problem of the rapid increase in ordering services for hospitalized patients that has occurred over the last several decades, and that appears to contribute considerably to the overall increase in hospital costs. They cite studies that reveal what is termed "flat of the curve medicine"—where many hospitals services are ordered for patients unnecessarily. It is recognized that physicians and hospitals are confronted with powerful personal, organizational, and economic incentives to constantly increase the ordering of hospital services. On the basis of their careful review of various strategies designed to modify physician ordering behavior, Myers and Schroeder conclude that audit, with feedback and education, appears to be more effective in reducing ordering than restrictions on ordering, or positive incentives to reduce use. Michael Redisch examines the physician's role in the hospital cost inflation process and the impact of hypothesized physician behavior on the expected relative success of alternative policies for containing hospital costs. He argues that the search for a single panacea to contain hospital and other health care costs is likely to be a futile one. Instead, the problem is one that will have to be solved (or at least partially alleviated) through a number of small discrete steps. Utilizing the physician as a lever to help contain hospital costs is suggested as one of those steps.

The second section concerns what some consider to be the number one problem affecting hospitals around the world: namely, the proliferation and adoption of medical technology. Judith Wagner and Michael Zubkoff discuss what the proliferation of medical technologies portends for hospital cost inflation. They are alarmed at the way new equipment, procedures or systems are introduced by hospital decision makers without knowledge of, or concern for, their relative effectiveness or efficiency. Technology, particularly hospital technology, is attracting increasing attention because of the convergence of three lines of criticism of the health care system. First, there is evidence that technology is directly linked to increased hospital costs (one study revealed that about 75 percent of the rise in hospital costs relative to the general economy can be attributed to increases in labor and nonlabor inputs per patient day). Second, there is evidence that many new medical services (perhaps a majority) have made little difference to any health outcome. Nonmedical factors (for example, nutrition, improvements in water supply, etc.) appear to have been more important in reducing both mortality and morbidity rates over the last fifty years or so. Third, programs designed to control hospital cost expenditures have generally been disappointing failures. One well-known program (Certificate of Need) appears to have shifted the composition of capital spending from investments in new beds to investments in sophisticated equipment. Wagner and Zubkoff provide a useful discussion of some aspects of the diffusion process and conclude that major gaps remain in our knowledge of both the process by which technologies become established and their real impact on social costs and benefits. Policymakers in the future will face difficult choices as they seek to determine where on the trade-off curve between health care costs and benefits we should be and how to ration the availability of those technologies that offer clear benefits. Arnold Kaluzny and his colleagues investigate the differential contribution of various organizational variables affecting the innovation of high-risk versus low-risk health service programs in two types of health care organizations—hospitals and health departments. They found that variables are differentially related to both the type of program and the type of organization. Organizational size was a critical factor in program innovation as it relates to high-risk services in hospitals and low-risk services in health departments. Excluding size, staff characteristics such as cosmopolitan orientation and training were prime predictors for both high- and low-risk programs in hospitals. The degree of formalization was the primary predictor of innovation of high-risk programs in hospitals. Cosmopolitan orientation of the administrator was a critical factor in the innovation of high-risk programs in both hospitals and health departments.

The third section draws together five papers that deal with a major consequence of the diffusion of medical technology among hospitals—the escalation of health care costs. Katharine Bauer reviews highlights in the state and regional experience with hospital rate setting as of 1975. After outlining the nature of rate setting and the impetus behind the movement, she examines some of the issues that implementation has brought to the fore. She notes the kinds of assumptions on which this demanding form of regulation is premised, the sometimes contradictory expectations held for it, the strengths and weaknesses of various types of structures for its administration and certain problems of methodology and information that handicap efforts of rate setting bodies to accomplish their intended purposes. She also discusses the kinds of risks and incentives that rate setting programs introduce to the hospital industry, sometimes intentionally, sometimes inadvertently, and often because of the still limited state of the art. Her arguments and descriptions are ably supported by case studies of major rate setting programs conducted or supervised by the author between 1973 and 1975.

In August, 1971, the federal government froze all wages and prices for a period of three months and then controlled increases in them through April, 1974. Special regulations were developed for health care providers because of unique characteristics of the health care industry. Paul Ginsburg shows that while the economic stabilization plan was quite effective in reducing rates of increase of hospital employees' wages, it was not effective with regard to hospital costs. In neither of the models he considers did input intensity decline as a result of controls. Ginsburg believes the program did not work because, first, the influence of the economy-wide controls over the design of health care controls created serious disincentives. Second, there was persistent and widespread confusion and ambiguity over the regulations. Third, there was a general expectation that the controls would be short-lived. James Blumstein discusses one fairly recent attempt to promote cost consciousness and ensure quality maintenance in federal medical programs—Professional Standards Review Organizations (PSROs) composed exclusively of licensed physicians in an area. A PSRO reviews medical care provided to federal beneficiaries under Medicare, Medicaid and maternal and child health programs. The author raises a number of doubts concerning the ability of PSROs to contain costs—especially because of the reliance on professionally developed norms of care. Blumstein considers the contribution, if any, that PSROs can make to hospital cost containment. Certificate-of-Need (CON) controls over hospital investment have been enacted in a number of states in the United States in recent years and the National Health Planning and Resources Development Act of 1974 provides incentives for the adoption of CON in additional states. Salkever and Bice review some questions that have been raised about the effectiveness of CON controls and then develop quantitative estimates of the impact of CON on investment. They show that CON did not reduce the total dollar volume of hospital investment, but altered its composition, retarding expansion in bed supplies but increasing investment in new services and equipment. They caution against any conclusion that CON controls should be broadened and tightened. Although focused on regulation of bed supply in nursing homes, the paper by Judith Feder and William Scanlon has obvious implications for such regulation in various types of hospital settings. Federal and state regulation of capital expenditures has been advanced as a major means both to ensure rational allocation of resources and to control costs. On the basis of evidence drawn from eight states, Feder and Scanlon suggest that limiting the supply of nursing home beds ("certificate of need") without refining conflicting standards of eligibility, quality control and reimbursement policies (Medicaid and "rate setting") discriminates against people who are most in need of medical care.

The fourth section concerns policy prescriptions for the future. John McMahon and David Drake, writing from the perspective of the American Hospital Association, argue forcefully that hospitals themselves are very much the victims rather than the cause of the current round of inflation in health care costs. They attempt to demonstrate through an analysis of the nature of long-run hospital inflation that the problems of inflation can be successfully approached only if the entire health care system or delivery network is examined for its contributions to and encouragement of inflationary tendencies. Cost-containment strategies directed exclusively at hospitals therefore are not only likely to fail permanently to reduce the rate of inflation in health care but will further discredit mechanisms to control costs. They propose and argue for national health insurance as a method of addressing the problems of systemic, or structurally induced inflation. Their paper represents a demurrer to the currently popular position that the enactment of national health insurance must await the discovery and attainment of effective controls on health care and hospital costs. They believe that a carefully constructed national health insurance plan may represent the only real opportunity for finding the elusive handle on health care costs.

Ralph Berry's final contribution to this volume outlines his thoughts on research needs for future policy concerning hospital cost containment. His review of experience to date does not inspire great confidence in the current capacity to contain such costs. Many complex issues await resolution: what are the prospects for hospital cost containment? Do such mechanisms as rate regulation, prospective budgeting and reimbursement, planning and certificate of need, utilization review, have the potential to control or contain cost inflation in the hospital sector? What is the structure of the hospital industry? What behavioral patterns are associated with varying market conditions? What are the dimensions of the problem of hospital cost inflation? What impact will various cost containment mechanisms have on structure, behavior, costs, and productivity? It is not Berry's intention to provide definitive answers, but rather to pose strategically important questions. He does not presume to offer specific research agenda. Rather, he views it as more appropriate and useful to reflect on a research strategy, to delineate the set of questions that should be asked in any research context and to consider some answers in the context of hospital cost containment.

John B. McKinlay

I General Issues

Milbank Memorial Fund Quarterly/*Health and Society, Vol. 57, No. 2, 1979*

Organizational Determinants of Services, Quality and Cost of Care in Hospitals

W. RICHARD SCOTT, ANN BARRY FLOOD, AND WAYNE EWY

Department of Sociology, Stanford University; Organizations and Mental Health Training Program, Stanford University; and Warner-Lambert/Parke-Davis Pharmaceutical Division

AFTER MORE THAN A DECADE of research on the structural features of organizations (Blau and Schoenherr, 1971; Pugh, Hickson, Hinings et al., 1968 and 1969), researchers are turning their attention from the determinants to the consequences of organizational structure. In particular, attention has recently been focused on the effects of structure on organizational effectiveness and efficiency (Child, 1974 and 1975; Goodman and Pennings, 1977; Price, 1972; Steers, 1977). Good examples of the latter variables are provided by quality (effectiveness) and cost (efficiency) of health care in hospitals. These variables are also of great interest to policy makers because of the recent rapid increases in hospital costs and uneven quality of hospital care in this country.

A large number of studies have examined factors associated with quality or cost of care in hospitals, but only a small number have examined both simultaneously, and an even smaller number have attempted to relate them to structural features of hospitals (Cohen, 1970; Morse, Gordon and Moch, 1974; Neuhauser, 1971; Rushing, 1974; and Shortell, Becker and Neuhauser, 1976). Results from these and related studies have not been clear or persuasive. Important limitations of previous work include: 1) a lack of effective techniques for taking into account differences among patients that

0026-3745-79-5702-0234-31/$01.00/0 ©1979 Milbank Memorial Fund affect both the cost and the quality of care observed; and 2) a lack of attention to the development of output measures that distinguish the outcome of care received from the quantity or costs of services delivered or from the potential to provide care implied by the elaborateness of facilities and the qualifications of health care personnel.[1] We designed our research approach to deal with both of these difficult issues. To handle the first issue, we adjusted the measures of services and outcomes for hospital patients to take into account variations due to the health status of the patients being treated. To handle the second issue, we developed independent measures of quality of care, quantity of services, costs of care, and structural measures of the potential of the organization to provide care, and examined their interrelationships. Based on this research, we examined in a related paper (Flood, Scott, Ewy et al., 1978) the relations among measures of the average quantity of services delivered and the average quality of outcomes achieved by patients in a hospital. In this paper we focus on a set of structural characteristics of hospitals as predictors of variations in the average intensity and duration of services provided to patients, the average amount of expenditure for patient care, and the average quality of outcomes experienced by patients in the hospital.

Methods

Data Sources

Data used in this study were drawn from 17 acute care hospitals. The hospitals had all previously participated in the prospective study of our research team concerning the organizational factors affecting quality of outcome following surgery (Stanford Center for Health Care Research, 1974). Although some of the data on organizational characteristics was used in our previous study, the patient data in our current study are based on a much broader spectrum of patients, including both surgical and medical patients, and employ information obtained entirely from abstracts of patient records. The study

---

[1]Strengths and limitations of the various classes of measures employed to assess care quality are discussed in Donabedian (1966) and Scott (1977).

hospitals were selected from a roster of 1377 hospitals participating as of 1972 in the Professional Activities Study (PAS) of the Commission on Professional and Hospital Activities (CPHA), a hospital abstracting system collecting and summarizing selected information on all patient discharges from its member hospitals. Thirty-two hospitals were selected randomly from a stratified sample of all short-term voluntary hospitals participating in PAS; of these 32, 16 agreed to participate in the research and a 17th, administratively linked to one of the 16, volunteered to participate at its own expense. Stratification variables included size, teaching status, and expenses. The 17 hospitals are not completely representative of all short-term acute care hospitals in this country. In particular, they do not include proprietary or federal short-term hospitals. Compared to hospitals of a similar type, their average size is greater than the national average (304 vs 164 beds).[2] Six of the study hospitals (35%) were affiliated with a medical school or had an approved and active house staff program, compared to 28% of comparable U.S. hospitals. Costs of care within the study hospitals were similar to the national average: $113 average cost per patient day for our study hospitals compared to $115 for U.S. hospitals. The goal of obtaining substantial variance within the sample along these important dimensions was achieved: for the sample, size varied from 99 to 638 beds, and average costs from $77 to $154 per patient day. Ten states and all major geographic regions within the continental United States were represented.

All patient data were based on information contained in the PAS abstract record, which was available for each of the approximately 670,000 patients discharged from the study hospitals during the period, May 1970 through December 1973. The final set of study patients numbered approximately 603,000; virtually all of the excluded cases were newborns. Data from the patient abstract provided the basis for our measures of services received and outcome, including the number and types of diagnostic and therapeutic services received during the hospitalization, the length of hospital stay and the measure of patient outcome, i.e., death in hospital. In addition, we used information from the patients' abstracts (by means of a procedure to be described below) to adjust the service and outcome

---

[2]Study hospital and national figures are based on 1973 data.

measures for differences in patient mix and in hospitalization experience.

Data on the organizational characteristics of the hospital and medical staff came primarily from our previous study on the quality of surgical care (Stanford Center for Health Care Research, 1974). For that study, interviews had been conducted during the spring of 1974 with key hospital and medical staff personnel who acted as expert informants, describing the structure and operation of their units. Questionnaires had also been administered to the staffs of the operating room, recovery room, and surgical wards, and to selected physicians providing primary care and selected ancillary services. Data on surgeons' training and experience had been collected from either hospital records or American Medical Association (AMA) records. In addition to these data from our earlier study, information was assembled on selected hospital characteristics from the American Hospital Association (AHA) annual survey for each of the 4 years studied.

Measures of Major Variables

The principal measures in this study may be grouped into four categories: 1) outcome of hospitalization; 2) amount and type of in-hospital services; 3) actual hospital costs; and 4) hospital structure.

Measure of the Outcome of Hospitalization. The indicator of quality of care is the rate of *in-hospital mortality* adjusted for patient characteristics—a measure emphasizing the quality of outcome of care for patients.

Measures of In-Hospital Services: Rates of Service Intensity and Duration. We developed indicators to estimate the number or amount of services of varying types received by a patient during a hospital stay. Although it is not feasible to assess all of the many types of services provided by hospitals, we measured seven types of important diagnostic and therapeutic services provided to inpatients. We also assessed the duration of the services, as measured by length of stay. For purposes of this analysis, we limited our attention to a composite measure of these seven services rather than to each service measured independently. An *Index of Service Intensity* reflects the amount and variety of diagnostic and therapeutic services provided to patients, as well as the relative cost of each of these different types of services.[3] An *Index of Service Duration* is based on length of stay. This measure weighs length of stay by the proportion of total hospital charges associated with routine nursing and hotel services provided to all patients regardless of any specific services consumed.[4] The two indexes, their component measures and weights, are summarized in Table 1.

The measures of outcome and of service intensity and duration were first computed at the patient level by detailed analysis of individual records for the 603,000 patients, to permit standardization for individual patient differences. General features of the approach are described in Appendix A; specifics are provided in Forrest, Brown, Scott, et al. (1977). Briefly, using a combination of classification by diagnosis (with 332 diagnostic groupings) and linear regression, and using indicators that characterized each patient's condition and treatment record, including diagnoses, operations, admission test findings, and socio-demographic characteristics, we computed the expected levels of service intensity, duration, and outcome for each patient, conditional on the patient's specific

---

[3]Categories of therapeutic and diagnostic services measured are reported in Table 1. Costliness of services was reflected in a weight assigned to each individual category before combining them into the composite measure. These weights were based on the average proportion of total charges for a hospitalization episode associated with each category of service. The weights were obtained from data on hospital charges supplied by a non-study hospital. Thus, they are not intended to reflect the actual variations in charges among study hospitals, but were uniformly applied to all hospitals. The intent was only to reflect differences in *relative* costliness among the various categories of services provided by hospitals.

Since we were able to assess not only whether a given category of service was used by a given patient but often the amount or numbers of such services consumed as well, the actual weights applied to each service used by a patient took into account these frequencies. Thus, the final weighting for each service consisted of the proportion of total charges for each category of services, as reported in Table 1, divided by the average amount of each type of service consumed by study patients during their hospitalization. For example, since the average number of operations for study patients was 0.545, the final weight assigned was $14.27/0.545 = 26.183$, which was applied to each operative procedure received by a given patient.

[4]For some analyses not reported here, these two composite measures were combined into an overall measure of services. For this reason, a weighting of length of stay was introduced. This weighting does not alter any of the results presented in this paper, but is included to allow a comparison of the relative costliness of specific services and routine care.

TABLE 1

Components of the Service Intensity and Duration Indexes and Their Weights

Items From the PAS Abstract for Patients	Class of Services Being Estimated	Proportion of Patient Charges for Class* (%)	Weighting Factor of PAS Item for Each Patient†
Components of Index of Service Intensity:			
Diagnostic services:			
No. of radiographic procedures performed	Radiological services	7.08	32.627 per procedure
No. of blood tests	Laboratory	8.48	12.676 per test
Therapeutic services:			
No. of operative procedures	Surgery	14.27	26.183 per procedure
Administration of any blood or blood parts	Laboratory	2.83	52.407 if any blood given
Physical therapy	Therapy	2.66	52.157 if physical therapy given
No. of classes of drugs	Medical supplies	8.52	7.992 per class of drugs
Use of intensive care unit	Special care units	4.21	56.892 if special unit used
	Subtotal	48.05	
Component of Index of Service Duration:			
No. of days in hospital	Hotel services Routine nursing care	51.95	6.185 per day
	Total	100.00	

*Based on the proportion of average patient's bill attributable to a given service class using 1973 figures from a non-study hospital.
†To obtain the weighting factor, the proportion of charges for the class is divided by the mean number of corresponding services on the PAS abstract actually used by patients in the study (see footnote 3).

characteristics and physical condition at admission. For each of the three types of measures based on patients—service intensity, duration, and outcome—the expected levels reflected the pattern of utilization or outcome obtained on the average in the set of study hospitals by patients with the same type of disease and physical condition. We then calculated difference scores for each patient, which reflected the difference, whether positive or negative, between the expected level of service intensity, duration, and outcome for a patient of that type and the actual level of service intensity, duration and outcome observed for that patient. To obtain a measure for a hospital, these difference scores were then averaged for the set of all patients treated in the hospital during the study period. Thus, our measures of service intensity, duration, and outcome for each hospital are summary measures of observed departures in the experience of individual patients from expected scores based on the typical experience of similar patients treated in all of the hospitals in our sample.

Measure of Cost Based on Actual Hospital Charges. Unlike the measures of services and outcomes, the measure of cost was not based on data obtained on individual patients and then aggregated to the hospital level, nor was it adjusted for differences in patient mix among hospitals. Data on actual expenditures on, or charges to, patients were not available. Instead, the cost measure was based on data obtained from the AHA's annual survey of 1973 and consisted of the total annual expenditures of each hospital divided by the number of patients treated during that year, which provides the *average expenditures per patient episode.* We attempted to correct this measure for regional differences in cost by dividing each hospital's score by the Medicare reimbursement index for the county in which the study hospital was located. Clearly, however, because our measure of cost does not take into account differences in patient mix, its usefulness is compromised, and it will not receive much attention in our subsequent analyses.

Measures of Hospital Structure. Measures of the structural characteristics of hospitals were grouped into two categories, capacity and control, as follows:

1. *Capacity* refers to those aspects of the hospital that represent its potential to supply services. Six types of measures were used. One obviously important measure was that of hospital size or scale. Since

hospitals are organizations heavily dependent on personal services, we used as our indicator of size the *total number of personnel employed.* (This indicator was correlated 0.93 with average daily patient census.) Second, to measure the elaborateness of the therapeutic and diagnostic facilities available, we assessed the *number of different types of facilities* and the *proportion of beds devoted to intensive care* in the hospital. The third set of measures examined the intensity of the staffing, indicated by the *ratio of all staff to the average daily census* and by the *ratio of direct care nurses to average daily census.* Fourth, the teaching status of the hospital was measured by the *ratio of residents to regular medical staff.* Fifth, the qualifications of the staff were determined by several types of measures indicating training, certification, and experience. These included the *ratio of registered nurses (RNs) to other types of nurses* e.g., licensed vocational nurses (LVNs); the *average number of years in nursing* for staff nurses; the *proportion of the surgical staff that was board-certified;* and the *average number of years in practice since residency* for surgeons. A final measure assessed the unused capacity or slack resources of the institution as measured by the *occupancy rate,* the ratio of occupied beds to total bed capacity. It should be noted that occupancy rate measured capacity used.

All of the above measures of the hospital's capacity to supply services were based on data supplied by the hospital administrator for each study hospital, with the following exceptions: information on facilities and intensive care beds was obtained from the AHA annual survey, and information on the average years of nursing experience was compiled from a questionnaire distributed to all ward staff nurses in the study hospitals (average return rate, 75%).

2. *Control* encompassed several features of the organization including the distribution of power or influence over decisions and mechanisms for the control and coordination of work activities. We assessed the distribution of influence among two major sets of actors within the hospital—administrators and staff physicians, coordination at several organizational levels, and controls exercised by the surgical staff over its own members. Brief descriptions of the variables used to assess these control features follow; more detailed information on the measures employed is provided in Appendix B.

Three measures of influence were developed on responses by key hospital informants to a set of hypothetical decision questions. One measure focused on the *hospital administrator's influence on decisions in the administrative area;* a second focused on the *chief of surgery's influence on decisions within his jurisdiction;* and a third examined the extent of *encroachment by physicians on administrative decisions.*

Coordination and control activities were assessed using measures of administrative intensity, clerical support, formalization, and frequency of communication with quality assurance personnel. Specifically, for the hospital as a whole, we assessed the *ratio of supervisory-to-direct care personnel.* At the nursing ward level, we measured the *average number of ward clerks and secretaries* present and, based on questionnaire responses from staff nurses, the *explicitness of general nursing policies.* To assess coordination by special professional units, we determined the *frequency of case discussions between physicians and pathologists* as reported by pathologists.

Finally, to assess the control exercised by the physician staff over its own members, we measured the extent of formalized *control exercised by the surgical staff over new members* as well as the *control exercised over tenured members.* These measures of formalized control were based on the rigorousness of the initial and continuing review of credentials, length of probation, and/or gradations of privileges. A third measure assessed the *proportion of contract (salaried) physicians* on the physician staff, an indicator favored by Roemer and Friedman (1971) as the best single measure of physician staff control.[5]

Predictions

In general, we expect organizational capacity to be positively associated with greater average service intensity and hence with higher average costs per patient episode. It should be noted that, since service intensity was adjusted to take into account differences in patient mix, the argument is not the conventional one that patients with more severe illnesses are more likely to be treated in larger and more elaborate facilities where they receive more services. Rather, we argue that patients served in more elaborate and more

---

[5]The data sources, the techniques employed to standardize service intensity, duration, and outcome measures, and all of the individual measures are described in detail in Forrest, Brown, Scott et al. (1977).

professionalized facilities are more likely to receive more services than expected, taking into account their specific condition. Such services are expected to be provided both because they are "more available" and because they contribute to other valued organizational and staff goals, such as teaching and research. There is no clear rationale for linking organizational capacity in general to duration of services, so no predictions are made concerning length of stay.

Hypotheses relating organizational capacity to quality of care are also somewhat problematic. Since the indicators of care quality vary considerably from one study to another, and since measures of structure, process, and outcome tend to be poorly correlated with one another (Brook, 1973), we restrict attention to outcome indicators of quality. There is some evidence to suggest that quality of outcomes is higher in larger hospitals (Kohl, 1955; Lipworth, Lee, and Morris, 1963; and the Commission on Professional and Hospital Activities, 1969). The relation between the average level of staff qualifications and surgical outcomes was investigated in an earlier prospective study of 9500 patients by the Stanford Center. In her analysis of these data, Flood (1976) reported that better surgical outcomes were associated with hospitals whose surgical staff had completed a greater average number of residencies (e.g., more varied postgraduate training) but, unexpectedly, poorer outcomes were associated with staffs having longer average residencies. Also unexpected was the finding that greater average specialization on the part of surgeons—measured by the types of operations actually performed—produced poorer outcomes, while the proportion of board-certified surgeons on the staff was not associated with quality of outcomes. The same study showed that better outcomes were associated with hospitals whose nursing staff had longer nursing experience, on the average.[6] Whether one should expect the average length of nurse and physician experience to be positively associated with better quality outcomes is unclear: a staff with a higher average level of experience signifies, on the one hand, more practice and exposure to varied medical problems but, on the other hand, increasing age and

---

[6]It should be emphasized that these results were observed at the aggregate level of analysis—i.e., using the average level of training and experience as the independent variables. Different results may be expected and have been observed when the level of analysis is shifted to the individual physician (Flood, 1976; and Flood, Scott, Ewy et al., 1977).

remoteness from training and, perhaps, from contemporary methods of care.

Turning to predictions involving control and coordination systems, we might expect to see greater controls exercised by administrators and physicians associated with reduced services to patients. Such an expectation is probably somewhat utopian since it is not at all clear that, given high influence, hospital administrators or the medical staff have much incentive to curb the services provided to patients and thus to contain the costs of medical care (Fuchs, 1974). Also, we should not expect both service intensity and service duration to be affected in the same manner by administrative and professional controls. Thus, our predictions with respect to hospital coordination and control systems and services are unsure, and we hope to learn from an examination of the empirical relations observed. By contrast, previous research suggests that better quality of medical care is positively related to administrative influence over decisions within its own domain (Flood and Scott, 1978), to coordination of work at the overall hospital and ward levels (Georgopoulos and Mann, 1962; Longest, 1974; and Neuhauser, 1971) and to the ability of the physician staff to regulate its members (Flood and Scott, 1978; Roemer and Friedman, 1971; and Shortell, Becker, and Neuhauser, 1976).

Strengths and Limitations

Before presenting the results, we should note the important strengths and limitations of the present data base and approach. Considerable confidence can be placed in our estimates of differences in services and quality of care among hospitals since they are based on a very large number of observations per hospital. Also, detailed measures of patient characteristics are used to standardize service and quality measures for differences among hospitals in patient mix. Further, unusually varied and detailed measures of the organizational characteristics of the hospitals and their medical staffs are available. These strengths are somewhat offset by several serious limitations. First, our indicator of quality of care—death in hospital—while highly reliable, is severely limited in reflecting only mortality experience. Had the data sources permitted, it would have been greatly preferable to include other outcome measures such as morbidity or return to function,[7] as well as to include information on patient condition after discharge. Second, although detailed measures of hospital and physician staff characteristics are available, there is some discrepancy in the time at which they are measured in relation to the patient data. As noted, patient information covers the period 1970 through 1973, while on-site collection of organizational data occurred in the spring of 1974. One must allow for the possibility that basic structural changes occurred within one or more hospitals during the period under study. A further limitation: since the original data were collected for a study of surgical care, most of the measures of physician staff are based on the characteristics of surgeons and the organization of the surgical staff. Surgeons constitute, of course, only a subset of the full medical staff. Third, although the measures of services and outcomes are based on the experience of a large number of patients, we have only a small number of hospitals on which to test predictions relating hospital characteristics to these dependent variables. Clearly, in presenting these results, our mode must be exploratory, and the results must be regarded as suggestive rather than definitive.

Results

Interrelation Among Service Intensity, Quality, and Cost

Before presenting the data relating to our predictions regarding organizational factors affecting services, cost, and quality of care, we note briefly the interrelations among these aggregated dependent variables. In all cases, except costs, results are based on the standardized measures. There exists a slight negative association between service intensity and service duration (-0.27):[8] hospitals delivering more services to patients than expected tend to exhibit shorter average stays than expected. Longer average service duration

---

[7]An attempt to include in-hospital complications as another indicator of care quality had to be abandoned due to the poor quality of data in this area.

[8]All correlations are Pearson product moment. The significance level adopted for these analyses is $p \leq 0.10$. For an n of 17 and a two-tailed test, an $r \geq 0.412$ is significant at this level.

was slightly associated with higher average costs per patient episode (0.37), while the average level of service intensity showed no association with average costs per patient episode (0.07). Most important, a higher than expected level of services within a hospital was significantly associated with a lower than expected mortality rate (−0.43), while longer than expected service duration was significantly associated with a higher than expected mortality rate (0.64).

Analyses of these relations reported in detail in a companion paper (Flood et al., 1978) reveal that both indexes of services and the outcome measure were strongly influenced by regional location of the hospital. When relations among these measures are examined for hospitals within regions, however, the negative association between service intensity and mortality persisted while the positive association between service duration and mortality tended to disappear. In short, it appears that the association between duration of services and poorer outcomes, which was observed for all study hospitals, is probably due to regional variations in medical practice rather than to hospital differences.

Effects of Organizational Capacity on Service Duration, Intensity, Quality and Cost of Care: Zero-Order Associations

Table 2 presents the zero-order correlations among the several measures of organizational capacity and the measures of service intensity and duration, quality, and cost of care. We note that larger hospitals having proportionately more residents and more elaborate facilities tended to provide more services than expected—both intensity and duration—and to be characterized by higher expenses per patient episode. On the other hand, these same measures of capacity were not associated with better than expected outcomes. The only exception to this general pattern was that hospitals having a higher proportion of their beds devoted to intensive care tended to exhibit shorter than expected lengths of stay and better than expected outcomes.[9] Higher labor intensity also was associated with better out-

---

[9]Since the indicator of quality of care used is the hospital's mortality rate adjusted for differences in patient mix, a negative correlation is indicative of better outcomes, hence, higher quality of care.

TABLE 2
Effect of Hospital Capacity on Service Duration and
Intensity, Quality and Cost of Care: Zero-Order Correlations*

Hospital Capacity:	Services		Quality: In-Hospital Mortality	Costs: Expenditures per Patient Episode
	Duration	Intensity		
Size:				
Total no. of staff	0.38†	0.41†	0.00	0.62†
Facilities:				
No. of different facilities	0.16	0.39†	0.02	0.65†
Percent of beds in ICU	−0.36†	0.54†	−0.32	0.29
Labor intensity:				
Ratio of total staff to ADC	−0.29	0.19	−0.44†	−0.05
Ratio of direct care nurses to ADC	−0.17	−0.22	−0.25	−0.48†
Teaching:				
Percent of residents	0.47†	0.18	0.09	0.71†
Qualifications:				
Ratio of RNs to LVNs	−0.31	0.29	0.05	−0.03
Average yrs of experience in nursing	−0.29	−0.31	0.30	−0.26
Percent surgeons with board certification	0.05	−0.08	−0.29	0.37†
Average yrs since residency	0.57†	−0.58†	0.60†	0.19
Extent capacity used:				
Occupancy rate	0.23	0.39†	0.22	0.30

*All measures of services and quality rates have been standardized to take into account patient mix of hospitals. Note that, since quality is measured by death rate, a negative correlation reflects a lower standardized death rate and thus better quality of care. *Abbreviations:* ICU = intensive care unit; RN = registered nurse; LVN = licensed vocational nurse; ADC = average daily census.
†Significant at ≤ 0.1 for one-tailed test; sample size of 17.

comes, but, at the same time, it was negatively associated with expenses.

The measures of qualifications were, in general, not related to services as predicted, or to quality of care. In general, training levels for both nurses (proportion RNs) and physicians (proportion board-certified surgeons) revealed little association with services and outcomes; costs tended to be higher in hospitals served by more board-certified surgeons. Nursing experience revealed no significant associations with services and outcomes, but length of practice for surgeons was strongly associated with longer service duration, lower service intensity, and poorer than expected outcomes. Finally, we had expected that lower occupancy rates—greater unused capacity—would be associated with higher levels of services and costs, but the data tended to be in the opposite direction: higher occupancy rates were associated with higher service intensity.

Effects of Organizational Control on Service Duration, Intensity, Quality and Cost of Care: Zero-Order Associations

The zero-order correlations among the indicators of influence, coordination, and control within the hospital and physician staff on the measures of services, quality and cost of care are presented in Table 3. Beginning with the measures of influence of administrators and the surgical chief and his staff, we note that higher influence of both groups tended to be associated with longer service duration and

TABLE 3

Effect of Hospital Control Factors on Service Duration and
Intensity, Quality, and Costs of Care: Zero-Order Correlations*

Hospital Control Factors	Services		Quality: In-Hospital Mortality	Costs: Expenditures per Patient Episode
	Duration	Intensity		
Influence:				
Administrative influence in own area	0.66†	−0.27	0.54†	0.37†
Surgical chief's influence in own area	0.33	−0.02	0.28	0.69†
Encroachment by medical staff	0.39†	0.26	0.16	0.31
Coordination within hospital:				
Ratio of supervisors to direct care personnel	−0.19	0.51†	−0.38†	−0.38†
Coordination within wards:				
No. of clerks on wards	−0.29	0.57†	−0.58†	0.06
Explicitness of nursing policies	−0.41†	0.41†	−0.19	−0.13
Coordination by professional units:				
Frequency of case discussions with pathologists	−0.64†	0.36†	−0.33	−0.26
Physician staff controls:				
Control over tenured staff	0.32	−0.61†	0.42†	−0.25
Proportion of contract physicians	0.41†	−0.27	0.38†	0.33
Control over new staff	−0.19	0.10	−0.28	−0.09

*All measures of services and quality rates have been standardized to take into account patient mix of hospitals. Note that, since quality is measured by death rate, a negative correlation reflects a lower standardized death rate and thus better quality of care.
†Significant at ≤0.1 for one-tailed test; sample size is 17.

with greater expenses per patient episode. This pattern was observed both for influence measures within each role group's domain of decision-making as well as for the measure indicating physicians' encroachment on administrative decisions. Administrative influence was also associated with poorer quality outcomes.

The several indexes of coordination also revealed a rather consistent general pattern. Higher levels of coordination within the hospital generally and in the patient care wards tended to be associated with shorter length of stay and lower expenses per patient episode but with a higher level of service intensity and better care outcomes. By contrast, two of the three measures of physician staff control indicated that a higher level of staff control over its own members tended to be associated with longer service duration, lower service intensity, and, unexpectedly, with poorer quality outcomes.

Combination Effects of Selected Measures of Hospital Capacity and Control on Service Intensity, Duration, Quality and Costs of Care: Multiple Regressions

Multiple regression analysis was employed to examine the combined effects of selected variables assessing both organizational capacity and control. Variables were selected in terms of their theoretical interest, the magnitude of their association with the dependent variable, and to provide breadth of coverage of the various types of factors considered. The results of one set of regressions are presented in Table 4. These results are representative of other regressions examined employing various combinations of factors and alternative indicators. Variables in Table 4 are listed in the order obtained in a step-wise regression. In addition to the zero-order association, this table reports the individual regression coefficients (B) for each variable, which are equivalent to their regression slopes partialling out the impact of the other variables in the equation, the standard error for B, and the standardized regression coefficients, or betas (β). Results of F tests are reported, which assess the significance of each partial coefficient as well as the significance of the combination of coefficients included within each prediction equation.

Table 4 *A.* reports results using the index of average-adjusted service duration as the dependent variable. Four variables stand out as very strong predictors of average length of stay: administrators' influence, average years of practice for surgeons, and proportion of

TABLE 4
Effect of Selected Measures of Hospital Capacity and Control on Service Duration and Intensity, Quality and Cost of Care: Multiple Regressions*

Selected Measure	r	β	B	Std. Error B	F
A. Service Duration					
Administrative influence in own area	0.66	0.38	0.96	0.18	27.40†
Average yrs since residency	0.57	0.80	0.35	0.04	78.77†
Total no. of staff	0.38	0.29	0.0006	0.0004	2.79
Control over new staff	−0.19	−0.60	−0.52	0.07	48.69†
Percent of beds in ICU	−0.36	0.59	52.45	9.59	29.90†
Explicitness of nursing policies	−0.40	−0.23	−0.59	0.20	8.15†
Percent of residents	0.47	0.35	4.87	2.61	3.49
Multiple R = 0.99		R² = 0.98		Overall F at final step 38.25†	
B. Service Intensity					
Average yrs since residency	−0.58	−0.03	−0.038	0.35	0.01
Total no. of staff	0.41	1.03	0.006	0.003	3.31
Percent of residents	0.18	−0.52	−19.24	22.73	0.72
Ratio of supervisors to direct care personnel	0.51	0.32	20.20	16.56	1.49
Percent of beds in ICU	0.54	0.47	114.35	85.61	1.78
Control over new staff	0.11	−0.24	−0.55	0.69	0.64
Administrative influence in own area	−0.27	−0.03	−0.20	1.57	0.02
Multiple R = 0.86		R² = 0.75		Overall F at final step 2.56	
C. Quality: In-hospital Mortality					
Average yrs since residency	0.60	0.73	0.0013	0.0006	4.70*
Administrative influence in own area	0.54	0.55	0.0056	0.0026	4.62*
Ratio of direct care nurses to ADC	−0.25	−0.33	−0.0067	0.0045	2.24
Control over new staff	−0.28	−0.38	−0.0014	0.0010	1.89
Percent of beds in ICU	−0.32	0.46	0.17	0.13	1.82
No. of clerks on ward	−0.58	0.08	0.0006	0.0024	0.07
Multiple R = 0.85		R² = 0.72		Overall F at final step 3.04	
D. Costs: Expenditures per Patient Episode					
Percent of residents	0.71	−0.09	−152.59	1432.32	0.01
Control over new staff	−0.10	−0.02	−2.44	43.27	0.003
Administrative influence in own area	0.69	0.48	151.58	100.57	2.27
No. of different facilities	0.65	0.47	12.29	15.39	0.63
No. of clerks on wards	0.06	−0.21	−47.28	68.08	0.48
Total no. of staff	0.62	0.28	0.076	0.17	0.20
Multiple R = 0.85		R² = 0.73		Overall F at final step 3.58†	

*All measures of services and quality rates have been standardized to take into account patient mix of hospitals. Note that, since quality is measured by death rate, a negative correlation reflects a lower standardized death rate and thus better quality of care. *Abbreviations:* ICU = intensive care unit; ADC = average daily census.
†Significant at ≤0.05.

17

beds in the intensive care unit (ICU) were strongly associated with longer than expected service duration; control over new staff was strongly associated with shorter than expected service duration. Explicitness of nursing policies was also significantly associated with shorter than expected duration of services. Of those variables significantly associated with service duration, only proportion of beds in the ICU changed the direction of its association, its zero-order relation being negative and its partial relation becoming positive. The combined effect of these variables was strongly significant. And, in combination, these variables accounted for 98% of the variance in the average service duration.

Table 4 *B.* reports a multiple regression with the index of average-adjusted service intensity as the dependent variable. Unlike the previous equation predicting service duration, in the equation predicting average service intensity none of the individual predictor variables reached significance nor was the combination of variables significant. The strongest individual predictor was size of staff, which tended to be associated with a higher than expected level of service intensity. Proportion of beds in the ICU was the next strongest measure. Both of these measures assess hospital capacity, and the direction of their association is as predicted. Although none of the individual variables was significant, in combination the variables accounted for 75% of the variance in the average service intensity.

Table 4 *C.* reports the regression of the measure of quality—standardized mortality rate—on selected measures of hospital capacity and control. Only two of the variables were significantly associated with average mortality: average years of practice for surgeons and administrators' within-domain influence were positively associated with adjusted death rate. Two other measures—of labor intensity and control over new surgical staff—were negatively associated with death rate (that is, positively associated with better outcomes) but neither association was strong enough to be significant. The overall F at the final step measuring the significance of the combination of predictive measures did not reach significance. The combined variables accounted for 72% of the variance in average-adjusted mortality.

Table 4 *D.* reports results of the regression of average expenditures per patient episode on selected measures of hospital capacity and control. No single predictor variable attained significance, but in combination the variables were significant at the 0.05 level. The strongest single predictor variable was administrators' within-domain influence, a measure positively associated with higher costs, but this relation was not statistically significant. The combined variables accounted for 73% of the variance in expenditures per patient episode.

Two measures tend to stand out in Table 4 and in similar regression equations examined but not reported here. They are average years of practice for surgeons and administrators' within-domain influence. Each merits further brief examination.

Average years in practice since residency for surgeons is a measure based on data obtained from the study hospital or from AMA records. To a surprising degree, this measure tends to be positively associated with both average-adjusted service duration and mortality. We should recall that these two measures were themselves strongly associated (0.64). Moreover, this measure tended to be negatively associated with a large number of indicators that were themselves negatively associated with both mortality and length of stay. These measures include frequency of case discussions with pathologists (-0.71), control over new surgical staff (-0.13), proportion of beds devoted to ICU (-0.38), ratio of total staff to average daily census (-0.29), ratio of supervisors to direct care personnel (-0.50), number of clerks on wards (-0.53), and a number of other indicators of control and coordination developed but not included in this report.[10] These indicators of control and coordination were not themselves highly intercorrelated, but the consistency of their negative association with average years of surgeon practice is striking. The question was raised earlier about the proper interpretation of this indicator: these data suggest that a higher average number of years of practice for physicians was associated with more lax control and coordination arrangements.

As described in Appendix B, the indicator of administrators' within-domain influence is based on a question assessing the relative power of hospital administrators to influence a decision regarding contracting for a service such as a laundry. Like years of surgeon ex-

---

[10]However, note that two measures of physician staff control are notably absent from this list: control over tenured physicians and proportion of contract physicians. These two measures were positively associated with years of physician experience (0.25 and 0.15, respectively) and, as reported in Table 3, were positively associated with service duration and mortality. As previously noted, these associations were unexpected.

perience, administrative influence was positively associated with both average-adjusted service duration and quality, even when the effect of related variables was taken into account. And like years of surgeon experience, administrative influence was negatively associated with variables that were themselves negatively related to both mortality and length of stay. For administrators, these variables included most of the measures of coordination within the hospital: administrative influence was negatively associated with ratio of supervisors to direct care personnel (−0.41), number of clerks on the wards (−0.51), explicitness of nursing policies (−0.46), and ratio of total staff to average daily census (−0.38). As might be expected, given the pattern of relationships just described, administrative influence was positively associated with years of experience for surgeons, but only moderately so (0.24). Thus, both the measure of administrators' influence and average years of surgeons' experience appeared to be related to larger complexes of coordination and control measures that help to explain their observed association with differences in average service duration and quality of care.

Summary and Conclusions

It is not easy to summarize these results relating hospital characteristics to measures of services, outcomes, and costs. The small number of hospitals studied—only 17—severely limits the confidence to be placed in any generalizations relating hospital characteristics to these dependent variables. Nevertheless, the opportunity to study structure (hospital characteristics), process (service intensity and duration), outputs (patient care outcomes), and costs in a single study encouraged us to carry out this exploratory analysis.

The prediction that hospitals characterized by greater capacity would tend to provide more services than expected received some empirical support in our analysis. Zero-order correlations showed that hospitals with larger staffs, a higher proportion of residents, and more elaborate facilities exhibited higher levels of average service intensity and duration. When the effects of other variables were controlled in multiple regressions, partials for ICU beds, and resident and staff size, tended to be associated with longer than expected service duration; and ICU beds and staff size were slightly associated with a higher than expected service intensity. For the most part, indexes of staff qualifications were unrelated to services, with one important exception: the average number of years since residency for surgeons was positively associated with service duration but negatively associated with service intensity.

Measures of capacity to deliver services showed only a slight association with quality of care as measured by standardized mortality rates. Measures of labor intensity tended to be slightly associated with better outcomes as assessed by both zero-order and partial correlations. Again, measures of qualifications were not associated with quality of care, with the exception of average years since residency for surgeons; this indicator was negatively associated with higher quality of care.

Measures of service capacity were positively associated with costs of patient care in zero-order analyses: staff size, facilities, proportion of residents, and proportion of board-certified surgeons were all positively associated with higher costs per patient episode. The only measure of capacity negatively related to costs was an indicator of labor intensity. When examined in multiple regressions, however, none of these measures remained significantly associated with costs.

Turning to measures of coordination and control, we find that most of the measures of coordination were positively associated with better quality care, as predicted. When the effect of other variables was controlled, however, few of these measures exhibited partials large enough to be significant. Contrary to expectation, two of the measures of physician staff controls—control over tenured staff and proportion of contract physicians—tended to be associated with poorer quality care.

No predictions were developed relating coordination and control to measures of average service intensity and duration. In general, coordination measures were negatively related to duration but positively related to service intensity. The two measures of physician staff control discussed above showed just the opposite pattern.

Finally, administrators' within-domain influence was positively related to service duration and higher costs but negatively associated with quality of care.

The negative association between control over tenured physicians and between administrators' influence and quality of care was not only unexpected but is contrary to the results of our earlier study using these same measures (Flood and Scott, 1978). Even though the hospitals and the measures of these independent variables are the same in these two studies, discrepant results are quite possible given differences in the patient populations and outcome measures employed: briefly, the earlier study was based on a small subset of surgical patients treated during 1973 and 1974 and included measures of morbidity as well as mortality in the outcomes assessed. Nevertheless, we were surprised by the inconsistent results in these two similar studies.

Although the specific associations revealed in these analyses were not as clear and consistent as we would have preferred, the general research approach employed, which combines measures of organizational structure, processes, and outcomes into a single design and which attempts to adjust process and outcome measures for differences in the types of clients served, seems to us promising. Indeed, the low and/or inconsistent associations observed among these three types of measures indicate the dangers entailed in using one type of measure as a surrogate for the others—a practice all too common in health services research specifically and, more generally, in research on organizational effectiveness.

We recommend that analyses of the type explored here be carried out in a larger sample of hospitals. Increased sample size would greatly assist in sorting out the complexities of associations that seem to characterize the relations among the types of variables considered. Of course, improved measures of costs that take into account differences in patient mix are essential. Finally, we hope that others will explore the uses of patient abstract data as a potential source of information on that most elusive of all measures in service organizations—the outcome experienced by clients.

References

Blau, P. M., and Schoenherr, R. 1971. *The Structure of Organizations.* New York: Basic Books.

Brook, R. H. 1973. *Quality of Care Assessment: A Comparison of Five Methods of Peer Review.* DHEW Publication HRA 74-3100 (July). Washington, D.C.: Bureau of Health Services Research and Evaluation.

Child, J. 1974 and 1975. Managerial and Organizational Factors Associated with Company Performance: Parts I and II. *Journal of Management Studies* 11: 175–189; 12: 12–27.

Cohen, H. A. 1970. Hospital Cost Curves with Emphasis on Measuring Patient Care Output. In Klarman, H. E., ed., *Empirical Studies in Health Economics*. pp. 279–293. Baltimore, Md.: The Johns Hopkins University Press.

Commission on Professional and Hospital Activities. 1969. *Cholecystectomy Mortality: A Study from PAS and MAP*. Ann Arbor, Mich.: Commission on Professional and Hospital Activities.

Donabedian, A. 1966. Evaluating the Quality of Medical Care. *Milbank Memorial Fund Quarterly/Health and Society* 44 (Part 2, July): 166–206.

Flood, A. B. 1976. Professions and Organizational Performance: A Study of Medical Staff Organization and Quality of Care in Short Term Hospitals. Unpublished Ph.D. dissertation, Stanford University, Department of Sociology, Stanford, Calif.

———, and Scott, W. R. 1978. Professional Power and Professional Effectiveness: The Power of the Surgical Staff and the Quality of Surgical Care in Hospitals. *Journal of Health and Social Behavior* 19 (September): 240–254.

———, ———, Ewy, W. et al. 1977. Effectiveness in Professional Organizations: The Impact of Surgeons and Surgical Staff Organizations on the Quality of Care in Hospitals. Paper presented at the meetings of the American Sociological Association, Chicago, Ill., September, 1977.

———, ———, ——— et al. 1978. The Relationship Between Intensity of Medical Services and Outcomes for Hospitalized Patients. Paper presented at the meetings of the Pacific Sociological Association, Spokane, Wash., April, 1978. (Revised, December, 1978.)

Forrest, W. H., Jr., Brown, B. W., Jr., Scott, W. R. et al. 1977. *Studies of the Determinants of Service Intensity in the Medical Care Sector*. Report to the National Center for Health Services Research, DHEW, under contract HRA 230-75-0169 (September). Stanford, Calif.: Stanford Center for Health Care Research, Stanford University.

Fuchs, V. R. 1974. *Who Shall Live? Health, Economics, and Social Choice*. New York: Basic Books.

Georgopoulos, B. S., and Mann, F. C. 1962. *The Community General Hospital*. New York: Macmillan.

Goodman, P. S., and Pennings, J. M. 1977. *New Perspectives on Organizational Effectiveness*. San Francisco, Calif.: Jossey-Bass.

Goss, M. E. W. 1970. Organizational Goals and Quality of Medical Care: Evidence from Comparative Studies of Hospitals. *Journal of Health and Social Behavior* 11 (December): 255–268.

Kohl, S. G. 1955. *Perinatal Mortality in New York City.* Cambridge, Mass.: Harvard University Press.

Lipworth, L., Lee, J. A. H., and Morris, J. N. 1963. Case-Fatality in Teaching and Non-Teaching Hospitals, 1956–59. *Medical Care* 1 (April/June): 71–76.

Longest, B. B., Jr. 1974. Relationship Between Coordination, Efficiency, and Quality of Care in General Hospitals. *Hospital Administration* 19 (Fall): 65–86.

Morse, E. V., Gordon, G., and Moch, M. 1974. Hospital Costs and Quality of Care: An Organizational Perspective. *Milbank Memorial Fund Quarterly/Health and Society* 52 (Summer): 315–345.

Neuhauser, D. 1971. *The Relationship Between Administrative Activities and Hospital Performance.* Research Series 28. Chicago, Ill.: Center for Health Administration Studies.

Price, J. L. 1972. The Study of Organizational Effectiveness. *The Sociological Quarterly* 13 (Winter): 3–15.

Pugh, D. S., Hickson, D. J., Hinings, C. R. et al. 1968. Dimensions of Organization Structure. *Administrative Science Quarterly* 13 (June): 65–91.

———, ———, ——— et al. 1969. The Context of Organization Structures. *Administrative Science Quarterly* 14 (March): 91–113.

Roemer, M. I. 1959. Is Surgery Safer in Large Hospitals? *Hospital Management* 87 (January): 35–37ff.

———, and Friedman, J. W. 1971. *Doctors in Hospitals.* Baltimore, Md.: The Johns Hopkins University Press.

Rushing, W. 1974. Differences in Profit and Nonprofit Organizations: A Study of Effectiveness and Efficiency in General Short-Stay Hospitals. *Administrative Science Quarterly* 19 (December): 474–484.

Scott, W. R. 1977. Effectiveness of Organizational Effectiveness Studies. In Goodman, P. S., and Pennings, J. M., eds., *New Perspectives on Organizational Effectiveness* pp. 63–95. San Francisco, Calif.: Jossey-Bass.

Shortell, S. M., Becker, S. W., and Neuhauser, D. 1976. The Effects of Management Practices on Hospital Efficiency and Quality of Care. In Shortell, S. M., and Brown, M., eds., *Organizational Research in Hospitals.* Chicago, Ill.: Blue Cross Association, Inquiry Book.

Stanford Center for Health Care Research. 1974. *The Study of Institutional Differences in Postoperative Mortality: A Report to the National Academy of Sciences-National Research Council.* Springfield, Va.: National Technical Information Service.

Steers, R. M. 1977. *Organizational Effectiveness: A Behavioral View.* Pacific Palisades, Calif.: Goodyear.

Appendix A
Rationale and Procedures Used to Standardize Services and Outcomes for Patient Health Status

The rationale and procedures for standardization are essentially the same for service intensity, duration, and outcome. To simplify this discussion, we use services as the primary example.

The Rationale for Standardization

Our approach makes the important assumption that patients with a given initial health status (including the disease for which they are being treated and their general condition at the time of admission) have a "need" for services which is (can be viewed as) constant across all hospitals. To estimate what types and amounts of services are needed by what types of patients, an empirical regression procedure is employed based on the experience of all patients in the study, ignoring in what hospital they are treated. Having determined what each patient "needs" in the way of services, we can also determine what services the patient has actually received in the study hospital under the assumption that the types and amounts of services hospitals actually provide will vary greatly. It is the discrepancy between what services a patient needs and what services are actually received that is the datum of primary interest.

How best to assess the need for services is a difficult question, both theoretically and empirically. Clearly, one of the most important determinants of the amount and types of services needed is the nature of the disease and the general condition of the patient on admission. A second important determinant, whether the patient undergoes surgery, increases the likelihood of receiving specific amounts and types of services—for example, the need for blood. A third determinant, complications that arise during the hospitalization (intermediate outcomes), also increases the likelihood of requiring additional services. A fourth determinant, leaving the hospital before complete recovery, clearly implies some "need" not only for more days of care but for specific types of services as well. Death in hospital is, of course, the extreme example of incomplete recovery and immediately ends the "need" for services.

To assess the four types of factors affecting need for hospital services, we defined four basic sets of standardization variables, incorporating over 40 different measures:

1. *Admission Status.* This set of variables included the major diagnosis explaining admission to the hospital using 332 diagnostic groups; several indicators of the patient's physiological status such as additional diagnoses, admission test findings, and severity of the disease; and several demographic characteristics such as age, sex, and a height-weight index.

2. *Surgical vs Medical Treatment.* For surgical patients, the indicators included the number of (non-diagnostic) operations and the severity of the operations undergone.

3. *Complications.* This set of variables included in-hospital infection as well as other complications.

4. *Discharge Status.* This set of variables included death at discharge, transfer to another facility, or discharge with incomplete recovery.

For most of the analyses reported here involving service intensity and duration, all four sets of standardization variables were used. The only exception occurred when the relation between services and outcomes was assessed and then, of course, the variables measuring death in hospital were excluded as predictors of services.

These four factors affecting the need for services were used to estimate the impact of a patient's health status on the amounts and types of services needed. But before detailing the standardization procedure, let us turn briefly to two additional considerations incorporated into our approach: the unit of analysis in assessing intensity of services, and the assumption of the independence of sets of services.

During a hospitalization episode, a patient can receive varying amounts of several different types of services. Some authors point out that the *rate* of services consumed during a single hospitalization is not constant, but varies by day of stay—usually being a higher rate at the beginning of the stay. We chose not to focus on the rate at which a patient consumed services, in defining the intensity of services. Instead, we examined two different measures summarizing the total amount of services received during the entire stay. We called the total amount of a given specific service consumed the "intensity" of that service delivered to the patient. The total length of stay we called the "duration" of routine services. The duration of services reflects the total amount of routine nursing and hotel services consumed. (Note that intensive nursing care is treated as a specific service and variations in nurse/patient ratios are examined as a capacity measure.)

The second assumption incorporated into our approach is the independence of services consumed, for purposes of defining the "need" of the patient for each service. In defining the seven specific medical services, we took care to group interdependent services to the extent possible. Thus, categories of drugs were grouped together as one type of service; radiographic examinations for diagnostic purposes were grouped, and so on. In this manner, we have assumed that the seven types of services can be delivered independently of the other classes of services. For example, we assume that the number of drugs does not depend on blood use, etc. Therefore, the "need" for each service can be derived independently. The one major exception to this assumption was the belief that surgery (a class of service) is interdependent with the other services so that, for example, the need for intensive care, blood, and drugs does depend on whether the patient underwent surgery. We handled this interdependence by using surgery as one of the predictor sets in assessing the need for other services.

Standardization Procedure

The standardization procedure involves assessing the needs of a patient for a given service by comparing that patient with other similar patients. The first step in determining what patients are similar is to group patients into one of the 332 diagnostic categories on the basis of their final diagnosis explaining admission. Within each diagnostic group, the standardizing variables (age, additional diagnoses, operation, discharge status, etc.) are used to predict the amount of service needed by each patient. It is important to note two consequences of this procedure. The assumption of independence of need for each service (except surgery) is made only for services supplied to the same diagnostic category of patients. And the impact of each standardization variable for predicting the need for each service can vary across diagnostic groups. For example, age could be a very important predictor of intensive care for gallbladder patients, but not so for cardiac patients. The standardization procedure described below was then performed for each of the seven specific services reported here and for duration of services separately for each of the 332 diagnostic categories, or $8 \times 332 = 2656$ times. The final index of specific service intensity was based on the seven independently adjusted measures, combined to reflect their relative costliness as detailed in the main part of this paper and in footnote 3.

In the standardization procedure, data obtained from the PAS abstracts of all 603,000 patients are pooled into one of 332 groups by final diagnosis explaining admission. Through linear regression, an estimate is obtained of the impact of each of the predictor variables on the amount of medical services of a given type received by a patient. Each estimate of the impact of the predictor variable (i.e., the unstandardized coefficient) is multiplied by the actual value of each predictor variable (e.g., age, diagnosis, number of operations, and so on) observed for a given patient. The sum of these products for a given patient provides an estimate of the amount of the service "needed" by that patient. The estimate of what is needed is based on the average experience of similar patients in the "standard hospital"—which, in this case, is simply all hospitals combined. Having determined the amount of service needed by (predicted for) the patient, we also assess the amount of service actually received. The estimate of services needed is used as the baseline for a given patient against which we can observe whether more or fewer services were actually received than expected on the basis of the patient's health status.

In a similar manner, the likelihood of dying in the hospital is calculated for each patient based on the experience of all patients having similar characteristics in the study hospitals combined, and is compared with information on whether the patient actually did die. Discrepancies are measured and, as with services, can occur in either direction. The greatest disparities occur, of course, when a patient with a low likelihood of dying actually does die and when a patient with a high likelihood of dying is discharged alive instead.

Since our primary interest is in examining the relation between structural features of hospitals and service intensity, duration, and outcome, the final step is to aggregate the standardized measures of each of these variables for all patients in each study hospital. In this paper, only a composite measure of the intensity of the specific services is examined. The composite, which combines the adjusted measures to reflect their relative costliness, is also aggregated for all patients in the study hospitals. The measures reflect whether patients in each hospital received more or fewer services than expected, remained in the hospital a longer or shorter time than expected, and experienced a better or poorer outcome than expected in comparison with other patients with similar characteristics but treated in different hospitals.

Appendix B
Measures of Hospital Control

Influence Measures

To determine the relative influence of the administrator and the heads of the physician staff in affecting various types of decisions in the study hospitals, we asked informants in each hospital to rate, on a five-point scale, the amount of influence exercised by a given position on a specific, hypothetical decision. Responses were obtained by interview or questionnaire from the following types of informants: hospital administrators, chiefs of surgery, chiefs of anesthesia, directors of nursing, ward supervisors, head nurses, and ward nurses. Positions rated include the hospital administrators, chiefs of surgery, the director of nursing services, and physicians as a group. Ratings from all respondents in the same position were first averaged; then these position scores were themselves averaged. Respondents within hospitals exhibited a very high degree of consensus in their assessments of the influence exercised by the various positions on specified decisions.

After combining the data from all hospitals, we observed that the distribution of influence by position, as expected, varied greatly by type of issue. Based on these profiles as well as on the content of the decision items, we distinguished between the "within-domain" influence of a role group and its "encroachment" into the decision terrain of other role groups. The decision item used to assess the within-domain influence of the hospital administrator was "a decision to purchase contract services, e.g., laundry." The average rating given by the respondents in each hospital to the administrator provided the hospital's score on this indicator. The same decision item also served to assess the extent of encroachment by the physicians on the terrain of the hospital administrator: the greater the reported influence of physicians as a group on this item, the higher the encroachment. To assess the within-domain influence of the chief of surgery, responses to three decision items were combined: "a decision to add a clinical service, e.g., an intensive care unit"; "a decision to add an ear-nose-throat specialty room in the operating suite"; and "a decision to terminate a major department head, e.g., the operating-suite nursing director." As before, responses from all respondents were combined into a single score for each hospital.

Coordination Measures

The ratio of supervisory to direct care personnel measures the number of supervisory and managerial personnel to the staff engaged in patient care activities. The latter group does not include physicians but does include all personnel engaged in technical support activities, such as in the laboratories. Data are drawn from a questionnaire completed by each hospital administrator. The measure of the average number of ward clerks and secretaries—a measure of coordination activities at the ward level—is based on data supplied by head nurses for each ward.

To assess the extent to which coordination was effected through use of formal rules, nursing respondents from each hospital were asked to rate on a five-point scale the degree to which explicit general nursing policies had been developed. The specific items included were dress or attire on the wards; returning to work after an illness; and conditions for which nurses could be requested to work overtime. For each hospital, average ratings were obtained from the ward supervisors as a group, the head nurses as a group, and from non-rotating staff nurses working on the day shift as a group. The ratings were then combined into a grand mean for each hospital.

Control Within the Physician Staff

To assess the extent of control exercised by the physician staff over new staff members, several questions were asked of the chief of surgery. The questions sought information on: 1) the existence of separately defined probationary periods for different surgical specialties; 2) the presence of any waivers of probationary period (no waivers receiving a higher score); 3) the number of groups or positions that must review applications for staff privileges; and 4) the length of the usual probationary period. Reponses to these questions were standard-Z-scored, and then added together to provide a composite index.

A similar approach was used to assess the control exercised by the physician staff over its tenured members. The questions provided information on: 1) restrictions on the surgical privileges granted to general practitioners; 2) the use—not simply the existence—of written procedures to review the surgical privileges already granted; 3) the number of years for which privileges are granted (item reversed so that shorter periods received higher scores); and 4) the existence of explicit criteria defining who can serve as the first assistant to the surgeon. As before, all information was obtained through an interview with the chief of surgery; items were standard-scored before being combined into a composite index.

Roemer and Friedman (1971) have argued that the proportion of contract physicians on the medical staff is a good indicator of the extent to which the physician staff organization is tightly organized. Information for this measure is provided by the administrator for each hospital.

The larger project of which this study is a part was carried out under Contract HRA 230-75-0169 with the National Center for Health Services Research, Health Resources Administration, Department of Health, Education, and Welfare.

The Commission on Professional and Hospital Activities (CPHA) of Ann Arbor, Michigan, collaborated with the Center to provide data for this study. These data were supplied by CPHA only at the request and upon the authorization of the hospitals whose data were used. Any analysis, interpretation, or conclusion based on these data is solely that of the Center, and CPHA expressly disclaims any responsibility for any such analysis, interpretation, or conclusion.

Acknowledgments: We are indebted to all our colleagues at the Stanford Center for Health Care Research at Stanford University. We particularly acknowledge the help of William H. Forrest, Jr., director of the Center; Byron William Brown, Jr., who contributed statistical advice; and Betty Maxwell, coordinator and administrative assistant, who provided innumerable support services.

Address correspondence to: Prof. W. Richard Scott, Department of Sociology, Stanford University, Stanford, California 94305.

Hospital Costs
and Quality of Care:
An Organizational Perspective[1]

EDWARD V. MORSE

GERALD GORDON

MICHAEL MOCH

Based on survey data gathered from 388 government non-federal and voluntary general service hospitals, this study examines the impact of several dimensions of organizational structure on indicators of hospital efficiency and level of adoption of new medical technology. Attention is focused on the degree to which resource allocation decision making is centralized and levels of visibility of medical and economic consequences. The evidence presented suggests that, in terms of efficiency, organizational structure is an important factor in determining whether gains in effectiveness outweigh expenses associated with the adoption of new medical technology.

Within a predictive framework this paper will deal with the relationships among several dimensions of organizational structure and performance and their impact upon the quality and cost of care provided by hospitals. An assumption often made is that modern medical technology is costly. Clearly hospital medical costs are rising with a large percentage of the rise due to increased delivery of new and improved medical services made possible by advances in medical technology.

However, it is less clear that new medical technology increases the cost for care. Indeed, the argument can be made that by increasing the ability to treat illness, technology which facilitates higher quality care may be reducing patient care costs. A major problem in dealing with the effect of technology on efficiency is the difficulty in employing econometric methods to non-profit areas such as health. Lave and Lave (1970b:294) state, "The difficulties in estimating hospital costs and production functions are overwhelming. . . ." As a result of the difficulties in assessing quality of care from an

[1]This research was supported, at different times, by U. S. Public Health Service Contract No. 8667268 and Social Security Administration Grant No. 10-P-56076/2/-02.

M M F Q / Health and Society / *Summer 1974*

economic perspective, many investigators have discussed medical cost reduction with little reference to the level of care provided. A consideration of both efficiency and quality measurements is necessary if we are to adequately deal with the question of the utility of expenditures for health care.[2] Further, to our knowledge little large-scale empirical research has been conducted on the impact hospital structure has on quality of care and efficiency. Two structural factors, the degree of centralization of decision making and the levels of visibility of medical and economic consequences in a hospital, are seen as having predictable impact on both quality of care and efficiency. Before presenting our theoretical framework, it will be useful to specify how both the independent and dependent variables have been conceptualized for purposes of this paper.

Quality of Care

Quality of care is an elusive factor to measure. It would appear at first easy to compare hospitals in terms of the morbidity and recidivism rates of a representative sample of patients. However, comparisons of hospitals in terms of mortality, morbidity, and recidivism cannot be related directly to quality of care.

First of all, hospitals differ in the facilities and services they offer to patients. Some have emergency rooms, intensive care units, outpatient units, etc., while others have none of these facilities. This complicates the comparative process, for the hospital with an intensive-care unit may receive many victims of accidents, heart attacks, etc., and consequently show a high mortality rate.

A second consideration implicit here is that hospitals are likely to develop exchanges of patients. The consequence of this is that one partner in such an exchange relationship may appear to obtain better results in its treatment of patients, but this is only because difficult cases are sent elsewhere.

Third, it is clear that medical science has made great advances

---

[2]Here efficiency is only being considered in terms of process. Ultimately it is felt a single index which considers both quality and process efficiency must be developed. Understanding how various organizational factors are related to both process efficiency and effectiveness is viewed as a first and necessary step in the development of such an index.

in the knowledge and technology used for diagnosing and treating disease, yet hospitals differ widely in the extent to which they have incorporated these new techniques into patient care. Acquisition of these techniques may alter the clientele of the hospital considerably, possibly increasing or decreasing the numbers of patients with serious illnesses.

An alternative to direct, comparative measurement of quality and, we believe, at the present a more viable strategy is to develop a set of criteria for an "effective" hospital. By an effective hospital, we mean one which has the ability to deliver high-quality patient care. Once variability in effectiveness has been specified, factors which help explain it can be isolated and anlyzed.

In attempting to provide a proxy measure or indicator of quality of care to meet our definition, we have developed a scale of institutional adoption of specific innovations in modern medical technology rated by a panel of experts as important for high-quality medical care within a defined area.[3] We have labeled this scale "adoption."

The fact that a hospital can treat the whole patient means that, in general, patients do not have to be transferred in order to receive emergency treatment and that facilities are available for handling complications associated with a particular disease; this appears to be fundamental to the concept of an effective hospital. Similarly, a hospital that lacks medical innovations deemed important by medical experts simply cannot deliver high-quality (i.e., effective) care by current standards.[4] Finally, because medical care involves economic goods or scarce resources, cost inefficiencies may function to deny services to those who need them and hence limit a hospital's effectiveness.

It is recognized that availability of technology is no insurance that it will be properly employed. However, without appropriate technology the potential quality of care delivered is likely to be at a lower level.

[3]We recognize this measure may not be appropriate for use with hospitals individually in determining effectiveness. However, we feel it does have validity on an aggregate analysis basis.

[4]These statements are made with reference to medical technology basic to the normal practice of medicine in a hospital and not with regard to technology required for the diagnosis and management of esoteric diseases which present themselves far less frequently.

Efficiency of Operation

While there are few who would disagree with the idea that all hospitals should have up-to-date facilities and deliver a high quality of medical care, economic realities of the nation's health care system necessitate considering quality of care in relation to efficiency of hospital operations. Given cost constraints, from a policy perspective the question becomes how to provide modern technology at the lowest possible cost. Before proceeding, it is important to explicate clearly the term "efficiency."

In asking how efficient a hospital is, three different and distinct questions are really being raised:

1. To what extent is the hospital utilizing the capacity of its *physical plant?*
2. How much *time* does it take to process a patient?
3. How much *money* does it cost to process a patient?

An indication of the extent to which a hospital is utilizing its physical plant can be inferred from its occupancy rate. A hospital's occupancy rate may be affected by a number of factors (Rafferty, 1971; Ingbar and Taylor, 1968; Lave and Lave, 1970a). But given that an unoccupied hospital bed producing no revenue costs about three fourths as much to maintain as one which is filled, underutilization of a facility clearly results in diseconomies (Lave and Lave, 1970a; Feldstein, 1961). These diseconomies must eventually be borne by the patient and third-party payers.

The second question is directed at the time dimensions of efficiency, a sense of which can be gained by calculating the average length of stay for a hospital's patients. Once again, it must be recognized that a number of factors not controlled for, particularly a hospital's case mix, may play a significant part in determining a hospital's average length of stay. Still, how long a patient remains in the hospital is not wholly determined on the basis of medical exigencies and thus is amenable to being affected by administrative as opposed to purely medical decisions. One example is the informal practice of some hospitals of holding patients over to reduce the likelihood of malpractice suits.

A third question raised deals with the expenses incurred by a hospital to process patients. How much a hospital expends to process a patient is a highly significant question—much more easily asked than answered. The difficulties stem basically from whether expenses should be measured in terms of admissions or patient days. Conceptually, using either unit of analysis would entail making a series of erroneous assumptions noted by Lave and Lave (1970b:295). Though seemingly an unlikely choice, the total expenses of a hospital were chosen to measure the monetary dimensions of efficiency. The rationale for using total expenses and the method of calculation are discussed in a later section of the paper.

Keeping in mind how quality of care (adoption) and efficiency have been conceptualized, the next thing to consider is how organizational factors affect both quality and efficiency. It is to this matter the paper now turns.

Organizational Variables

Centralization/Decentralization

We believe that certain organizational factors affect both adoption and efficiency. Our perspective derives from the work of Becker and Gordon (1966) who postulate that formal organizations are developed to coordinate scarce resources to achieve given goals in as efficient a manner as possible. Coordination, however, limits the organization's ability to change. All organizations thus face a dilemma posed by the desire to maximize the benefits of coordination and the necessity for change in response to environmental demands. According to this perspective, the best organizational structure reflects a balance between the gains to be accrued from coordination and the need to adjust to environmental changes. The general premise is that the lower the level within an organization at which procedures are specified, the less requirements for coordination inhibit organizational change.

For example, in assembly-line manufacturing, specified procedures are spelled out to determine the flow of resources from the time the raw materials enter the plant gate to the end of the assemblage process. The end product (e.g., in automobile production) is highly standardized, with limits placed on the variation allowed to meet unique demand requirements. Highly coordinated centralized authority structures are postulated as most effective when external conditions are relatively stable and uniform.

Most organizations, however, deal with heterogeneous environments. Often, as a means of handling diverse environments, multiple authority structures will be established within the same organization. The occurrence of units with different authority patterns within the same organization can best be understood in terms of what we have referred to as the organizational dilemma: the desire to maximize the gains of coordination and yet respond to environmental demands. One way to resolve this dilemma is to divide the organization into component elements, some with centralized authority patterns facilitating coordination and others with decentralized authority patterns responsive to change.

Hospitals are prime examples of organizations with multiple organizational structures. Characteristically the administrative group in a hospital operates under a different authority pattern from the doctors: the administrators have an executive authority pattern while the doctors operate on a collegial basis with some degree of unit autonomy. By decentralizing decision making in the larger organization to smaller semi-autonomous units, each having responsibility for dealing with a limited sector of the environment, coordination can be accomplished with fewer hierarchical levels. This not only reduces the number of hierarchical levels that must decide upon change but permits independent unit change.

As with all administrative structures, advantages gained in one area incur costs in other areas. Decentralization through the development of semi-autonomous units leads to duplication of administrative functions, difficulties in over-all coordination, and limits economies of scale. On the other hand, decentralization facilitates resource change—that is, the introduction of new and different resources into the organization.

Thus, if the board of directors of a hospital retains most decision-making prerogatives over resource allocation (indicating a centralized structure), the benefits of coordination would be maximized. On the other hand, to permit maximal response and resource flexibility, a hospital would decentralize decision making down to the lowest possible level. However, for most organizations, moving to either extreme compromises overall ability to perform.

This has specific bearing on the question of the impact of organizational structure on adoption and cost. Adoption reflects the ability of an organization to change. But if the ability to change is associated with a lack of coordination in areas in which such coordination is desirable, costs associated with change will be high.

Visibility of Consequences

Given these assumptions, the fundamental question is what factors tend to lead to a hospital structure with a balance between coordination and responsiveness to change? One of the most important factors affecting organizational structure is the basis upon which decisions are made. The assumption underlying this postulate is quite simple, namely that knowledge of cause and effect in terms of goal attainment (e.g., quality of care) leads to the selection of organizational practices that facilitate goal achievement at lowest costs. Going one step further, it is predicted that in the absence of knowledge about goal-related cause and effect, organizational structure will reflect whatever criteria are used to assess performance. Often, where information regarding goal performance is lacking, the organization assesses performance in terms of relative costs (Thompson, 1967).

Visibility of consequences is considered to range from highly visible, where an organization gathers information on the results of its past performance, to low visibility, where it is not possible or no information on performance is gathered. In the case of hospitals, it is useful to distinguish between two different types of visibility, one related to medical consequences, the other to economic consequences of the hospital's behavior. The sheer presence of either type of information would not be expected to have a direct relation with either a hospital's level of adoption, or its efficiency, since information in and of itself is assumed to have little or no impact until acted upon. The relation of centralization of resource decision making to a hospital's level of adoption and efficiency is expected to be affected by the type and level of information available upon which to base decisions.

Data Base

To collect data to test the relationship between cost and adoption as well as other organizational variables, a random sample of 1,021 hospitals was drawn from the population of United States hospitals for detailed study. Separate questions were sent to each hospital's chief administrative officer and medical officer.[5] Sixty-seven per-

[5]This not only enabled us to obtain a wide range of information but also provided two sources of data on which to base an analysis of the reliability of the instruments. Although space limitations preclude a delineation of our reliability analyses, we can say that, for each hospital, the amount of agreement between the medical officers, the administrative officers, and, for the intensively studied hospitals, our field site researcher, was high. For the questions concerning the presence or absence of each technological item within the hospital, for example, the medical and administrative officers agreed 75 percent of the time. Furthermore, for these items, the administrative officer agreed with study researchers who performed 17 intensive case studies 77 percent of the time and the medical officers agreed with our researchers 79 percent of the time.

cent of the administrative officers ($N = 678$) and 67 percent of the medical officers ($N = 669$) returned the questionnaire. Forty-seven percent of the hospitals returned both questionnaires, and 86 percent responded with at least one of the two instruments.

We also compared our data with the 1968 American Hospital Association annual survey data to determine possible sources of bias. Aside from a tendency for proprietary and federal hospitals to be slightly under- and overrepresented respectively, the two populations appeared similar. In an effort to reduce introduction of factors which might obscure testing the principle thrust of the analysis, the study was limited to a sample of government non-federal general service hospitals and voluntary general service hospitals. Limiting our frame to these hospitals enables us to perform our analysis in the context of hospitals with similar functions. The primary function of these hospitals is to treat a wide range of diseases without limitations due to profit motive or social characteristics of the patient. Since voluntary and government non-federal general service hospitals account for 60 percent of the hospitals in the United States, to a large degree generalizability is not compromised. Limiting our analysis to these classes of general service hospitals leaves us with a sample of 388 hospitals.

Operationalization of Variables

In selecting a measure of adoption it was decided, for purposes of comparison, to concentrate on a limited area of medical care. The criteria in selecting the area for study were:

a. That the medical area be relatively broad and relevant to the over-all quality of medical care provided in a hospital;

b. That the area be one where significant progress has occurred, but where serious problems remain;

c. That the innovations in the area reflect many different aspects of medical technology (e.g., drugs, equipment, operating procedures);

d. That the area include a large group of medical experts competent to evaluate the innovations.

The area selected was respiratory disease. Modern technology in this area seemed sufficient to provide a general measure of technological innovativeness. Besides occurring fairly frequently, respiratory disease often complicates other illnesses. Furthermore, respiratory technology is very often applied in anesthesiology and in postoperative-care illnesses entirely unrelated to respiratory disease itself. It was felt that the ubiquitous nature of respiratory disease technology in health care delivery made it an appropriate focus for study.

To measure the level of adoption of a hospital, a scale was constructed by counting the number of items from a list of twelve innovations[6] each hospital reported having purchased, leased, or rented. The scale constructed can take on values ranging from "0" (no adoption) to "12" (high adoption).[7]

The three dimensions of efficiency are measured using data taken from the 1968 American Hospital Association annual survey. The dimensions of physical plant utilization and time are operationally defined in terms of average occupancy rate and average length of stay respectively. Directly measuring the third dimension, expenses incurred to process patients, gives rise to some conceptual difficulties as previously discussed. An indirect indication of hospital expenses, however, can be constructed. It was reasoned that a hospital's total expenses are affected by both the number of patients it admits and its number of patient days. In turn, both of these factors should be a function of hospital bed size. Analysis of the data showed that size was correlated + .98 with number of ad-

[6]In order to identify technological innovations in this disease area, Dr. Robert Anderson, then Medical Director of the American Thoracic Society, and Dr. Lewis B. Clayton, Director of Medical Statistics for the National Tuberculosis Association, selected from the ranks of the American Thoracic Society 75 physicians who were thought to be experts on respiratory disease. The experts were split into two panels, one to generate a list of technical innovations, the other to rate these innovations in terms of various criteria including the initial and current importance of the innovation for diagnosis and treatment. From the initial list generated of over 200 ideas and discoveries, 12 items were selected for study. Many factors, such as importance, availability of records, and risk, influenced the selection of the 12 items. In each case, however, the items selected were rated to be of at least some importance for the diagnosis or treatment of respiratory disease. An additive index, we felt, was justifiable in this case because the items form a Guttman Scale.

[7]The items selected for inclusion were: Macroaggregated[131], Venti Mask, Blood Gas Electrode, Esophageal Balloon, Plethsmograph, Spirometer, Ethambutol, Nacetylysteine, Ultrasonic Nebulizer, IPPB Unit, Mediastinoscope, and LDH Determination. For the sample the 12 form a Guttman Scale with a coefficient of reproducibility of .92.

missions and + .95 with number of patient days. The high correlation with size means that if the effects of size were controlled for in the data analysis, variation in the hospital's total expenses attributable to its number of admissions and patient days would also be controlled for. This is done for the analysis presented by mathematically regressing each independent variable on the variable bed size and extracting the residual for each independent variable. Hence, it should be noted that in the presentation of findings, the independent variables will all be residuals of the variable size. The mathematical treatment of the measure results in it being independent of size and, therefore, analogous to hospital expenses per bed.

Measures of the extent of centralization-decentralization and visibility of consequences were derived from responses to the questionnaires sent to the chief of medicine and hospital administrator.

The survey questionnaire sent to each hospital included an item designed to determine the locus of discretion for five representative resource allocation decisions. To build an index of centralization/decentralization, the responses given for each of the five decisions were coded to reflect the relative frequency with which each decision was made by the board of the hospital, the chief subunit officer (hospital administrator or chief of medicine), or lower levels of the medical staff. Responses were combined to provide an over-all measure of the number of decisions made at each of the three organizational levels. The final measure constitutes an index ranging from "0" (decentralized) to "10" (centralized) which is taken as an indicator of the extent to which the locus of resource allocation decision making is predominantly situated at the board level, the chief officer level, or at the level of the medical staff.

The index of visibility of medical consequences is based on four factors: a hospital's autopsy rate, the number of times a year a hospital's credentials committee met, the percentage of time the chief of medicine devoted himself to the administration of the medical staff, and the percentage of time the hospital administrator devoted to administration of the medical staff. The index of medical visibility was constructed by first ipsitizing the responses to correct for response set. The standardized responses were then weighted by their respective factor loadings generated by a principal components analysis and summed for each hospital.

The index of economic visibility was built by summing the numerical responses hospitals made to two questions regarding the extent to which the governing body of the hospital was actually involved in decisions about how money is to be spent (i.e., specifications of budget categories) and examination of expenditures within budget categories.

Other Factors Included for Analysis

Although the primary thrust of this study focuses on the impact of centralization-decentralization and visibility of consequences on hospital adoption behavior and efficiency, a series of other factors felt likely to affect either adoption behavior or efficiency was introduced into the analysis as control variables. The series of factors includes: demographic (rural-urban) location of hospital, affiliation with medical schools, presence of outside funds for research, number of full-time non-medical personnel, number of full-time physicians, and number of services available in the hospital. Since, however, a multiple-regression technique will be employed in analyzing the data, an advantage is gained in that any control variable can also be examined in terms of its independent impact on the dependent variables.

The Relationship Between Efficiency and Adoption

As a first step in understanding the impact of organizational structures on efficiency and adoption, it is essential to examine the nature of the relationship between the three measures of efficiency and adoption. From the statements made in the introduction to the paper, two contradictory hypotheses may be advanced:

1. Modern technology is expensive and increases the costs of care in an absolute sense.
2. The costs associated with adoption of modern technology are more than offset by the savings resulting from higher-quality (i.e., more efficient) treatment associated with such technology.

If the first hypothesis is correct, we would expect costs of processing a patient to increase with adoption. A finding that adoption is associated with lower costs would not, in and of itself, indicate that the costs associated with adoption are offset by an increase in efficiency. However, if such a decrease were associated with a reduc-

TABLE 1

Zero-Order Correlations Between Adoption
and Three Measures of Efficiency

Total expenses (per bed)[a]	.18[b]
Average length of stay	−.12[b]
Average occupancy rate	.04

a   Each variable is a residual of the variable bed size
b $< .05$

tion of time spent in a hospital, support would increase for the second hypothesis. If, in addition, the occupancy rate were found to be associated with adoption, there would be some indication that where choice is possible the medical profession is channeling its patients to what it feels are better hospitals. Controlling for bed size, the following zero-order correlations were found:

Although the relationships are not large, the findings provide support for both hypotheses—there is a relationship between cost and adoption, but there is also support for the effectiveness hypothesis. The smallness of the relationship and its contradictory nature leads one to suspect that other factors may be affecting the efficiency/adoption relationships.

Centralization, Adoption, and Efficiency

Following from the "organization dilemma" discussed earlier, decentralization of decision making was associated with adoption and increased effectiveness, and centralization with increased efficiency. Thus, two hypotheses are posited:

1. The less centralized a hospital's decision-making structure, the greater its rate of adoption of medical technology.
2. The more centralized a hospital's decision-making authority structure, the more efficient it will be in its health care delivery as measured by average length of stay, average occupancy rate, and total expenses.

To investigate the impacts of centralization on adoption and the three measures of efficiency, a series of multiple regressions was

43

TABLE 2

Regression Estimates of the Impact of Centralization
and Other Organizational Factors on Adoption

Explanatory Variables	*Adoption* [a]
Centralization of decision making	−.13[b]
Urban/rural (urban = 1, rural = 0)	.36[b]
Hospital affiliated with medical school	.08
Years since founding	.09
Outside funds for research	.26[b]
Other assets	−.09
Number of full-time physicians	−.01
Number of different specialists on staff	+.06
Number of full-time non-medical personnel	−.02
Number of services	.07
Visibility of economic consequence	.00
Visibility of medical consequence	−.07

$MR = .64$ $N = 388$.
a Values reported are Beta weight.
b Beta greater than twice its standard error, significant at .05 level.

performed. Turning to the data presented in Tables 2-5, it is seen that when the direct effect of centralization is taken into account, hospitals which adopt more modern technology have higher occupancy rates, lower average lengths of stay, and no higher level of total expenses. Table 2 presents the results of the multiple regression of adoption on a series of variables. The negative Beta = − .13 supports the hypothesis that centralization of decision making has an inverse effect on a hospital's level of adoption. This finding supports the proposition that concentration of decision making, with regard to resource allocation, tends to result in the hospital's incorporating fewer advances in medical technology. Conversely, when the discretion to make resource decisions is held by members of the medical staff, the hospital is more likely to acquire technological advances in medicine and thus have more up-to-date medical facilities.[8] If, as stated earlier, having a modern medical facility is a prerequisite to delivery of a high quality of medical care, then the data suggest that consideration be given to developing mechanisms which increase physician participation in the resource allocation decisions of hospitals. The positive and negative consequences which might arise as a result of involving

[8]In the 10 percent of hospitals where the hospital administrator is a physician, it is expected that the impact of centralization on adoption would be modified.

TABLE 3

Regression Estimates of the Impact of Centralization
and Other Organizational Variables on Occupancy Rate

Explanatory Variables	*Average Occupancy Rate* [a]
Centralization of decision making	−.10[b]
Adoption	.13[b]
Urban/rural (urban = 1, rural = 0)	.10[b]
Delay in admission	.34[b]
Hospital affiliation with medical school	.05
Other assets	−.04
Number of full-time physicians	.00
Number of different medical specialists on staff	.06
Number of full-time non-medical personnel	.02
Number of services	−.04
Visibility of economic consequence	−.01
Visibility of medical consequence	−.14[b]

MR = .46   *N* = 388.
a Values reported are Beta weight.
b Beta greater than twice its standard error, significant at .05 level.

physicians in the process of resource allocation decisions are important considerations worthy of empirical study.

Given the second hypothesis, though, an equally critical problem is posed: what happens to the level of efficiency with which care is delivered if decision making is decentralized? Tables 3, 4, and 5 show the impact of centralization-decentralization and the organizational factors on the three dimensions of efficiency: the average occupancy rate, average length of stay, and total expenses.[9] A hospital's level of adoption is retained in the analyses of efficiency, since interest lies with the impact of centralization on the efficiency with which a hospital processes patients at a given level of quality.

Table 3 shows that centralization of resource decision making has a negative relation (Beta = − 10) to occupancy rate, indicating that utilization of a hospital's physical facilities is not facilitated where decision-making powers rest with the head of the organization, as hypothesized. On the contrary, the data suggest that more

[9]Although our primary theoretical concern is with the effect of centralization on adoption, significant impact of geographic location and outside funds for research can also be seen. Further comment on the independent impact of these factors will be deferred until a later point.

complete use of beds occurs where physicians at the patient-care level are themselves directly involved in the administration of resource allocation decisions in the hospital. Why this is the case is possibly clarified if one notes that the relation of level of adoption to occupancy rate is significant and positive (Beta = .13), keeping in mind that centralization of decision making was found to have a negative relation to adoption. This suggests that hospitals which adopt more medical innovations tend to experience higher rates of utilization of their facilities. A possible explanation for this finding is that hospitals with modern medical facilities are more medically attractive to both patients and physicians and thus experience greater demand for their beds. The plausibility of this explanation is supported in part by the significant relation between delay in admission and occupancy rate (Beta = .34). Thus, contrary to what might have been expected, having modern medical facilities may in fact lead to greater efficiency of health care delivery in terms of the more complete utilization of the facility. The direction of causality could, however, work in the opposite direction. That is, fully utilized hospitals would be more likely to have the resources needed to adopt new medical technology. Obviously, longitudinal data are required to determine directionality. However, regardless of the direction of causality, the analysis suggests that the nature of the association of adoption and occupancy rate does not directly contribute to hospital inefficiency.

It can be seen from Table 4 that centralization does not have a significant impact on a hospital's average length of stay, as hypothesized. Taking account of other variables, whether the owner of the hospital maintains tight control over decisions himself or lets the medical staff make decisions has little impact on expediting the process of treating patients. As was the case in Table 3, however, a hospital's level of adoption does appear to bear significantly on the average time it takes to treat a patient (Beta = −.11). To the extent that a hospital's level of adoption can be taken as an indicator of the hospital's over-all ability to provide modern medical facilities, the data suggest that adoption contributes to efficiency by reducing the average length of time taken to treat patients.

Of further interest, it is noted from Table 4 that while the number of non-medical personnel (presumably available to treat patients) appears to have the effect of reducing average length of stay (Beta = − .14), the magnitude of a hospital's outside funds for research (Beta = .10) and its number of full-time attending physi-

TABLE 4

Regression Estimates of the Impact of Centralization
and Other Organizational Factors
on Average Length of Stay

Explanatory Variable	*Average Length of Stay* [a]
Centralization of decision making	.05
Adoption	−.11[b]
Urban/rural (urban = 1, rural = 0)	.01
Delay in admission	.01
Hospital affiliated with medical school	.01
Outside funds for research	.10[b]
Other assets	.00
Number of full-time physicians	.18[b]
Number of different medical specialists on staff	−.06
Number of full-time non-medical personnel	−.14[b]
Number of services	−.03
Visibility of economic consequence	.05
Visibility of medical consequence	−.02

$MR = .29$ $N = 388.$
[a] Values reported are Beta weight.
[b] Beta greater than twice its standard error, significant at .05 level.

cians (Beta = .18) are related to an increasing average length of stay. These fundings raise the question of whether teaching hospitals, which normally have both large numbers of full-time attending physicians and large quantities of outside research funds, tend to keep patients for longer periods of time. It would be of interest to examine the implications of these findings with regard to the relation between the quality of patient care received and the use of patients for teaching purposes in such hospitals.

Finally, Table 5 shows that centralization of decision making appears to have an inverse effect on a hospital's total expenses (Beta = − .08), as predicted.[10] If the causal sequence is as predicted, in terms of monetary dimension of efficiency, this means that greater cost savings are realized by hospitals which have resource decision-making authority vested at the top than in hospitals

---

[10]The reader is reminded that by using variables in the analysis where the effect of hospital bed size, total number of admissions, and total number of patient days have been controlled for, the variable "total expenses" can be taken as a measure of expenses per bed.

TABLE 5

Regression Estimates of the Impact of Centralization
and Other Organizational Factors on Total Expenses

Explanatory Variables	*Total Expenses* [a]
Centralization of decision making	−.08[b]
Adoption	.03
Urban/rural (urban = 1, rural = 0)	.27[b]
Cost of manpower	.03
Delay in admission	.17[b]
Hospital affiliated with medical school	.14[b]
Years since founded	.16
Outside funds for research	.33[b]
Average occupancy rate	.03
Average length of stay	.08[b]
Other assets	.04
Total visits—outpatient services	.03
Number of full-time physicians	−.04
Number of different medical specialists on staff	−.16[b]
Number of full-time non-medical personnel	.18[b]
Number of services	−.09[b]
Visibility of economic consequence	−.05
Visibility of medical consequence	−.03

$MR = .81$ $N = 388$.
[a] Values reported are Beta weight.
[b] Beta greater than twice its standard error, significant at the .05 level.

where responsibility for resource allocation decisions lies with the medical staff.

Further, it is seen from Table 5 that a hospital's level of adoption does not, as is often assumed, appear to exert any influence on total expenses.[11] Care must be taken, however, in interpreting this finding. It would be in error to conclude from this that the costs of operating a modern medical facility are not increased, particularly where, in conjunction with adoption of a new innovation, a hospital must hire technical support personnel to operate it. Analysis by Andersen and May (1972) of factors contributing to increasing costs of hospital care strongly suggests that increased labor costs are a major cause of rising hospital expenses. Looking at the impact of the number of full-time non-medical personnel on total expenses (Beta = .18) would appear to support such a contention. For this argu-

[11]Since staff size is an independent variable in our multiple regression, the effect of adoption on total expenses is independent of its contribution to increases in staff size.

ment to hold, though, there would have to be a strong relation between level of adoption and number of full-time non-medical personnel. The correlation between adoption and number of full-time non-medical personnel, however, is only $r = .03$ (data not shown), suggesting that the relation between adoption of medical technology, labor costs, and total expenses is much more complex than previously conceived of in the literature. Insight into the nature of this series of relationships will be presented in Table 9.

Total expenses, however, are only one way of looking at monetary efficiency. As has already been reported in Tables 2 and 3, hospitals with high adoption rates have a shorter average length of stay and a higher occupancy rate. Thus, while the technologically modern hospital may have higher costs per patient day, it processes more patients in fewer days, with the result that the cost per patient stay may be lower for higher-quality care.

Thus, from Tables 2-5 it is seen that while the impact of centralization-decentralization of resource decision making on a hospital's level of adoption is as was predicted, its impact on efficiency is not as clear. It was hypothesized that centralization would facilitate efficiency of health care delivery, but this appears to be the case only with regard to total expenses. In terms of the time it takes the hospital to process patients, it seems to make little difference at which level resource allocation decisions are made in the organization. On the other hand, hospitals with decentralized decision-making authority do show a higher rate of utilization of bed capacity. Taken together, these findings emphasize the underlying complexity of factors which must be understood in order to deal with the problems of increasing hospitals' efficiency of health care delivery.

Further, in Table 5 it can be seen that geographical location (urban), delay in admissions, affiliation with a medical school, age of facility, amount of outside funds for research, average length of stay, and number of full-time non-medical personnel all contribute to higher total expenses for hospitals. However, as will be seen shortly, the impact of some of these factors is variable when the availability of information to decision makers (as measured by visibility of consequences) is taken into account.

Having examined the effect of who in the hospital makes decisions (centralization), the next question to raise is how the presence or lack of information (medical/economic visibility of consequences) concerning the organization's activities modifies the impact of adoption on efficiency under varying degrees of centralization-decentralization of decision-making authority.

The Basis of Decision

The data presented thus far provide support for the contention that who makes decisions in a hospital has differential effects on how well the organization is able to handle the problem of keeping down the cost of care and maintaining up-to-date medical facilities. Following this lead, the next thing asked is whether having available information or knowledge of past consequences on which to base decisions facilitates these trends.

Distinguishing between medical and economic visibility of consequences led to the formulation of two hypotheses:

1. Decentralized hospitals with high visibility of medical consequences would adopt more new medical technology than decentralized hospitals having low medical visibility.
2. Centralized hospitals with high visibility of economic consequences would be more efficient than centralized hospitals with low visibility.

Further, it was expected that the predicted relations between adoption and centralization of resources decision making and the three measures of efficiency and centralization would be enhanced when either type of visibility was high. Operating under conditions of high visibility of either type, it was felt, would have the general effect of facilitating decision makers' awareness of issues, thus enabling them to find ways to improve the hospital's quality of care when resource decision making was decentralized and improve efficiency of delivery when decision making was centralized.

To test the hypotheses, it is necessary to dichotomize hospitals twice: first on the basis of high or low visibility of medical consequences, and second on high or low economic visibility.[12] Tables 6-9 display the results of this analysis.[13]

A comparison of the beta values for centralization across conditions of visibility of consequences in Table 6 indicates two points.

[12]The correlation between economic and medical visibility of consequences is $r = -.05$.

[13]For reasons already explained, the variables used are corrected for hospital bed size.

TABLE 6

Regression Estimates of the Impact of Centralization and Other Organizational Factors on Adoption Controlling for Levels of Economic and Medical Visibility of Consequence

EXPLANATORY VARIABLE	ADOPTION [a]			
	Visibility of Economic Consequence		Visibility of Medical Consequence	
	High	*Low*	*High*	*Low*
Centralization of decision making	-.20[b]	-.11[b]	-.20[b]	-.09[b]
Urban/rural (urban = 1, rural = 0)	.28[b]	.45[b]	.31[b]	.30[b]
Hospital affiliated with medical school	-.03	.16[b]	.05	.09
Outside funds for research	.22[b]	.31[b]	.30[b]	.29[b]
Other assets	-.17[b]	-.02	-.03	-.08
Number of full-time physicians	.20[b]	-.08[b]	.02	-.03
Number of different medical specialists on staff	.02	.09[b]	.14[b]	.03
Number of full-time non-medical personnel	-.16[b]	.01	.09[b]	-.17[b]
Number of services	.10[b]	.06	.07	.02
Visibility of economic consequence			-.09[b]	.03
Visibility of medical consequence	.03	-.13[b]		
MR =	.64	.72	.67	.64
N =	205	170	156	184

[a] Values reported are Beta weight.
[b] Beta greater than twice its standard error, significant at the .05 level.

First, the negative signs of all four beta weights for centralization mean that, regardless of the type or level of visibility of consequences present in a hospital, centralization of resource decision-making authority has a negative relation to a hospital's level of adoption. Conversely, in situations where authority has been delegated to the medical staff, the hospital tends to keep the facility up to date medically. Secondly, the decentralized structure appears to facilitate adoption more when visibility of either medical or economic consequences is high. This finding tends to support the general contention that having information regarding the past performance of the hospital provides a basis for assessing anticipated courses of action and acts as an impetus on decision makers to improve medical performance.

Relevant to the above point are findings from a further analysis done on the same data base (Gordon, Tanon, and Morse, 1974). There hospitals were categorized into one of four groups on the basis of whether they exhibited high or low economic and medical visibility of consequences. A comparison of the mean level of adoption of each group supported the prediction that hospitals having a high level of medical visibility and a low level of economic visibility would adopt more medical innovations ($\bar{X} = 5.9$) than hospitals having high economic visibility and low medical visibility ($\bar{X} = 4.5$).

Returning to the present analysis, however, a more complex picture emerges when the direct effects of economic and medical visibility of consequences are examined. Under the condition of low economic visibility of consequences, the higher the level of medical visibility the lower the level of adoption (Beta $= -.13$). Similarly, under conditions of high visibility of medical consequences, the higher the level of economic visibility the lower the adoption. Further examination of the impact of other variables indicates that geographic location (urban) and amount of outside research funding have the most significant and consistent impacts on adoption. The differential impact of the number of full-time physicians and number of full-time non-medical personnel under different types and levels of visibility of consequences is a further indication of the complex relationship among information, structure, and adoption. The interrelationship among these variables clearly indicates that further research is warranted in this area.

Turning to the impact of centralization on efficiency, for occupancy rate, under all conditions of visibility (Table 7), the negative beta weights suggest that centralized decision making is associated with underutilization of a hospital's bed capacity.

TABLE 7

Regression Estimates of the Impact of Centralization and Other Organizational Factors on Average Occupancy Rate Controlling for Levels of Economic and Medical Visibility of Consequence

| | AVERAGE OCCUPANCY RATE [a] | | | |
| | Visibility of Economic Consequence | | Visibility of Medical Consequence | |
EXPLANATORY VARIABLE	High	Low	High	Low
Centralization of decision making	-.10	-.17b	-.11b	-.04
Adoption	.08	.20	.05	.16b
Urban/rural (urban = 1, rural = 0)	.07	.12b	.07	.10
Delay in admission	.40b	.28b	.40b	.30b
Hospital affiliated with medical school	.01	.09	.03	.05
Other assets	-.07	-.02	.01	-.16b
Number of full-time physicians	.01	.03	.00	-.03
Number of different medical specialists on staff	.03	.07	.11b	.06
Number of full-time non-medical personnel	.00	.03	.02	.08
Number of services	.01	-.13b	-.06	-.06
Visibility of economic consequence	-.05	-.26b		
Visibility of medical consequence			+.01	-.13
MR =	.47	.52	.53	.45
N =	205	170	156	184

[a] Values reported are Beta weights.
[b] Beta greater than twice its standard error, significant at the .05 level.

Further, this tendency is facilitated somewhat when the staff is operating in a situation where medical performance is being evaluated (high medical V of C) (Beta = − .11) or when the governing body of the hospital is not as cognizant of the hospital's economic circumstances (low economic V of C) (Beta = − .17). These patterns in the data suggest, contrary to the hypothesis, that allowing physicians more freedom in and responsibility for determining how and when to utilize the bed capacity of the hospital facilitates use of the physical plant.

Looking at the direct effect of adoption on average occupancy rate under different types and levels of visibility of consequences, it appears that adoption only has a positive influence when either economic or medical visibility is low. It also seems apparent from looking at the other variables in Table 7 that a hospital's delay in admission is most directly interrelated with its occupancy rate.

Table 8 shows the relation of centralization and other factors to the second dimension of efficiency, average length of patient stay. It was predicted that under the condition of high visibility of economic consequences, centralization would have a significant influence on reducing patients' average length of stay. The exact opposite is evidenced in the data.

The importance of introducing the factor of visibility of consequences into the analysis is made particularly evident in this instance. The reader will recall that Table 4 indicated that who made decisions had no significant impact on a hospital's average length-of-stay statistics. However, a very different conclusion is drawn when comparing the relation of who makes decisions under conditions of high and low economic visibility to average length of stay. Centralization of authority has the impact (Beta = .08) of increasing the average length of stay when visibility is high. There is a suggestion in the data, although not significant (Beta = − .07), that centralization only facilitates a lower average length of stay where awareness of the hospital's economic state is low. Why might this be the case?

The measure of economic visibility, it will be recalled, is based on the extent to which the governing body of the hospital participates in the budget allocation and review processes. Given this fact, the data indicate that if persons at the top of the organization retain administrative control over the hospital's activities, they are more apt to establish procedures and follow courses of action which give priority to economic rather than medical considerations when they are cognizant of the economic state of the system

TABLE 8

Regression Estimates of the Impact of Centralization and Other Organizational Factors on Average Length of Stay Controlling for Levels of Economic and Medical Visibility of Consequence

EXPLANATORY VARIABLE	AVERAGE LENGTH OF STAY [a]			
	Visibility of Economic Consequence		Visibility of Medical Consequence	
	High	*Low*	*High*	*Low*
Centralization of decision making	.08[b]	-.07	.03	.08
Adoption	-.12[b]	-.13[b]	-.12[b]	-.07
Urban/rural (urban = 1, rural = 0)	-.02	.09	.08	.02
Delay in admission	-.02	.08	.06	-.04
Hospital affiliated with medical school	.13[b]	.06	.06	-.10[b]
Outside funds for research	-.02	.07	.13[b]	.20[b]
Other assets	.22[b]	.04	.02	-.05
Number of full-time physicians	-.04	.24[b]	.21[b]	.18[b]
Number of different medical specialists on staff	-.21[b]	-.10[b]	-.08	-.15[b]
Number of full-time non-medical personnel	-.02	-.13[b]	-.11[b]	-.17[b]
Number of services		-.07	-.04	.03
Visibility of economic consequence			-.04	.05
Visibility of medical consequence	-.03	-.06		
MR =	.33	.39	.40	.33
N =	205	170	156	184

a Values reported are Beta weight.
b Beta greater than twice its standard error, significant at the .05 level.

55

than when they are not. This is not meant to imply that in such instances persons intentionally made decisions disregarding the medical needs of the hospital's patients. However, the economic realities of delivery of hospital care, if given priority over medical considerations, are less likely to result in decisions favorable to the patient.

For the most part, hospitals follow a policy of billing patients a fixed charge per day, regardless of how many days they remain in the hospital. In reality, though, a hospital incurs more expenses to process a patient at the time of admission and for a period thereafter than it charges the patient. As the patient stays longer, however, the price charged exceeds the expenses of services delivered, enabling the hospital to recover its costs. Thus as it now stands, given the billing policies which hospitals must presently follow if they are to be reimbursed by the major third-party payers, the economically aware rational head is likely to favor decisions which extend or do not reduce the average length of time a patient stays in the hospital.

A change in the present nationwide billing policy to allow hospitals to charge patients on the basis of a decreasing sliding scale would reduce or eliminate the economic constraints now operating and thus encourage hospitals to keep patients for a shorter period of time. Though such a policy would not presumably reduce the total charged a patient, by lowering the hospital's average length of stay, a hospital would be able to serve more patients with the same number of beds. Given the expanding demand for hospital inpatient care and the high cost of building new bed facilities, such a change seems warranted.

Returning to Table 8, it may be seen that, as was the case in Table 4, the number of non-medical personnel has the effect of reducing average length of stay, whereas the magnitude of a hospital's outside research funds and its number of full-time attending physicians have the effect of increasing average length of stay. It would appear then that the trends previously discussed remain even under different conditions of visibility of consequences.

The final dimension of efficiency considered, total expenses (Table 9), is seen to be inversely influenced by centralization under all four types and levels of visibility of consequences. Looking at the impact of other factors, it can be seen that geographic location, the time since the hospital was founded, and amount of outside research funds all have a positive impact on a hospital's total expenses. Adoption of medical technology has a differential impact on total expenses, depending upon the nature of a hospital's visibility of consequences. Under conditions of low economic visibility or high medical visibility, adoption has a positive impact on total expenses; but when economic visibility is high or medical visibility is low, a hospital's level of adoption has no effect. The interrelationship between types and levels of visibility of consequences as they impinge upon the impact of adoption on total expenses warrants further investigation. In line with this, there are several other indications from the data in Table 9 of the differential impact of various organizational factors on total expenses under varying conditions of availability and use of information in the hospital (i.e., visibility of consequences). For example, with high visibility of economic consequences, the greater the number of full-time nonmedical personnel the lower the total expenses. However, the reverse is true under conditions of low economic or high medical visibility of consequences. Thus, in reference to the previous discussion of the relation among level of adoption, labor, and total expenses, it can be seen that whether labor has an impact on total expenses depends upon the nature of the organization's information system. Similarly, where visibility of economic consequences is low, medical school affiliation has a positive relation to total expenses, whereas when economic visibility is high, such an affiliation appears to have no effect on total expenses. Interestingly, with high visibility of medical consequences, the use of outpatient services has a positive relation to total expenses but holds no relation under other conditions of visibility.

Looking at the effects of economic visibility of consequences itself on total expenses, only when visibility of medical consequences is low does it have a negative effect. On the other hand, there is no effect of visibility of medical consequences on total expenses under either level of visibility of economic consequences. These findings raise the serious question of the circumstances under which various medical and economic information systems contribute to improved performance of the hospital.

To a large extent, information regarding past performance can be thought of as value-free. While it can form the basis of a series of decisions, it does not determine the nature of the decisions themselves. Today, top officials of hospitals face myriad pressures from the public and private sectors of society to keep costs down. Thus it is understandable that their decisions would reflect a

TABLE 9

Regression Estimates of the Impact of Centralization and Other Organizational Factors on Total Expenses Controlling for Levels of Economic and Medical Visibility of Consequence

EXPLANATORY VARIABLE	TOTAL EXPENSES [a]			
	Visibility of Economic Consequence		Visibility of Medical Consequence	
	High	Low	High	Low
Centralization of decision making	-.13[b]	-.14[b]	-.21[b]	-.04[b]
Adoption	-.03	.12[b]	.08[b]	-.02
Urban/rural (Urban = 1, rural = 0)	.21[b]	.31[b]	.19[b]	.22[b]
Cost of manpower	.04	.00	.02	.00
Delay in admission	.19[b]	.14[b]	.16[b]	.19[b]
Hospital affiliated with medical school	-.03	.27[b]	.14[b]	.12[b]
Years since founding	.16[b]	.14[b]	.16[b]	.13[b]
Outside funds for research	.43[b]	.28[b]	.32[b]	.37[b]
Average length occupancy rate	.06	-.01	-.07	.06[b]
Average length of stay	.04	.03	.01	.10[b]
Other assets	.13[b]	-.09	.05	.00
Number of full-time physicians	.06	-.05	.04	-.38[b]
Total visits—outpatient services	.06	-.04	.11[b]	.01
Number of different medical specialists on staff	.00	-.32[b]	-.10[b]	-.17[b]
Number of full-time non-medical personnel	-.09[b]	.26[b]	.30[b]	.00
Number of services	-.01	-.16[b]	-.12[b]	-.14[b]
Visibility of economic consequence			.02	-.08[b]
Visibility of medical consequence	.00	-.03		
MR =	.84	.89	.86	.91
N =	205	170	156	184

[a] Values reported are Beta weights.
[b] Beta greater than twice its standard error, significant at the .05 level.

stronger concern for the monetary aspects of health care delivery. On the other hand, physicians are more likely to concern themselves with the quality of care they deliver to their patients. Thus simply increasing the level of awareness of economic and medical past performance in a hospital as a means of improving the quality and efficiency of health care delivery without concern for who is going to use the information is likely to result in wasted efforts. While this may appear to be a rather obvious point, it is the case that hospitals have in the past and are presently being pressed to institute programs and procedures for evaluating both their economic and medical performance. In at least two instances, findings of this study suggest that information-collecting programs have, as yet, little positive impact on hospital behavior. Specifically, we are referring here to a hospital's accounting system, and second, to whether a hospital participates in the Medical Audit Procedures (M.A.P.) program.

Though developing and maintaining an elaborate accounting system necessarily requires a sizable expenditure of funds, pressure at a national level has been placed on hospitals to improve their accounting practices. One possible rationale behind doing so is that having a sophisticated accounting system will provide a hospital with the kind of financial information needed to effectively control, if not reduce, its costs of delivering care. In a similar vein, encouraging hospitals to utilize the services of M.A.P. can be seen as a way a hospital can gain an increased awareness of its medical staff's performance relative to other hospitals. Conceivably, such information could provide a strong impetus to improve the quality of care they deliver. One indicator of this would be the frequency with which they adopt new medical technology. Since there is a great variation in the sophistication of hospitals' accounting systems, and less than half of them subscribe to M.A.P., it was possible to test whether in fact these two mechanisms for raising levels of visibility were having any effect.

The relation between hospitals' sophistication level of accounting techniques and the three dimensions of efficiency was found to be almost nil. Similarly, whether or not a hospital participated in M.A.P. showed no relation to the frequency with which it adopted new technology.

Hence, using the criteria of increasing efficiency on the one hand or stimulating the adoption of new medical technology on the other, neither of these techniques appears to work. But why shouldn't they, at least potentially, lead to increased information being available in the organization upon which to base decisions?

The answer may lie with a point raised earlier. Simply increasing the quantity and/or quality of information a hospital has concerning its past performance with regard for who is going to make use of the information may be a fruitless endeavor. Without question, an elaborate accounting system can provide decision makers with a great deal of information, but effective use of it can only be made if a hospital has someone on hand with the expert knowledge of accounting theory to interpret the figures. To the extent that decision makers in the hospital lack such expertise or access to it, a more sophisticated accounting system is only producing information which no one knows how to apply. It might be more judicious in terms of reducing expenses to refrain from pressuring hospitals any further on this front until such time as they are also required to retain on their administrative staffs the experts needed to adequately interpret the information.

Likewise, a hospital which participates in M.A.P. receives aggregated information regarding its past medical performance. While such information could be potentially useful, in the hands of individuals who are not oriented to it and who work in an environment which requires them to deal with one patient at a time, it may have no significant value. It is likely that such information can only be effectively utilized by persons sensitive to the complex issues involved in organizing health care delivery systems. Suffice it to say, it is unlikely physicians in most cases are prepared to use the statistics generated by M.A.P.

To the extent that what has been found in the two instances can be generalized to other mechanisms for generating information in hospitals, it would seem imperative to evaluate more fully the circumstances surrounding the intended use of the information produced before requiring hospitals to invest money and manpower to institute such mechanisms.

Conclusion

As stated in the introduction to the paper, our major concern was with clarifying the effects of various organization factors surrounding the relationship between level of adoption of new medical technology and the costs of hospital services. The data presented support the contention that who makes decisions in a hospital has a differential effect on how well the organization is able to handle the problem of keeping down the costs of care and maintaining up-to-date medical facilities. Decentralization of decision making appears to facilitate a hospital's adoption of modern medical technology. Conversely, centralization of decision making is associated with lower total expenses. Further, contrary to what is often thought, it was found that a high level of adoption has the effect of reducing average length of stay and increasing average occupancy rate while having little direct impact on a hospital's total expenses. The evidence indicates that in terms of efficiency, organizational structure is an important factor in determining whether gains in effectiveness outweigh expenses associated with the adoption of new technology.[14]

When the level of economic and medical information available (visibility of consequences) in hospitals is taken into consideration, the impact of centralization on adoption behavior and efficiency is found to be far more complex than initially predicted. These findings, in concert with the lack of effect of a hospital's sophistication level of accounting techniques on total expenses and the lack of effect of participation in M.A.P. on adoption behavior, suggest the importance of increasing our understanding of the relationships between information systems, decision making, and organizational structure in hospitals.

[14]While this paper has focused on the impact of internal organizational structure on hospital efficiency and effectiveness, a relatively consistent relation of hospital location (rural-urban) to the dependent variables is also apparent. Though only a global indicator of the nature of a hospital's external environment, the data suggest that a more refined examination of the impact of environmental characteristics on hospital behavior may be fruitful.

Edward V. Morse, PH.D.
Department of Sociology
Tulane University
New Orleans, Louisiana 70118

Gerald Gordon, PH.D.
New York State School of Industrial and Labor Relations
Department of Sociology
Cornell University
Ithaca, New York 14850

Michael Moch, PH.D.
Department of Sociology
University of Michigan
Ann Arbor, Michigan 48104

References

Andersen, Ronald, and J. Joel May
1972   ''Factors associated with increased costs of hospital care.'' The An-
         nals of The American Academy of Political and Social Science
         (January):62-72.

Becker, S., and G. Gordon
1966   ''The entrepreneurial theory of formal organizations, part I: patterns
         of formal organization.'' Administrative Science Quarterly, 2, number
         3:315-344.

Carr, J., and P. Feldstein
1967   ''The relation of hospital cost to size.'' Inquiry 4:45-65.

Feldstein, M.
1967   Economic Analysis for Health Service Efficiency. Chicago: Markham.

Feldstein, P.
1961   An Empirical Investigation of the Marginal Cost of Hospital Services.
         Chicago: University of Chicago Press.

Gordon, G., C. Tanon, and E. Morse
1974   ''Professional power, hospital structure, and innovation.'' Paper pre-
         pared for the American Sociological Association Meeting, Montreal,
         Canada.

Ingbar, Mary Lee, and Lester Taylor
1968   Hospital Costs in Massachusetts. Cambridge: Harvard University
         Press.

Klarman, H.
1965   The Economics of Health. New York: Columbia University Press.

Lave, J.
1966   ''A review of the methods used to study hospital costs.'' Inquiry
         3:57-81.

Lave, Judith R., and Lester B. Lave
1970a   ''Hospital cost functions.'' The American Economic Review (June):
         379-395.

1970b   ''Economic analysis for health service efficiency: a review article.''
         Applied Economics 1:293-305.

Mann, J., and D. Yett
    1968   ''The analysis of hospital costs: a review article.'' Journal of Business 41:191-202.

Rafferty, John
    1971   ''Patterns of hospital use.'' Journal of Political Economy 79 (January-February): 154-165.

    1972   ''Hospital output indices.'' Economic and Business Bulletin 24 (Winter): 21-27.

Rogers, Everett M.
    1962   Diffusion of Innovation. New Yori: Free Press of Glencoe.

    1967   Bibliography on the Diffusion of Innovation. East Lansing, Michigan: Michigan State University.

Rosner, Martin M.
    1968   ''Economic determinants of organizational innovation.'' Administrative Science Quarterly 12 (March): 614-625.

Thompson, James D.
    1967   Organizations in Action. New York: McGraw-Hill.

Cost and Efficiency in the Production of Hospital Services

RALPH E. BERRY, JR.

This paper summarizes the general findings of a research effort designed to complete a .detailed analysis to identify and measure the effects of factors which significantly affect the cost and efficiency of the short-term general hospital system in the United States.

The empirical analysis involved data on approximately 6,000 hospitals for the years 1965, 1966, and 1967 and involved a model which expressed hospital cost as a function of the level of output, the quality of services provided, the scope of services provided, factor prices, and relative efficiency. The statistical analysis does provide insight to the factors affecting hospital cost: hospital services are produced subject to economies of scale but the absolute magnitudes are rather insignificant; on the basis of the exceedingly limited data available it can be concluded that quality does affect costs; medical education is a significant factor affecting hospital costs; and product mix has a significant impact on costs.

Three separate analyses are summarized specific to the product mix difference aspect of the production of hospital services, its effect on hospital cost analysis, and techniques that can be employed to account for product mix.

Finally, an analysis of the characteristics of high cost and low cost hospitals is summarized.

Introduction

This paper, like the others in this issue, is intended to summarize the general findings of a specific research effort supported by the Social Security Administration (Berry and Carr, 1973). The primary purpose of the research effort was to complete a detailed analysis to identify and measure the effects of factors which significantly affect the cost and efficiency of the short-term general hospital system in the United States.

The rapid inflation of hospital costs is a well-known phenomenon. Hospital cost inflation is of particular concern to the Social Security Administration because of the less than subtle impact on the Medicare budget. Given its responsibility for the payment of a significant proportion of total expenditures for hospital services, and its responsibility for insuring that these funds are used as effectively as feasible, the Social Security Administration has

M M F Q / Health and Society / *Summer 1974*

both a factual and policy interest in the cost and efficiency of the production of hospital services. Thus the research effort was addressed to an area of signal public importance and concern.

Factors Affecting Hospital Cost

The empirical analysis of the factors affecting hospital cost involved data on approximately 6,000 short-term general hospitals for the years 1965, 1966, and 1967. The basic model utilized in the analysis was of the form:

$$C = f(O, Q, M, P, E)$$

where
  C = cost of hospital services
  O = level of output
  Q = quality of services
  M = product mix (complexity of scope of services)
  P = factor prices
  E = efficiency

i.e., hospital cost is a function of the level of output, the quality of services provided, the scope of services provided, factor prices, and relative efficiency. The estimated cost equations summarized in Table 1 are for 1966 and are representative of the general results of the analysis.

The statistical analysis of the cost of providing short-term general hospital care in the United States does in fact provide insight to the factors affecting hospital cost. A number of inferences can be drawn concerning the relationships among average costs, output, quality, product mix, factor prices, and relative efficiency.

Output, Cost, and Returns to Scale

The specific form of the equation estimated was chosen in order to form the basis for testing various hypotheses concerning returns to scale in the production of hospital services. A careful analysis of the results obtained indicates that hospital services are produced subject to economies of scale initially and decreasing returns to scale eventually. More specifically, since the dependent variable is average cost, hospital services are produced subject to decreasing costs initially and increasing costs eventually. In essence, the

TABLE 1

Summary of Average Cost Regression Equations
for Short-Term General Hospitals in 1966

	Coefficients a			
Variable	*All Hospitals*	*Voluntary Hospitals*	*Government Hospitals*	*Proprietary Hospitals*
Constant	−10.2802	−8.4397	−7.9165	−20.5254
Output				
ADC	−0.0162	−0.0164	−0.0372	−0.0952
	(0.0039)	(0.0048)	(0.0082)	(0.0931)
ADC^2	0.00001	0.00002	0.0001	0.0002
	(0.000002)	(0.000003)	(0.000003)	(0.0004)
Quality				
Hospital	2.7909	4.6002	1.6393	1.5212
accredited	(0.5481)	(0.7249)	(0.9244)	(2.3858)
Product mix				
Cancer	−0.7590	−0.3538	−0.1675	2.3120
program	(0.6055)	(0.6206)	(1.6197)	(7.5211)
Residency	2.5473	2.3647	5.5635	6.5105
program	(0.8661)	(0.8799)	(2.7210)	(9.3173)
Internship	1.5290	−0.2437	6.8730	−6.1715
program	(0.9242)	(0.9345)	(2.7986)	(15.9282)
Medical school	−0.3192	−0.1472	0.7693	b
affiliation	(0.9759)	(0.9848)	(2.7061)	
Member, Council of	6.2301	3.2337	10.9965	b
Teaching Hospitals	(1.1415)	(1.2124)	(2.5436)	
Nursing	−0.4611	−0.8683	1.3350	2.8359
school	(0.7412)	(0.7906)	(1.7691)	(22.7373)
Practical	0.1816	−0.2057	−0.5232	1.5362
nurse program	(0.7736)	(0.8642)	(1.5388)	(6.5094)
Blood	1.3621	1.1191	1.2159	2.4005
bank	(0.4378)	(0.5227)	(0.8220)	(2.1937)
Clinical	2.1404	2.5371	1.3799	−7.3122
laboratory	(1.6394)	(2.0359)	(2.7402)	(8.3226)
Pathology	1.7586	2.8678	0.9460	−2.0463
laboratory	(0.5410)	(0.6689)	(0.9598)	(2.3387)
Electroenceph-	1.5403	1.6305	1.5748	−0.6628
alography	(0.4782)	(0.5299)	(1.0662)	(2.7218)
Dental	−0.3575	−0.9276	1.2310	−1.8709
facilities	(0.4155)	(0.4558)	(0.9209)	(2.3393)

a Standard errors are in parentheses.
b There were no proprietary hospitals with medical school affiliation and no proprietary hospitals were members of the Council of Teaching Hospitals.

TABLE 1—*Continued*

	Coefficients a			
Variable	*All Hospitals*	*Voluntary Hospitals*	*Government Hospitals*	*Proprietary Hospitals*
Pharmacy with pharmacist	3.0279 (0.5100)	2.6857 (0.6408)	2.5382 (0.9206)	9.8480 (2.0455)
Occupational therapy	0.9518 (0.7148)	0.6844 (0.7541)	1.7027 (1.6757)	9.3659 (6.2890)
Physical therapy	0.8826 (0.4656)	0.7268 (0.5554)	1.6738 (0.9186)	1.8944 (2.0352)
Premature nursery	−0.1977 (0.4196)	−0.0859 (0.4997)	−1.6412 (0.7853)	2.3422 (2.0709)
Emergency room	−0.3732 (0.8745)	−1.4028 (1.0776)	1.4202 (2.0252)	−0.0178 (2.6988)
Home care program	4.4726 (0.8450)	2.4143 (0.8957)	9.2165 (1.9844)	12.9343 (6.3169)
Operating room	2.0646 (1.9123)	1.3471 (2.3695)	9.4138 (4.1142)	9.4971 (8.2515)
Obstetrical delivery room	−4.1893 (0.9316)	−3.1266 (1.0908)	−11.6384 (2.8794)	−5.7794 (3.0453)
Postoperative recovery room	1.7292 (0.5279)	1.7256 (0.6710)	1.6688 (0.9166)	1.9797 (2.2767)
Social work department	1.7197 (0.9652)	2.1561 (1.0311)	2.0916 (2.3645)	0.4175 (6.4436)
X-ray diagnostic	0.3081 (2.1182)	0.3502 (2.7003)	0.5894 (3.3828)	4.2781 (11.5529)
X-ray therapeutic	−0.7554 (0.5748)	−0.2971 (0.6345)	−1.6945 (1.2971)	−6.1921 (2.6898)
Radioisotope therapy	2.0788 (0.5731)	2.3032 (0.6143)	3.0758 (1.3569)	−1.4691 (3.5486)
Hospital auxiliary	0.9697 (0.5046)	0.7783 (0.6769)	1.0518 (0.8140)	2.4512 (2.4198)
Psychiatric inpatient unit	−1.4540 (0.6068)	−0.9399 (0.6597)	−4.1494 (1.2936)	4.6078 (6.6739)
Rehabilitation inpatient unit	0.5605 (0.7798)	−0.1052 (0.8085)	3.8620 (1.9009)	9.5832 (8.6649)
Cobalt therapy	2.0280 (0.6372)	1.9045 (0.6612)	1.2640 (1.6330)	6.1452 (5.8678)
Radium therapy	−0.1203 (0.5727)	−0.7905 (0.6148)	1.5616 (1.3619)	5.5161 (3.1854)
Outpatient department	−0.6007 (0.4024)	0.1017 (0.4719)	−1.6412 (0.7853)	−4.2913 (2.0606)
Routine chest X-ray on admission	−0.1322 (0.3865)	−0.6626 (0.4381)	0.5111 (0.7957)	0.6390 (2.2207)

TABLE 1—*Continued*

	Coefficients a			
Variable	All Hospitals	Voluntary Hospitals	Government Hospitals	Proprietary Hospitals
Routine blood sugar on admission	−0.2481 (0.4600)	0.3803 (0.5183)	−0.6441 (0.9418)	−6.3044 (2.5032)
Average length of stay	−0.7674 (0.0581)	−0.7695 (0.0747)	−1.3652 (0.1362)	−1.5037 (0.4938)
Obstetric inpatient days/inpatient days	8.0007 (2.5627)	0.3803 (0.5183)	5.7629 (4.8873)	2.0952 (8.5610)
ICU inpatient days/ inpatient days	−0.4799 (3.4578)	2.1904 (5.9049)	−1.1651 (4.7007)	7.9239 (11.6626)
Outpatient visits/ inpatient days	1.6334 (0.1629)	1.7601 (0.2938)	1.2078 (0.1989)	3.8775 (0.9079)
Student nurses/ ADC	0.8327 (1.2676)	1.4124 (1.3689)	0.0794 (2.9102)	−3.6205 (12.5698)
Interns and residents/ADC	31.5818 (4.4895)	54.9247 (5.8928)	5.6487 (8.2197)	−100.9583 (127.0582)
Other Trainees/ ADC	0.7868 (1.4881)	1.0264 (1.4552)	−6.5405 (5.0839)	−30.5541 (22.6756)
Factor Prices				
Predicted annual wage rate	0.0130 (0.0005)	0.0125 (0.0006)	0.0109 (0.0010)	0.0160 (0.0023)
Predicted construc- tion cost index	−0.0808 (0.0336)	−0.1048 (0.0384)	0.0466 (0.0654)	0.0474 (0.2370)
Other Variables				
Empty beds	0.4715 (0.3648)	1.5165 (0.7681)	−0.1578 (0.4276)	−12.1822 (3.0475)
Output change 1965 to 1966	−3.3091 (1.1146)	−1.2953 (1.3399)	−5.5310 (2.8283)	−17.5889 (4.9627)
Output change 1966 to 1967	4.9848 (0.8295)	7.1727 (1.1406)	1.8509 (1.2405)	12.0419 (4.3978)
Government dummy	−0.0752 (0.4887)	—	—	—
Proprietary dummy	3.6050 (0.7949)	—	—	—
$\bar{R}^2$	0.57	0.59	0.58	0.69
Degrees of freedom	2678	1752	647	134

a Standard errors are in parentheses.

average cost curve of hospital services was found to be "U" shaped.[1]

Although the results are statistically significant, perhaps a more important question is how significant are the absolute magnitudes of the economies of scale? In effect, given that the average cost curve is "U" shaped, how steep or how shallow is the "U"? In fact, the average cost curves are rather shallow—the absolute magnitudes of the economies of scale are rather insignificant. A few straightforward calculations can serve to put the cost-output relationship into perspective. Thus, for example, the equations in Table 1 imply the following four cost-output relationships for 1966:[2]

(1)	All hospitals	$AC = 44.56 - .0162\,ADC + .00000967\,(ADC)^2$
(2)	Government hospitals	$AC = 42.11 - .0372\,ADC + .0000146\,(ADC)^2$
(3)	Voluntary hospitals	$AC = 45.46 - .0164\,ADC + .0000191\,(ADC)^2$
(4)	Proprietary hospitals	$AC = 48.93 - .0952\,ADC + .000168\,(ADC)^2$

These relationships in turn provide the basis for comparing average costs at various levels of output. The data outlined in Tables 2 and 3 indicate the relative insignificance of the absolute magnitude of economies of scale in the production of hospital services.

In Table 2, the comparisons are delineated in terms of the mean average daily census and the optimal average daily census. The mean ADC is the actual mean that prevailed in 1966. The optimal ADC is that level of output which corresponds to minimum average cost. In each case it would require a several-fold increase in the level of output to bring about minimum average costs. Further, the

[1]The equations estimated were cost equations of the form:

$$AC = a \pm b_1\,ADC \pm b_2\,(ADC)^2 \pm b_i X_i$$

where the factors other than output are represented by the vector X. The relationship between average cost and the level of output is then represented by the sign and statistical significance of b_1 and b_2. In fact the sign of b_1 is negative in each case while the sign of b_2 is positive in each case. The level of significance for both b_1 and b_2 is greater than .01 in all cases except that of proprietary hospitals.

[2]These equations are derived from those in Table 1 by assigning the mean values for each of the independent variables other than the output variables.

TABLE 2

Summary of Comparative Cost and Output at Mean Average Daily Census
and Optimal Average Daily Census

	Output			Average Cost at		
	Mean ADC	*Optimal ADC*	*% Increase in Output*	*Mean ADC*	*Optimal ADC*	*% Decrease in Cost*
All hospitals	128	838	555	42.64	37.78	−11.4
Voluntary hospitals	146	429	194	43.48	41.94	−3.5
Government hospitals	108	1274	1080	38.26	18.42	−52.9
Proprietary hospitals	50	283	466	44.59	35.44	−20.5

TABLE 3

Summary of Comparative Cost and Output at Mean Average Daily Census
and 110 Percent of Mean Average Daily Census

	Average Cost at		Decrease	
	Mean ADC	*110 % of Mean ADC*	*Dollars*	*%*
All hospitals	42.64	42.47	0.17	0.40
Voluntary hospitals	43.48	43.32	0.16	0.37
Government hospitals	38.26	37.89	0.37	0.97
Proprietary hospitals	44.59	44.20	0.39	0.87

minimum average cost in most cases is not much below the prevailing average cost.

Since the optimal sizes are so much larger than the mean sizes, the comparisons are delineated in Table 3 in terms of the mean average daily census and an average daily census 10 percent larger than the mean. In each case a 10 percent increase in the level of output would result in less than a 1 percent decrease in average cost. Hence, albeit hospital services are produced subject to economies of scale, the absolute and relative magnitudes of the potential savings are such that they probably do not provide much of an incentive for exploitation. In fact, these cost estimates are exclusively in terms of internal money costs and take no account of travel costs or the costs associated with inconvenience to patients, attending physicians, or visitors. Since travel costs and inconvenience would necessarily increase if hospitals were larger and consequently served a larger catchment area, it would seem that the relative insignificance of the magnitude of economies of scale may explain the large number of relatively small hospitals.[3]

The relative changes in output from 1965 to 1966 and from 1966 to 1967 were included in the 1966 equations outlined in Table 1 to assess the impact on costs of short-term output changes. The results indicate that an increase in output from the previous year to the current year is associated with lower current average cost. Conversely, an increase in output from the current year to the succeeding year is associated with higher current average cost. If these relative changes in output are indicative of random short-run variations, then the results are consistent with decreasing costs but not consistent with either constant costs or increasing costs (see Berry and Carr, 1973: 45-47). If these relative changes in output are indicative of growth in output over time, then the results are probably a reflection of the discontinuities that are characteristic of additions to capacity, particularly additions to the physical plant.[4]

Empty beds as a proportion of the average daily census were included in the analysis to assess the effect of unused capacity on average cost. One would expect, a priori, that unused capacity would tend to raise average cost. The results reflected in Table 1 appear mixed. Empty beds do lead to higher average costs for voluntary hospitals and for all hospitals—the latter undoubtedly because voluntary hospitals dominate in the all hospitals equation. But empty beds lead to lower average costs for proprietary hospitals and government hospitals. In the case of government hospitals the result is not statistically significant, but it is quite significant in the case of proprietary hospitals. A difference in the relative magnitude of the effect of unused capacity on average costs

[3]In fact, if travel costs and costs associated with inconvenience rise more rapidly than internal costs fall, then hospital services are produced subject to increasing *total* costs.

[4]Thus, the lower current average cost associated with an increase in output from the previous year may be a result of the inability to increase all inputs proportionately (e.g., the capital may be used more intensively in the current year); while the higher current average cost associated with an increase in output from the current year to the succeeding year may be a consequence of the current addition of relatively fixed inputs in anticipation of future growth.

between voluntary and proprietary hospitals would be expected because of the rather significant difference in their respective capital intensities, but a difference in the direction of the effect is difficult to explain.

Quality and Cost

The quality of hospital services is a factor of signal importance. Unfortunately, there is little information that is empirically useful concerning the quality of hospital care. It is to be expected that higher-quality services are more costly to produce than lower-quality services, but there is no index of quality available that can be employed to derive the relationship between quality and cost directly.

The accreditation status of each hospital was included in the regression analysis and allows a first approximation of the quality-cost relationship.

In addition, there are a number of facilities and services that tend to enhance the quality of basic hospital services rather than to expand the complexity of the scope of services offered. These services and facilities include a blood bank, pathology laboratory, postoperative recovery room, premature nursery, and a pharmacy with a registered pharmacist.

A certain insight into the relationship between quality and cost can be gained from the data in Table 4. These data summarize the relationship between average cost and certain quality-related variables. Hospitals which are accredited have higher average costs, other things equal. To the extent that accreditation reflects quality, there is a positive relationship implied between quality and average cost. The relationship is generally statistically significant. Of course accreditation status is a dichotomous variable and quality is undoubtedly a continuous variable, but the results do allow a first, albeit rough, approximation to the quality-cost relationship.

The several relationships between average cost and the several quality-enhancing services and facilities are generally positive and often statistically significant. In fact, with the exception of the premature nursery, the pattern is consistent and significant, particularly for voluntary hospitals and all hospitals.

On balance, on the basis of the exceedingly limited data available, it seems reasonable to conclude that quality does affect hospital costs—higher-quality hospital services cost more to produce than lower-quality services.

TABLE 4
Summary of the Relationship Between Average Cost
and Certain Quality-Related Variables

| | "t" Statistics [a] | | | |
Variable	*All Hospitals*	*Voluntary Hospitals*	*Government Hospitals*	*Proprietary Hospitals*
Hospital accredited	5.09c	6.34c	1.77b	0.64
Blood bank	3.11c	2.14b	1.48	1.09
Pathology laboratory	3.25c	4.29c	0.99	−0.88
Pharmacy with pharmacist	5.94c	4.19c	2.76c	4.81c
Premature nursery	−0.47	−0.17	−2.09b	1.13
Postoperative recovery room	3.28c	2.57c	1.82b	0.87

[a] For regression results in Table 1.
[b] Significant at the .05 level.
[c] Significant at the .01 level.

Product Mix and Cost

The product mix of hospitals varies in two important dimensions. First, hospitals may engage in the provision of patient care, teaching, and research. Second, the complexity of the scope of services provided varies among hospitals. These product differences affect hospital costs. Hospitals are in fact an extreme case of multiproduct firms and, unfortunately, a classic example of firms for which it is virtually impossible to differentiate completely among the several services produced.

Some forty approvals, facilities and services available, and other product-mix related variables were included in the average cost-regression equations to account for product mix and to allow for an assessment of the effect of product-mix differences on hospital costs. Some insight to the relationship between product mix and cost can be gained from the data in Tables 5 and 6. The data in Table 5 summarize the relationship between average cost and teaching activities. The data in Table 6 summarize the relationship between average cost and the scope of services provided.

Albeit certain care must be exercised in interpreting the results, the data in Table 5 clearly indicate that average costs are higher in those hospitals that are involved in medical education.

TABLE 5

Summary of the Relationship Between Average Cost
and Certain Variables Related to Teaching Activities

	"t" Statistics [a]			
Variable	All Hospitals	Voluntary Hospitals	Government Hospitals	Proprietary Hospitals
Residency program	2.94[d]	2.69[d]	2.05[c]	.070
Internship program	1.65[c]	−0.26	2.46[d]	−0.39
Interns and residents/ADC	7.04[d]	9.32[d]	0.69	−0.80
Medical school affiliation	−0.33	−0.15	0.28	[b]
Member, Council of Teaching Hospitals	5.46[d]	2.67[d]	4.32[d]	[b]
Nursing school	−0.62	−1.10	−0.76	0.13
Student nurses/ADC	0.66	1.03	0.03	−0.29
Practical nurse program	0.24	−0.24	−0.34	0.24
Other trainees/ADC	0.53	0.71	−1.29	−1.35

[a] For regression results in Table 1.
[b] There were no proprietary hospitals with medical school affiliation and no proprietary hospitals were members of the Council of Teaching Hospitals.
[c] Significant at the .05 level.
[d] Significant at the .01 level.

The first five variables listed in Table 5 are all related to medical education, and the results should be interpreted collectively rather than individually.[5] On balance, these data suggest medical education as a significant factor affecting hospital costs.

The results imply that other types of teaching do not have a significant effect on costs. The existence of a professional nursing

[5]Thus, for example, the variable Member of Council of Teaching Hospitals is undoubtedly picking up the variation that might in its absence be picked up by the variable Medical school affiliation. Similarly, Internship program is very significant for government hospitals but very insignificant and actually negative for voluntary hospitals, while Interns and residents per ADC is very significant for voluntary hospitals but insignificant for government hospitals. It appears most likely that the Internship program variable is picking up the variation for government hospitals that Interns and residents per ADC is picking up for voluntary hospitals.

school has a negative but insignificant effect on costs. The number of student nurses per patient has a positive but insignificant effect on costs. The other relationships are mixed and all insignificant.

The data in Table 6 are indicative of the relationship between average cost and the scope of services provided. A number of factors are implicit in these data. First, some of the facilities and services which represent an expansion in the complexity of the

TABLE 6

Summary of the Relationship Between Average Cost
and Certain Variables Related to the Scope
of Services Provided

	"t" Statistics a			
Variable	All Hospitals	Voluntary Hospitals	Government Hospitals	Proprietary Hospitals
Electroencephalography	3.22c	3.08c	1.48	−0.24
Dental facilities	−0.86	−2.04b	1.34	−0.80
Physical therapy	1.90b	−1.31	1.82b	0.93
X-ray therapeutic	1.31	−0.47	−1.31	−0.23
Radioisotope therapy	3.63c	3.75c	2.27b	−0.41
Cobalt therapy	3.18c	2.88c	0.77	1.05
Radium therapy	−0.21	−1.29	1.15	1.73b
Psychiatric inpatient unit	−2.40c	−1.43	−3.21c	0.69
Occupational therapy	1.33	0.91	1.02	1.49
Home care program	5.29c	2.70c	4.65c	2.05b
Social work department	1.79b	2.09b	0.89	0.07
Rehabilitation inpatient unit	0.79	−0.13	2.03b	1.11
ICU inpatient days/ inpatient days	−0.14	0.37	−0.25	0.68
Outpatient visits/ inpatient days	10.03c	5.99c	6.07c	4.27c
Average length of stay	−13.20c	−10.31c	−10.02c	−3.05c

a   For regression results in Table 1.
b   Significant at the .05 level.
c   Significant at the .01 level.

scope of inpatient services provided have significant positive relationships with average cost, as would be expected. ECG, physical therapy, radioisotope, and cobalt therapy are all associated with higher average cost. Second, some of the variables which are characteristic of a hospital engaged in community medical services in addition to strict inpatient activity have significant positive relationships with average cost. The most characteristic and the most significant in this context is the number of outpatient visits as a proportion of total inpatient days, but the availability of a home care program and a social services department display a similar relationship. It would appear that in general, more complex inpatient services and the provision of community medical services are significant factors affecting hospital costs.

Finally, the results summarized in Table 6 also imply a significant length of stay effect on hospital costs. Some types of patient care are less expensive per day to provide on average than other types of patient care. This phenomenon is explicit in the significant negative relationship between average cost and psychiatric inpatient care and undoubtedly implicit in the significant negative relationship between average cost and average length of stay. Also, of course, the significant negative relationship between average length of stay and average cost is indicative of the well-documented fact that for any given type of patient care the early days of hospitalization are generally more expensive to provide than the later days of hospitalization.[6]

Factor Prices and Costs

In all the analysis undertaken, the wage rate was consistently the most significant variable in terms of explaining average cost. In essence the results outlined in Table 1 are representative of the relative significance of the wage-rate/cost relationship. In fact differences in wage rates across hospitals explain a significant part of the differences in average costs across hospitals.

Wage rates may vary for a number of reasons. Hospitals in different labor markets may face different wage rates as a result of local labor market differences, for example. Further, the labor in-

---

[6]Of course, this result does not imply that longer lengths of stay are less expensive, only that the average cost per day of a longer stay is lower. The total cost depends on both the cost per day and the number of days. Unnecessary extra days undoubtedly add to total hospital costs even though their impact on average cost is to lower it.

put requirements may differ for differences in quality, scope of services, and complexity of services.

The wage-rate variable in the equations outlined in Table 1 represents a predicted average annual wage. The wage rate for each hospital was estimated as a function of the proportion of personnel in various occupational categories, geographic location, size of the standard metropolitan area, hospital size, product mix, union status, and market structure. These predicted wage rates are intended to represent differences in wages associated with labor-market differences and product-mix differences. Again, the results are quite consistent and very significant.

Construction-cost indexes were estimated as a function of geographic location and the size of the standard metropolitan area and included as a surrogate for the cost of capital in the equations outlined in Table 1. The results indicate that differences in construction costs are not consistently significant in explaining differences in average cost; in fact, the indicated relationships are quite mixed.[7] On the one hand, the relationship between the predicted construction cost and average cost is positive but statistically insignificant in the cases of government hospitals and proprietary hospitals. On the other hand, the relationship is negative and significant in the case of voluntary hospitals. The same general result obtains for all hospitals undoubtedly because of the dominance of voluntary hospitals in the all hospitals equation.

Interpretation of these results is a complex matter and inferences should be drawn with some care. First, of course, these predicted construction-cost indexes represent construction costs that prevail in the geographic proximity of each hospital. Hence they would reflect differences in the cost of capital in instances of additions to the physical plant, but they would not necessarily reflect differences in the cost of capital equipment. Further, differences in construction costs would only have a direct effect on average costs if construction were in fact undertaken. Thus, for example, the results obtained for voluntary hospitals would be consistent with a set of circumstances where relatively high construction costs were a disincentive to capital accumulation such that where capital costs are high, lower-cost services are produced—lower-cost services in the sense of lower-quality services, less complex services, and a narrower scope of services. The effect of this phenomenon might be exaggerated for voluntary hospitals which

[7]On balance, it must be obvious that the predicted construction cost index is at best an imperfect surrogate for the cost of capital.

are often in receipt of a fixed amount of funds from philanthropic sources, especially for additions to the physical plant. Any increase in construction cost must necessarily reduce proportionately the quantity that can be funded with a fixed sum.

In fact, when separate regressions were run for groups of hospitals producing different product mixes, the negative relationship between average cost and predicted construction cost occurred only for the groups of hospitals producing the more basic services. The groups of hospitals producing more complex services and a broader scope of services were characterized by a positive relationship between average cost and predicted construction cost.

Differences in wage rates are consistently significant in explaining differences in average costs among hospitals; differences in construction costs are not. This is consonant with the fact that wage rates vary more than capital prices in general or the predicted construction cost indexes in particular.[8]

Hospital Control and Cost

The results in Table 1 provide some insight into the effect of hospital control on hospital costs. Dummy variables were included in the all-hospital equation for government and proprietary control. The regression coefficients on these dummy variables indicate the effect on average cost of government and proprietary control, respectively, relative to voluntary control. The regression coefficients and "*t*" statistics were:

	Coefficient	"*t*" Statistic
Government	−0.0752	−0.17
Proprietary	3.6050	4.54

[8]The relative variation of the factor price variables are as follows:

	Relative Variation[a]			
Variable	*All Hospitals*	*Voluntary Hospitals*	*Government Hospitals*	*Proprietary Hospitals*
Predicted average annual wage rate−1966	11.47	9.93	12.72	17.01
Predicted construction cost index−1966	6.98	6.44	7.65	7.75

[a] The standard deviation as a percentage of the mean.

Thus, the effect of government control relative to voluntary control is to lower average cost very slightly, but the result is quite insignificant statistically. The effect of proprietary control relative to voluntary control is to raise average cost by some $3.61, other things equal, and the result is statistically very significant.

Given the fairly common assumptions that proprietary hospitals (a) operate more efficiently, and (b) select relatively lower-cost patients for admission, this result may seem unexpected. In fact, however, the result is quite consistent with a hypothesis that proprietary hospitals produce hospital services at lower total cost.

The results imply that costs in proprietary hospitals are $3.61 higher per day than they are in voluntary hospitals, other things equal. But, in fact, the mean average length of stay in proprietary hospitals is some 1.11 days shorter than the mean average length of stay in voluntary hospitals.[9]

It was noted above that the relationship between average cost and average length of stay was negative in part because earlier days of hospitalization were more likely to be more expensive than later days of hospitalization. In this context, most of the product-mix measures included in the equations indicate the availability of facilities and services but not their level of utilization. It is quite likely that proprietary hospitals utilize their facilities more intensively per patient per day and consequently incur a higher cost per patient day but a lower total cost per patient, other things equal. This conclusion has been questioned. J. Pettengill (1973: 349) states "for-profit hospitals have higher expenses per day and per admission." His conclusion is apparently based on comparisons of for-profit and voluntary hospitals of similar size in 1971. Two points are worthy of note. First, "other things equal" in our analysis includes more than size. Second, the data don't completely support Pettengill's conclusion—in fact, of the six size categories he reports, cost per admission is higher for for-profit hospitals in four categories but lower in two. Further, the data reported by the American Hospital Association (1971) imply that cost per admission is higher for for-profit hospitals in three size categories, lower in three size categories, and approximately the same in one

---

[9]The mean average lengths of stay are:

All Hospitals	— 7.63 days
Voluntary hospitals	— 7.79 days
Government Hospitals	— 7.52 days
Proprietary hospitals	— 6.68 days

size category. In 1966, cost per admission in for-profit hospitals was higher in three size categories and lower in three size categories.

Product Differences

The nature of the hospital industry is such that product-mix differences are of particular importance. Whatever else may be characteristic of them, the units of production in the hospital industry certainly do not produce a homogeneous product.

Since hospitals should be viewed as multiproduct firms in both the sense of patient care-teaching-research and the complexity of each, a considered attempt was made to deal with the phenomenon of product differences. The available data representative of product-mix differences in hospitals were analyzed in order to ascertain whether or not the multidimensional character of hospital output could be rationalized. The results of the analysis provided additional insights into the product-mix phenomenon.

Three separate albeit related analyses were undertaken specific to the product-difference aspect of the production of hospital services, its effect on hospital cost analysis, and techniques that can be employed to account for product mix. The results of these analyses were consistent and reinforcing. They serve to emphasize the importance of product mix and the implications of product differences.

First, a factor analysis served to delineate the dimensions of product mix in hospital output. This factor analysis is described in detail by Berry (1970: 67-75) and also by Berry and Carr (1973: 48-55). Eight common factors were generated that explained a significant proportion of the variation in the variables related to product mix. Among the more significant factors identified were: a medical school factor; a basic services factor; a complex services factor; a length of stay factor; and an outpatient activities factor.

This factor analysis has a number of implications. Primarily, it provides evidence that the approach to adjusting for product mix employed in the regression analysis of this study was certainly reasonable. Further, the factors identified provide a basis for reducing significantly the dimensionality of the problem of adjusting for product mix. Finally, since the factors are orthogonal, the extent of multicollinearity may be significantly reduced in further regression analysis.

Second, an analysis of the available data served to indicate that there is a systematic pattern to the expansion of facilities and services in short-term general hospitals (Berry, 1973; or Berry and

Carr, 1973: 55-68). There is such a thing as a basic-service hospital. As hospitals add facilities and services there is a strong tendency to first add those that enhance the quality of the basic services. Only after the services that enhance the quality of the basic services have been acquired do short-term general hospitals display a tendency to expand the complexity of the scope of services provided. The final stage of the expansion process for certain hospitals occurs when they add those facilities and services that essentially transform them from inpatient institutions to community medical centers.

The results of this analysis of the pattern of expansion of facilities and services contain a number of implications. It would seem that the results of this analysis support the contention that there are significant differences among short-term general hospitals and indicate that it is possible to identify groups of similar hospitals. The groups of hospitals formed in the analysis are distinct, they cover the range of services provided, and they seem to have a significant intuitive appeal.

The range of services provided in hospitals extends from the most basic services provided in a small institution with exceedingly limited facilities, through a somewhat higher quality of essentially basic services, through the more complex services, to the services provided in a hospital which serves as a community medical center in addition to its role as an inpatient institution. Different patients presumably need different services. For some the services of the basic service hospital would be quite appropriate. Others need higher-quality basic services or more complex services. Still others can only be treated adequately in a community service hospital. This is related to the question of the appropriate mix of available capacity—what is the optimal mix of types of hospitals? The importance of this question is emphasized by the significant differences in average cost per patient day among the four types of hospitals. The cost dimension of the issue is representative of the implications of this analysis and indicative of the potential value of the analysis.

Indeed, the cost implication was the primary concern of a third analysis specific to the product difference aspect of the production of hospital services. A comparative analysis was made of the extent to which hospital costs are explained by what hospitals have the capacity to provide and by what they actually do provide for a sample of hospitals for which diagnostic data were available. This analysis is described in detail in Berry and Carr (1973: 68-76). The diagnostic information for a sample of New England hospitals was gathered as part of a study entitled "International Comparative

Study of Medical Care,'' under the direction of Osler Peterson, Gerald Rosenthal, and others, sponsored by the Division of Hospitals and Medical Facilities of USPHS (NIH 00237-01). The results indicated that the capacity to provide services explains hospital costs better than the actual services provided explains them.

This result has significant policy implications. The result is not profound, or even surprising, but it does lend support to the position that hospital costs depend more on what hospitals "gear up to do" than on what they actually end up doing. It would seem that much more attention needs to be paid to the question of what the appropriate mix of available capacity is and how public policy might best control that mix.

Much hospital cost analysis has been preoccupied with the question of what is the optimal size of hospitals. A more fundamental question is what is the optimal mix of complexities of scope of services or what is the optimal mix of types of hospitals.

Characteristics of High-Cost and Low-Cost Hospitals

The primary empirical analysis of the factors which affect hospital costs involved the regression equations designed to measure the influence of such factors as output, quality, product differences, and factor prices on hospital costs. The estimated cost equations, however, provided the basis for additional considerations.

Since the estimated equation takes output, quality, product mix, and factor prices into account, an analysis of the residuals of the equation was employed as a mechanism to identify hospitals with unusually high or unusually low costs after allowance for these several factors. This analysis of residuals provided insight to certain characteristics of such high-cost or low-cost institutions. This analysis is described in detail in Berry and Carr (1973: 89-95).

In essence, the estimated equation provided a predicted cost for each hospital on the basis of its output, quality, product characteristics, and factor prices. This predicted cost was compared to the actual cost for each hospital. In fact, an analysis was undertaken of those hospitals with the 50 highest and 50 lowest relative residuals where relative residual is defined as the difference between actual and predicted cost as a proportion of the predicted cost. Comparisons among such characteristics as the qualifications of administrators, regions of the country, the ratio of personnel expense to total expense, occupancy rate, and bed size, were made. The implications of this analysis are of some interest, and they can be summarized briefly.

First, with respect to the administrative background of administrators, the results indicated that low-cost hospitals were more likely to have administrators with medical qualifications (M.D., D.D.S., R.N.). It is of some interest to speculate on this phenomenon in terms of the probable interests, abilities, and goals of the various groups and the alternatives available to them.

Since physicians (and dentists), generally, form a very competent and highly motivated group, it may be that only those with exceptional interest and ability in administration would be willing to give up the earnings and other benefits available to most practicing physicians. Registered nurses usually attain the position of administrator only after advancing through the administrative hierarchy of the nursing department. The initial pool of candidates is usually large, and comparisons can be made among individuals in comparable administrative positions, resulting in a highly competitive situation.

In contrast, the nonmedical administrator group appears to consist generally of those who have drifted into the hospital field after indifferent success in other endeavors. This even appears to be true among hospital administration program graduates.

Another possible explanation for lower cost in hospitals with medical administrators is that those with medical knowledge and authority may be able to interact with the medical staff to some administrative advantage. Thus, for example, it is quite likely that medical administrators are able to resist the demands of the medical staff for additional equipment and the like in certain instances when their nonmedical counterparts would not be able to do so.

A second characteristic considered involved regional differences. There was a significant difference among the proportions of high- and low-cost hospitals in the nine Census Divisions of the United States. This difference, of course, was that existing after regional and urban-rural differences in factor prices had been taken into account. The New England and Pacific states tended to be high-cost and the southern states low-cost. It is possible to speculate on the likely causes of these regional differences, and perhaps some research effort should be directed to this apparent phenomenon in the future.

The third characteristic was indicative of differences in factor intensities in the production process. It is of considerable interest that the ratio of personnel expense to total expense was higher in low-cost hospitals than in high-cost hospitals. The mean ratio for low-cost hospitals was 0.656 while for high-cost hospitals the mean ratio was only 0.558. This difference in apparent labor intensity may be related to the fact that the cost of capital is abnormally low for voluntary, and, possibly, government hospitals. Hospitals which face lower than market prices for capital may be expected to use too much capital for optimum efficiency. The inefficient capital intensity could well be reflected in higher than expected average costs.

Fourth, hospitals with relatively high occupancy rates were found to have lower costs. The median occupancy rate for low-cost hospitals was 70.7 percent and for high-cost hospitals 64.5 percent. Since these cost differences were observed after the number of empty beds had been taken into account in the regression equation, it appears likely that occupancy rate was acting as a surrogate variable for other factors peculiar to very high- and very low-cost hospitals. In other words, the low-cost hospitals all may have been operating near an optimal occupancy rate of 70 percent while the high-cost hospitals were operating over a suboptimal lower range.

The fifth characteristic considered was bed size. As expected, there was no significant difference in the proportion of high- and low-cost hospitals by bed-size category, since size had already been taken into account in the regression equation. However, there appeared to be some tendency for low-cost hospitals to group around the middle of the size range. This may reflect a phenomenon similar to that discussed with respect to occupancy rate.

Some degree of care must be exercised in interpreting the results of the residual analysis. The residuals should be interpreted in the perspective of the regression analysis which generated them. In fact, the original regression equation included surrogates for output, quality, product factor prices, and certain other variables. If the surrogate included to account for each of the several factors did in fact do its job, that is, if it picked up the influence of the factor it was intended to represent, then the residuals would be distributed randomly over that factor. Thus, for example, a dummy variable was included to represent hospital control. In fact, an analysis of the residuals indicated that neither the high-cost group nor the low-cost group was characterized by disproportionate numbers of any of the three hospital control types (voluntary, government, or proprietary).

On balance, the residual analysis is a useful mechanism for identifying hospitals which have relatively high or relatively low costs. Given the institutions identified by the analysis of the residuals it is possible to identify certain characteristics which high-cost or low-cost hospitals have in common. In the last analysis, of course, further research would be necessary in order to test any hypotheses that might be suggested by the analysis of residuals.

In Sum

The primary purpose of this research effort was to complete a detailed analysis to identify and measure the effects of factors which significantly affect the cost and efficiency of the short-term general hospital system in the United States. The empirical analysis did serve to delineate in some detail the interaction of many factors with one another and with hospital costs. Further, the analysis of the product-mix phenomenon, its effect on hospital cost analysis, and certain techniques that can be employed to some advantage in dealing with product mix should prove useful in future hospital cost and production research. Finally, the identification of certain characteristics of particularly high-cost and particularly low-cost hospitals may provide the basis for further research.

It is hoped that the analysis outlined in this report will make some contribution to the general understanding of the hospital cost phenomenon.

Ralph E. Berry, Jr., PH.D.
Harvard School of Public Health
677 Huntington Avenue
Boston, Massachusetts 02115

The analysis presented in this paper was supported in part by Grant No. 10-P-56002 from the Social Security Administration, DHEW.

References

American Hospital Association
1971   Hospital Statistics.

Berry, Ralph E.
1970   "Product heterogeneity and hospital cost analysis." Inquiry 7, 1 (March):67-75.

1973   "On grouping hospitals for economic analysis." Inquiry 10, 4 (December).

Berry, Ralph E., and W. John Carr, Jr.
  1973   Efficiency in the Production of Hospital Services.

Pettengill, J.
  1973   ''The financial position of private community hospitals, 1961-71.''
           Social Security Bulletin (November):349.

Repeated Hospitalization for the Same Disease: A Multiplier of National Health Costs

CHRISTOPHER J. ZOOK,
SHEILA FLANIGAN SAVICKIS,
and FRANCIS D. MOORE

Public Policy Program, Kennedy School of Government,
Harvard University;
Department of Surgery, Harvard Medical School,
Peter Bent Brigham Hospital

MEDICAL SUCCESS (SHORT OF CURE) AND FAILURE (short of death) favor patient recidivism, or repeated hospitalization for treatment of the same disease. This phenomenon has become a remarkably prominent factor in the national cost of illness, in the utilization of general hospitals, and in the future plans of many patients and families. It is a reflection of both bioscience advance and public expectation.

For example, the birth of a child with major congenital defects brings a social mandate for prolonged, repetitive, and expensive therapy once the child has survived the first few hours after birth. In end-stage chronic renal failure, kidney dialysis requires lifelong, repetitive therapy, and even kidney transplantation will sometimes lead to repeated hospitalization. By the same token, total hip replacement, if successful, leads the patient directly to repair of the other hip as soon as it becomes symptomatic; if unsuccessful, complications of total hip replacement can be among the most expensive episodes in orthopedic surgery. Other such repetitive, and therefore predictable, illnesses include cirrhosis of the liver in chronic alcoholism, poorly

Milbank Memorial Fund Quarterly/*Health and Society*, Vol. 58, No. 3, 1980
© 1980 Milbank Memorial Fund and Massachusetts Institute of Technology
0160/1997/5803/0454-18 $01.00/0

controlled diabetes, cancer, degenerative vascular disease, intractable anemia, chronic obstructive lung disease, and mental disease. In all, a superior science has made possible the first step, yet the sequelae continue to demand medical resources. These are the substrates on which American medicine spends so many billions of dollars. These—not the episodic cancer or chest trauma on a respirator—are the high-cost users.

A previous study (Zook and Moore, 1980) found that a comparatively small fraction of hospital patients, about 13 percent, utilized over half of hospital resources in a year. This finding held true across widely differing hospital populations. Yet, high-cost patients were not predominantly those in intensive care after major trauma, or "brain death" patients in terminal condition. Rather, the typical high-cost patient experienced multiple hospitalizations for the same disease, often a disease from which death is not even likely in the short term. Analysis beyond a single year revealed an even more significant cost of repeated hospitalization for the same disease (RHSD).

Gruenberg (1977) emphasized the importance of long-term illness in the national medical budget and suggested that its frequency was increased by improvements in medical procedures. Reduction of mortality from severe or chronic illness lengthens the average duration of the illness and increases its frequency in the total population. Over time, these RHSDs can be extremely demanding of medical resources. The maintained treatment posture (with neither cure nor death) is a remarkable cost-multiplier that can be ascribed to a small group of patients.

In this paper we examine the fiscal and clinical nature of repeated hospitalization for the same disease, in several different types of short-stay hospitals. The data were developed from a random sample of 2,238 medical records in six contrasting hospital populations. Because previous research has often underestimated the full long-term cost of an illness by failing to link repeated admissions of the same patient over time, each record was linked across earlier hospitalizations for the current illness to provide a longitudinal profile of repeated admissions.

Hospital recidivism has three principal implications for public health policy. First, if there are predictable, high-cost groups of "repeater" patients with particular illnesses (e.g., renal failure) or traits (e.g., alcoholism or extreme obesity), public health policies targeted at such groups might well achieve major economies. One such program of vigorous follow-up and increased medical compliance for diabetics reduced the incidence of hospital readmission in that group by 56 percent (Miller and Goldstein, 1972).

Second, medical recidivism has implications for the design of major-risk health insurance. If many high-cost patients suffer illnesses with predictably high utilization rates spread over years, a one-year eligibility definition will be inequitable, and will fail to provide financial incentives for more effective modes of long-term, preventive, or follow-up care. In addition, greater attention needs to be paid to the use of premium design and coinsurance to channel recidivist patients down the most cost-effective, long-term track of care.

Third, unusually high rates of readmission by certain hospitals, doctors, or communities might signal possible provider accountability or overuse of medical resources. Financial incentives in health insurance should be structured to discourage costly hospital readmissions when preventive programs and low-cost alternatives are available.

Method

Data and Definitions

Medical records for 2,238 patients were selected on the basis of a random sample of hospital discharges in 1976 from six diverse hospital populations in Massachusetts. Hospital A was a large teaching and referral hospital for adults. Hospitals B1 and B2 were, respectively, the medical-surgical service and the spinal-cord injury center of a Veterans Administration (VA) hospital. Hospital C was a suburban community hospital. Hospital D was a large teaching and referral hospital for children. Hospital E was a tax-supported municipal hospital.

In each hospital we selected records of patients discharged on particular days in 1976. These days were chosen by a randomized scheme that ensured an adequate representation of holidays, seasons of the year, and days of the week, since patient-discharge mix varies greatly over time. The sample as a percent of all discharges in the year was chosen to vary across hospitals, because of the wide range of institutional sizes. These sampling characteristics are summarized in Table 1.

TABLE 1
Sample of Patient Discharges from Six Hospitals in 1976

Hospital	Type	Number of Beds	Hospital Discharges Recorded by Hospital	Number of Records Sampled	Sample Fraction of All 1976 Discharges
A	Adult teaching-referral hospital	330	10,450	576	5.5%
B1	Veterans hospital (medical-surgical)	160	2,820	305	10.8
B2	Veterans hospital (spinal cord injury)	100	540	86	15.9
C	Community suburban hospital	275	9,110	455	5.0
D	Children's teaching-referral hospital	340	13,170	410	3.1
E	Tax-supported municipal hospital	190	6,790	406	5.9
		1,395	42,880	2,238	5.2%

The retrospective nature of these data means that the illness experiences are truncated, and understate the amount of lifetime readmission for any one patient and illness because the future is still unknown. Our data do not include readmissions throughout the entire illness, only the experience to date. However, sampling on the basis of discharges does provide aggregate evidence on the long-term importance of RHSD. The significance of RHSD can be assessed by comparing the number of readmissions with the number of first admissions for each disease category.

Billing data were obtained from a random sample of 30 percent of the indexed hospitalizations in each hospital, except for the VA hospital where bills are not computed. (The administrative cost of obtaining these old bills restricted the study to a sample that was sufficiently large to permit precise statistical estimation of the others.) To estimate missing billings for the indexed hospitalizations, a day-rating scale was developed. This represented five different degrees of complexity of care in a hospital day. The five groups ranged from a "1-day," a low-intensity day of dwelling or only the most minor testing, to a "5-day," a high-intensity day of emergency intensive care or full life-support services.

Observations were reweighted individually to account for proportional oversampling of repeating patients.[1] For instance, in estimating frequencies, data from patients seen twice in a hospital in 1976 were weighted by one-half, as compared with patients seen only once. In the absence of this reweighting, patients who experienced multiple admissions would be overrepresented in any frequency estimates for the patient population. For further details of the record review and data retrieval, see Zook and Moore (1980).

Each of the 2,238 records had every day of its indexed hospitalization fully characterized by this scale. Thus, a five-day stay might have the pattern: 2, 3, 2, 1, 1. For each hospital, the average billing for each day category was estimated from billing data for 30 percent of patients. This was done by regressing the total bill for each patient on the number of days in each category. The regression weights can be

---

[1] Several studies have found, in fact, that the most variable components of utilization across regions of the country (Gornick, 1977), across types of insurance plans (Luft, 1978), and across cost strata (Zook and Moore, 1980) are hospital admission and readmission rates, as opposed to length of stay or cost per day.

interpreted as the average charge for each category of day. Multiplying these five weights by the number of days in each category and summing yields an estimate for billings that has a .94–.98 correlation with the actual bills available. For days in categories 1 through 5 at Hospital A, these weights were, respectively, $216, $271, $426, $914, and $1,447. Combining this with the day rating profile 1, 1, 3, 2, 1, for instance, would yield an average bill of $1,345 (216 × 3 + 271 + 426). The scale and more detail on estimation are available upon request from the authors. Charges at the VA hospital, where no bills are computed, were estimated by combining day ratings, the average cost per occupied patient day (about $200), and the relative day weights for Hospital A. The average charge per day at the VA hospital was constrained to equal its $200 average.

Repeated hospitalization for the same disease was defined by a diagnostic classification system containing nineteen principal categories (listed in Table 3). All repeated hospitalizations in the years before the sampled hospitalizations were coded, whether at that or at another hospital. Multiple (different) illnesses were not studied; data collection was limited to treatment of the illness causing the current (index) admission.

Repeated hospitalizations were determined through page-by-page reading of the complete medical record, including all previous admissions at that hospital, all physician notes, patient histories, referral letters, and copies of discharge summaries from other facilities.

Results

The Frequency of RHSDs

Patients with repeated hospitalizations for the same disease were found frequently in each hospital population. (Reference to patients, as opposed to single hospitalizations, implies that data frequencies were corrected by a simple adjustment factor for oversampling of repeatedly hospitalized individuals.) Of our total sample of 2,238 hospital discharges in 1976, 1,170 (52 percent) were RHSDs. Between 40 percent at Hospital C and 70 percent at Hospital B1 of single hospitalizations were RHSDs, and in the spinal-cord injury center the proportion rose as high as 97 percent (Table 2).

TABLE 2

Fraction of All Single Hospitalizations That Are RHSDs, over Retrospective
Time Intervals

Hospital	Retrospective Time Intervals				
	One Year	Two Years	Five Years	Ten Years	All Years
A	39.5%	45.6%	53.0%	55.3%	55.6%
B1	44.3	60.4	68.0	69.3	70.2
B2	69.9	90.7	94.2	96.5	96.5
C	25.3	32.1	37.6	38.9	39.6
D	37.6	43.4	47.8	49.7	50.5
E	26.6	34.7	38.9	40.6	40.7

Long-term illness was surprisingly frequent in these "short-stay" hospital populations. At least five previous hospitalizations for the same disease were experienced by 27 percent of patients seen in 1976 in the VA hospital (B1), 14 percent in the children's referral hospital (D), 8 percent in the small, suburban community hospital (C). The spinal-cord injury center had a rate of 69 percent. If readmissions were of very short duration, as compared with first admissions, they might be of secondary cost-importance; on the contrary, however, readmissions were above average both in duration and in unit cost.

Patients with repeated hospitalizations had their first hospitalization an average of six years before the indexed discharge. This range is shown (Table 2) as the percentage of repeated hospitalizations within various retrospective time periods (one, two, five, ten, and all years). The proportions for one year ranged from 25 percent in Hospital C, to 44 percent at Hospital B1, to 70 percent at Hospital B2.

Costs of RHSDs

RHSD accounted for approximately 60 percent of all hospital charges. Repeated hospitalizations were generally more expensive than the first hospitalization. Across hospitals, repeated hospitalizations were from 24 percent (Hospital E) to 55 percent (Hospital B1) more expensive than first admission. Even in the suburban community hospital, Hospital C, repeated hospitalizations accounted for 48 percent of total billings and were 42 percent more expensive per incident than nonrepeated hospitalizations. Consequently, repeated hospitalizations accounted for a disproportionate share of total hospital charges, ranging from 46 percent at Hospital E to 79 percent at Hospital B1.

The frequency distribution of billings for repeated and nonrepeated hospitalizations showed that, on average, the cost of repeated admissions had a higher overall mean ($3,111 versus $2,040, in 1976 dollars) and greater density in the upper tail of the unit-cost curve. The proportion of single hospitalizations with billings over $2,000 ranged from 17 percent (Hospital C) to 46 percent (Hospital A), as compared with the proportion of repeated hospitalizations, which ranged from 28 percent (Hospital E) to 64 percent (Hospital A). RHSDs accounted for a majority of hospitalizations and of hospital resources.

To determine whether this might be due to some intervening variable, such as diagnosis, an additional calculation was made. For each major diagnostic group a regression equation was fitted, with billing as the dependent variable, and patient sex, hospital, age, personal habits indicated in the record, race, secondary diagnosis, and employment status, as independent variables. An indicator as to whether or not that hospitalization was a repeat was also included. The coefficient on this variable can be interpreted as the billing premium associated with repeated hospitalization.

By this regression method, repeated hospitalizations were found to cost substantially more than first hospitalization for gastrointestinal disease (by 45 percent), orthopedic disorders (by 16 percent), infectious disease (by 24 percent), peripheral vascular disease (by 56 percent), and for all other illnesses together (by 30 percent). Repeated hospitalizations were found to be *less* costly than the first admission for vascular disease of the heart and for spinal cord injury. There was no statistical difference with first admissions for cancer, lung disease, and endocrine-metabolic disease.

Diagnostic Categories Where RHSD Was Frequent

The long-term, repetitive nature of an illness is reflected in the frequency of RHSD, shown in Table 3. (Some might question whether more categories, refined from the nineteen here, would also show high RHSD rates or whether, in some sense, this is an artifact of the method. To examine this, we refined the system to fifty-five groups and found similar results.) If, for example, the number of first and repeated admissions in our sample were equal, then the average case of that illness would have two expected admissions over its duration. Each first hospitalization would be matched by a repeated hospitalization; an illness with a ratio of 3:1 would therefore have four admissions during its average course.

Table 3 gives the ratio of repeated to nonrepeated hospitalizations by diagnosis for all hospitals pooled together. Our sample was not large enough to give precise disease-by-disease estimates separately for each hospital, though the most repetitive illnesses tended to be the same ones across hospitals. The actual level of hospitalizations per illness was slightly greater in the teaching and the VA hospitals. For instance, repeated hospitalizations in vascular disease varied from 56 percent in the municipal hospital, to 64 percent in the adult teaching hospital, to 80 percent in the VA hospital. For trauma, these percentages were, respectively, 29, 33, and 37 percent. For cancer, they were 53, 75, and 73 percent.

Illnesses that accounted for the most repetitive hospitalizations were spinal cord injury, renal failure, cancer, congenital defects, diseases of the blood, benign lung disease, and chronic degenerative vascular disease. In the tertiary referral hospitals, illnesses requiring repeated and regular life-maintenance therapy (e.g., dialysis for renal failure or transfusion therapy for sickle cell anemia) were frequent among RHSD. Life maintenance accounted for 8 percent of repeated hospitalizations for the same disease in Hospital A and for 18 percent in Hospital D.

In all the hospitals except B2 (the spinal-cord injury center), the seven diagnostic categories listed above accounted for 56 percent of RHSDs, but for only 21 percent of nonrepeated admissions. At the other extreme, patients in eight diagnostic groups accounted for 66 percent of all nonrepeated admissions, but for only 27 percent of RHSD. Illnesses with few repeat episodes included genitourinary disease (male), gynecological disease (female), diseases of the eye, infectious disease, minor orthopedic disorders, pregnancy and related disorders, trauma, and a miscellaneous category of disorders and symptoms.

TABLE 3
Ratio of Repeated to First Hospitalization by Diagnostic-Related Group for All Hospitals Together*

Diagnostic Category	Proportion (P) of Hospitalizations That Were Repeated†	Ratio of Repeated to Nonrepeated Hospitalizations‡ (P/1-P)	Average Number of Stays per Illness Episode (1/1-P)	Number in Sample
Spinal cord injury	95.3% (2.3)	20.50 (13.3, 40.7)	21.50	86
Renal failure	94.7 (3.6)	18.00 (10.2, 57.8)	19.00	38
Alcohol-related gastrointestinal disease	80.0 (10.3)	4.00 (2.3, 9.3)	5.00	15
Disease of the blood	78.1 (7.3)	3.57 (2.4, 5.8)	4.57	32
Cancer	73.8 (3.5)	2.82 (2.4, 3.5)	3.82	157
Benign lung disease	70.9 (5.8)	2.44 (1.9, 3.3)	3.44	61
Chronic or degenerative vascular disease	70.8 (2.3)	2.43 (2.2, 2.7)	3.43	399
Congenital defects	68.8 (4.0)	2.21 (1.8, 2.7)	3.21	135
Endocrine/metabolic disorders	62.2 (6.7)	1.65 (1.3, 2.2)	2.65	53

Neuromuscular disease	62.1 (8.0)	1.64 (1.2, 2.3)	2.64	37
Mental disease	61.5 (5.5)	1.60 (1.3, 2.0)	2.60	78
Benign bowel disease	50.2 (4.1)	1.01 (.9, 1.2)	2.01	145
Orthopedic conditions	41.1 (4.0)	.70 (.6, .8)	1.70	148
Gynecological disorders	37.9 (6.8)	.61 (.5, .8)	1.61	58
Disease of the eye	35.5 (6.0)	.55 (.4, .7)	1.55	62
Trauma	33.8 (3.2)	.51 (.4, .6)	1.51	220
Genitourinary disease	24.8 (8.8)	.33 (.2, .5)	1.33	24
Infectious disease	24.8 (8.8)	.33 (.2, .5)	1.33	24
Other illnesses	19.4 (2.4)	.24 (.2, .3)	1.24	228

* The sample size by disease did not permit precise estimates for each hospital.
† Standard deviation in parentheses.
‡ Range shown is for recidivist proportion ± 1 standard deviation.

Potentially Harmful Habits of the Repeaters

Certain groups of patients, especially those with potentially harmful personal habits, were much more likely to be repetitive in their use of the hospital for that illness than were other groups. Table 4 shows the ratio of repeated hospitalizations to first hospitalizations for several contrasting groups of patients.

Substantial diversity existed across hospital populations. Patients treated at the VA hospital had the highest rate of repeated hospitalization, followed by the tertiary referral hospitals, and finally by the community hospitals. Patients over 70 years of age had more repeated admissions than others at Hospital C and Hospital D, but fewer at Hospital A and Hospital B1. Males also had a slightly higher rate of repeated hospitalization than females, except at Hospital D.

TABLE 4
Ratio of Total Repeated to Nonrepeated Hospitalizations in 1976 by
Category of Hospital and Patient

Patient Group	Hospital				
	A	B1	C	D	E
All hospitalizations	1.25	2.35	.65	1.02	.68
Age:					
Over 70	1.50	2.09	1.08	—*	1.35
Under 70	1.19	2.38	.56	1.02	.60
Sex:					
Males	1.31	2.38	.78	.88	.82
Females	1.19	—*	.52	1.27	.61
Potentially harmful personal habit noted in the record:†					
Habit-illness link	1.19	4.00	2.00	—*	2.00
Other	1.11	1.54	.45	1.01	.53
History of chronic alcoholism:					
Alcoholic problem	1.93	3.00	3.60	—*	2.82
Other	1.21	2.22	.60	1.02	.58

* Insufficient number in group.
† Possible association of illness with alcohol abuse, heavy smoking, obesity, or drug abuse as noted by physician comments or patient's history in the medical record.

Unhealthy personal habits such as alcohol abuse, drug abuse, extreme obesity, or heavy smoking were especially associated with a high ratio of repeated hospitalization. Patients with a history of chronic alcoholism had a ratio of repeated to first hospitalizations that ranged from 1.9 at Hospital A to 3.6 at Hospital C. The ratio for persons with no alcoholism noted in their history ranged from only .6 in Hospital E to 2.2 in Hospital B1. Patients who were judged on the basis of the medical record to have a potential link between illness and habit had ratios of repeated to first hospitalization that ranged from 1.2 in Hospital A to 4.0 in Hospital B1. Patients whose record showed no such possible link had an average rate that ranged from .5 in Hospital C to 1.5 in Hospital B1.

Regression analysis was used to check whether unhealthy personal habits indicated in the patient's medical record were associated with repeated admission for the same disease even within a diagnostic-demographic category.[2] To examine this we regressed the number of past readmissions on indicators of employment status, marital status, race, age, hospital attended, secondary diagnosis (present or not), sex, and a possible unhealthy habit indicated in the record (yes or no).

Using such an analysis of all diseases together, as well as for single illness groups, we still found readmission much more frequently among patients with an unhealthy habit. On average, the heavy smoker with a benign pulmonary disease had 65 percent more readmissions than other patients who suffered from the same illness. Patients with endocrine metabolic disease, who also were severely obese or alcoholic, had an average of 47 percent more readmissions than those without obesity or alcoholism. For benign gastrointestinal disease the excess share was 59 percent. In virtually every set of calculations—by hospital, by illness, and for all patients together—those with recorded adverse lifestyle factors had more readmissions for their present disease than other patients.

---

[2] These regressions were estimated by a Tobit maximum-likelihood procedure. Tobit analysis is appropriate when the dependent variable (hospitalizations) is truncated at a point of significant density (no patients have zero, but many have only one hospitalization). Without explicitly modeling this truncation, ordinary least-squares methods would lead to biased estimates. By explicitly modeling the limited data range, bias can be corrected. Tobit analysis was first introduced by Tobin (1956) to estimate regressions for unemployment rates, also a truncated variable.

Discussion

Importance of Long-Term Illness in Short-Stay Hospitals

Repeated hospitalizations for the same disease accounted for more than half of hospitalizations and for nearly 60 percent of total hospital charges. We estimate that a 20 percent reduction in rates of readmission for treatment of the same disease might save well over $11 billion in hospital costs. This special segment of high-cost users deserves special attention by scientists, clinicians, epidemiologists, and economists. Here is the "big expense" area of the budget where small fractional gains have large overall impact.

The few studies that focus upon this phenomenon confirm our findings. Roemer and Myers (1956) found that although 12 percent of middle-aged males under the Canadian National Health System used the hospital in any one year, only 33 percent used it over a period of five years, suggesting a large amount of recidivism. Gornick (1977) found that over a two-year period the share of Medicare patients who had multiple hospitalizations ranged from a low of 29 percent in Maryland to 45 percent in North Dakota. Patients who experienced multiple admissions accounted for 61 percent of all discharges during those two years. Other research in California by Schroeder et al. (1979), and in England under the Oxford Record Linkage Project (Acheson and Barr, 1965) has also found repeated hospitalizations and linked episodes of illness to be of substantial importance in their study populations.

RHSD is a highly nonrandom phenomenon that clusters in certain long-term diagnostic and patient groups. The frequency of medical recidivism has been obscured in previous research on "catastrophic illness," which has focused on annual or short-term, episodic, or partial single-insuror data rather than upon linked record data (Birnbaum, 1978; Trapnell, 1977; Meyer, 1976).

Implications of RHSD for Design of Health Insurance Plans

"Catastrophic health insurance," or insurance to pay for large medical expenses, has been proposed as a low-cost, politically acceptable alternative to complete national health insurance. The typical "high-cost illness" for which these plans are designed (with benefits based on one-year expenditure levels) is the sudden trauma or heart attack requiring intensive care and, often, accompanied by a high short-term mortality rate. Attention has not focused on the repeaters, who may survive for many years and may consume even more medical resources. Our results suggest that, in fact, patients with RHSD may be a more dominant high-cost group than has been heretofore recognized.

Many of the patients with high readmission rates also had notes in their medical records that indicated a potentially harmful habit. When insurance covers the expenses of illness whose incidence and treatment costs are beyond human control or influence, the "moral hazard" of excessive utilization is low. When insurance covers an event that can be influenced by the patient, in part, the "moral hazard" distortion is a more present danger. Components of both types appear among the high-cost patients and should be identified and dealt with separately.

Financial incentives need to be applied to change future behavior, not to punish for the past. Coinsurance to reduce moral hazard could take such forms as premium reductions for nonsmokers and persons at optimal body weight. It should also be possible to introduce premium increases for persons with early signs of an illness related to a current habit. Stoppage of the habit or participation in an educational program could be rewarded by premium reduction. In fact, it is true that stopping smoking even after a long period as a smoker can substantially reverse or retard the course of pulmonary disease (Ebert, 1979).

Companies that fund group plans might be offered financial reward for providing educational and incentive plans in the workplace. Although we do not at present know the exact location of the most promising leverage points, we do know that great opportunity exists. Even relatively mild educational campaigns such as the Stanford Heart Disease Project have induced significant changes in eating and smoking habits.

As we have shown, prevalence rates and the costs of long-term illness are high and are increasing over time. The percentage of persons in the population unable to carry on any major activity increased by 40 percent in the eight years from 1967 to 1974 (2.3 percent to 3.3 percent) and the percentages of persons with some major chronic limitation of daily living increased by 23 percent (11.5 percent to 14.1 percent) (Department of Health, Education, and Welfare, 1977). Failure to build appropriate long-term incentives into insurance reimbursement, to study specific tracks of long-term illness, and to highlight recidivism as a major cost factor will miss major opportunities for economies and improvements in the health care of the American people.

Our analysis focused primarily upon variations in readmission rates by disease and patient characteristics. However, as we noted earlier, large geographic variations in readmission rates also exist. To understand reasons for regional variations, one would need to look beyond illness mix and patient characteristics to different insurance structures, distances to the hospital, and income levels, to name a few factors. Our analysis is directed to "within-region" variation as opposed to "among-regions" variation. The large cost impact of even small changes in readmission probabilities in a region suggests that efforts be directed towards better understanding of these causes of medical recidivism.

Directions for Future Research

The "hidden" component of repeated hospital utilization demands greater attention. Debate over catastrophic health insurance will require fuller understanding of these recidivist patient groups who consume such large quantities of the national medical resources. In any single year, they may not fall into a "catastrophic" category, but over time they can be among the most expensive of all patients. Moreover, as medicine achieves mortality reduction in persons with these long-term, repetitive illnesses, there will be an increase in their prevalence and total medical costs.

For instance, before 1930 the mortality for spinal cord injury was near 100 percent; now the life table for paraplegics and quadriplegics is converging toward that of the overall population (although with much greater use of the health services). As a result, the number of persons in the population with a spinal cord injury has risen from near zero at the beginning of this century to over 600,000 today. This striking success in medicine is also the cause of higher cost (Smart and Sanders, 1976).

Children with extrophy of the bladder demonstrated a 25 percent ten-year mortality rate in the 1950s; now the mortality rate is only 2 percent (MacFarlane et al., 1979). Similar advances have occurred in cystic fibrosis, Down's syndrome, pneumonia in old age, childhood leukemia, and other long-term illnesses. More elaborate models of these illnesses are needed to chart their demographic trends and to predict future high-cost utilization for patients in identifiable clinical categories.

Failure to understand these relations was responsible, in part, for original underestimates in 1971 of the cost of the kidney disease amendments of the Social Security Act. In 1972 the Department of Health, Education, and Welfare projected that the cost of the program in 1976 would be $395 million; the actual total was $573 million, rising later to over $1 billion. This 45 percent underestimate (in the comparatively short time of four years) can be traced to underestimation of the effect of an increased number of surviving renal patients on the total number of those patients over time, a failure to appreciate the cost importance of repeated hospitalization for the same disease.

References

Acheson, F.D., and Barr, A. 1965. Multiple Spells of In-patient Treatment in a Calendar Year. *British Journal of Preventive and Social Medicine* 19:182–191.

Birnbaum, H. 1978. *The Cost of Catastrophic Illness.* Lexington, Mass.: D.C. Heath.

Department of Health, Education, and Welfare. 1977. *Limitation of Activity Due to Chronic Conditions.* Public Health Service Publication, Series 10, No. 111.

Ebert, R. 1979. Cessation of Cigarette Smoking and Pulmonary Disease. *Journal of the American Medical Association* 240:2159.

Gornick, M. 1977. Medicare Patients: Geographic Differences in Hospital Discharge Rates and Multiple Stays. *Social Security Bulletin,* June:22–41.

Gruenberg, E.M. 1977. The Failures of Success. *Milbank Memorial Fund Quarterly/Health and Society* 55 (Winter):3–24.

Luft, H.S. 1978. How Do the Health Maintenance Organizations Achieve Their Savings? *New England Journal of Medicine* 296:1336–1343.

MacFarlane, M., Lattimer, J., and Hensle, T. 1979. Improved Life Expectancy of Children with Extrophy of the Bladder. *Journal of the American Medical Association* 242:442–444.

Miller, L., and Goldstein, J. 1972. More Efficient Care of Diabetes in a County Hospital Setting. *New England Journal of Medicine* 286:1388–1391.

Meyer, M.F. 1976. *Catastrophic Illnesses and Catastrophic Health Insurance.* Washington, D.C.: The Heritage Foundation.

Roemer, M., and Myers, G. 1956. Multiple Admission to Hospital. *Canadian Journal of Public Health* 47:469–481.

Schroeder, S.A., Showstack, J.A., and Roberts, H.E. 1979. Frequency and Clinical Description of High Cost Patients in 17 Acute Care Hospitals. *New England Journal of Medicine* 300:1306–1309.

Smart, C., and Sanders, C. 1976. *The Costs of Motor Vehicle-Related Spinal Cord Injuries.* New York: Insurance Institute for Highway Safety.

Tobin, J. 1958. Estimation of Relationships for Limited Dependent Variables. *Econometrics* 26:12–24.

Trapnell, G. 1977. *The Rising Cost of Catastrophic Illness.* Falls Church, Va.: Actuarial Research Corporation.

Zook, C.J., and Moore, F.D. 1980. The High Cost Users of Medical Care. *New England Journal of Medicine* 302:996–1002.

Acknowledgments: This study was supported by grants from the Henry J. Kaiser Family Foundation, the Robert Wood Johnson Foundation, the William F. Milton Fund, Harvard Medical School, General Research Support Grants of the Peter Bent Brigham Hospital, the Medical Foundation, and the Walnut Medical Charitable Trust Fund.

We are grateful to each of the hospital executive committees and medical record departments for cooperating in this project. We also thank Richard Nesson, Lindsey Parris, Donald Shepard, David Willis, David Wise, and Richard Zeckhauser for helpful comments on this paper; and Arthur Finnegan for manuscript preparation.

Address correspondence to: Dr. Francis D. Moore, Department of Surgery, Harvard Medical School, 10 Shattuck Street, Boston, MA 02115.

Physician Use of Services for the Hospitalized Patient: A Review, with Implications for Cost Containment

LOIS P. MYERS and
STEVEN A. SCHROEDER

Institute for Health Policy Studies,
School of Medicine,
University of California, San Francisco

RESSURES TO SLOW THE RATE OF INCREASE IN hospital expenditures, especially the threat of federal regulation of hospital costs, have sparked concerted efforts toward cost containment. Among these is the present Voluntary Effort, in which participating hospitals and physicians voluntarily strive to stem the rapid growth in hospital costs (McNerney, 1980). Hospitals account for 40 percent of the national health care bill, which in 1979 amounted to $212 billion or 9 percent of the gross national product (Gibson, 1980). Expenditure increases can be attributed partially to price inflation and population growth but, as managers of patient care, physicians bear major responsibility for determining levels of hospital expenditure. They admit and discharge patients from the hospital and order for patients such hospital services as laboratory tests, X-rays, nursing services, pharmaceuticals, critical care, and surgery. Yet, because their role in managing patient care and influencing expenditures is central to the health care industry, they also offer an opportunity for judicious control of medical care costs.

Given the growing tendency of states to impose limits on hospital reimbursement (Biles et al., 1980), pressures to reduce physician use of hospital services will be felt by hospital administrators and others

Milbank Memorial Fund Quarterly/*Health and Society*, Vol. 59, No. 4, 1981
© 1981 Milbank Memorial Fund and Massachusetts Institute of Technology
0160/1997/81/5904/0481-27 $01.00/0

responsible for hospital finances. It thus becomes increasingly important to understand the determinants of physician use of hospital services and the ways in which physicians' behavior may be modified. In this paper we explore the ordering behavior of physicians in the hospital setting—its nature, determinants, and problems—and, through a critical review of the research, assess various strategies for modifying physician ordering. We present data that support the thesis that a reduction in use of hospital services can be effected without endangering quality of care. We then outline factors that encourage physicians to order increasing amounts of hospital resources, and examine the hospital's role in promoting resource use. On the basis of research to date, we evaluate four major strategies that could be employed to reduce unnecessary ordering, with regard both to their relative effectiveness and to their comparative feasibility.

Although this review focuses on care of patients who are already hospitalized, we emphasize that the decision to hospitalize a patient in the first place is the most costly one a physician makes. Further, we concentrate largely on the teaching hospital and on ordering of diagnostic laboratory and radiologic procedures by physicians in training, since these have been the most commonly studied. Where possible, however, we include assessments of physician determination of hospital stay, surgery, nursing, pharmaceuticals, and other hospital services. The studies reviewed range from methodologically sound endeavors to studies marred by inadequate experimental designs. In combination, they nevertheless provide a preliminary insight for those who seek to control medical expenditures by moderating patterns of physician ordering.

This review is addressed to medical educators and others, such as hospital administrators, physicians in private practice, and state and federal policy makers, who are concerned about the physician's role in the rising cost of medical care. It exemplifies a common policy dilemma: action to rectify a problem often must be taken before the problem is fully understood and before solutions are adequately evaluated. In the case of the pattern of physician ordering, despite an abundance of published research, its nature and magnitude elude precise definition; and sporadic attempts to trace its roots or to modify it yield suggestions more than prescriptions. Despite the inadequacy of such information, however, few quarrel with the need to change ordering behavior and thereby to slow the rise in hospital costs.

Physician Ordering, Quality of Care, and Cost Containment

Use of specific clinical services for hospitalized patients has increased markedly and steadily during the last two decades, becoming an important contributor to the general increase in hospital costs. For certain illnesses, the average number of some diagnostic and therapeutic services provided per patient grew by over 500 percent between 1951 and 1971, while length of stay dropped by as much as 40 percent (Scitovsky, 1979). Laboratory procedures and radiologic services alone now account for up to 25 percent of total bills at some hospitals (Griner and Liptzin, 1971; Schroeder and O'Leary, 1977; Smith et al., 1979). Patients and physicians alike have come to equate more intensive medical care with better care, thereby making it difficult to contain costs by reducing services.

The law of diminishing returns, applied to the relation between intensity of service use and outcome of patient care, demonstrates the weakness of a "more is better" approach. Every unit of care provided has a relative clinical value for that patient. Yet as increasing amounts of an input are employed in a production process, all other things being held constant, each additional unit of input, in general, will yield a relatively smaller benefit. The "improvement" of the product associated with the addition of one more unit of input may actually be reduced to nothing or even become detrimental.

The concept of diminishing returns applies both to multiple use of a single service and to use of multiple services for a patient. For example, in the first instance, an initial chest X-ray can yield valuable clinical information for the diagnosis and monitoring of pneumonia. Once the diagnosis is made and treatment initiated, however, daily chest films will provide little additional data beyond what the physician can learn through physical examination and patient interview. Since changes in the pneumonia usually will not be apparent on a chest X-ray from one day to the next, the benefit from each daily chest film will in most cases be negligible. In an example of multiple service use, an abdominal mass can be located and its size estimated through use of an X-ray, sonogram, radionuclide scan, or computerized tomography (CT) scan, each yielding differentially accurate information. When the four are used sequentially in diagnosis, each duplicates in part the information gained from the previous test, and the relative gain in knowledge may decline with each procedure (Showstack et al., 1981).

Figure 1 illustrates a marginal benefit curve where health is the "outcome" and medical services or expenditures are "inputs." Early in a diagnostic or treatment process (point 1 in the figure), the application of a specific medical service, such as a chest X-ray or a day in the hospital, may have a sizeable impact on patient care in either confirming a suspected diagnosis or providing basic nursing and custodial support. At some point in the patient's care (point 3), however, the treatment may be well under way and an additional

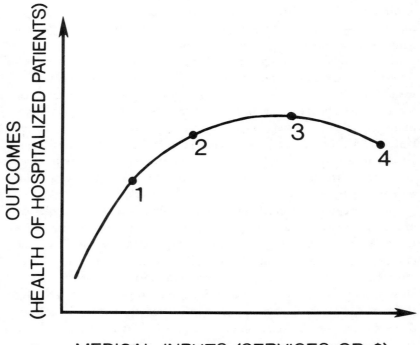

FIG. 1. Marginal benefit curve showing relation between medical services or expenditures (inputs) and patient health (outcomes). At point 1, provision of a specific service will produce a certain and dramatic improvement in health. At point 2, additional services do not add greatly to the patient's health. At point 3, no gain in health results from additional services. Finally, at point 4, additional care does more harm than good.

chest X-ray or an extra day in the hospital will add nothing to the patient's health. This is what John Bunker and Alain Enthoven call "flat-of-the-curve medicine" (Enthoven, 1978). For instance, previously recommended long hospital stays have been found to be unnecessary for uncomplicated myocardial infarction and postdelivery patients, adding nothing to patient recuperation (Hutter et al., 1973). Beyond this flat of the curve, additional care may be detrimental to patients (point 4). For example, needless surgery, excessive medications, or invasive procedures may cause iatrogenic disease and extended periods of hospitalization (Schimmel, 1964; Rogers, 1975; Seidl et al., 1966; Knapp et al., 1980; Schroeder et al., 1978). Unnecessary tests also can be detrimental: false positive results can misdirect physicians and patients into clinical wild goose chases through more unnecessary tests, diagnostic procedures, and in some instances even surgery (Barkin et al., 1977). Although the figure portrays a hypothetical curve, marginal benefit analysis can be applied to clinical situations, albeit not easily. Actual curves would vary according to service, patient, and disease. Similar marginal benefit curves, applied in the aggregate, can illustrate, for example, the relation between the frequency of a surgical procedure, such as a coronary artery by-pass, and health outcomes for a defined population.

Studies on diminishing returns of hospital services suggest that when increasing numbers of services are provided to patients, neither quality of care nor patient outcome necessarily shows a corresponding improvement (Table 1). For instance, hospitalized patients at the Strong Memorial Hospital in Rochester, New York, with one of two diagnoses, diabetic ketoacidosis or pulmonary edema, who received substantial increases over time in the use of laboratory test procedures or intensive care, showed no greater improvement in relation to length of stay or mortality than did a retrospective control group not receiving this additional treatment (Griner and Liptzin, 1971; Griner, 1972). A similar study of patients with myocardial infarctions yielded the same result (Martin et al., 1974). These studies may underestimate the effectiveness of added diagnostic or therapeutic services, however, because they rely on retrospective control groups, do not control vigorously for case severity, and use relatively insensitive indicators of outcome—length of stay and mortality. These methodologic flaws not only reflect the difficulty of conducting this type of study but also demonstrate the need for further research in this area. Despite

TABLE 1
Summary of Studies on Impact of Increased Physician Ordering

Setting	Patient Diagnosis	Findings
Hospital	Diabetic ketoacidosis	Observed increased use of laboratory tests for patients in 1969 compared with those in 1966. Found no difference in length of hospitalization (Griner and Liptzin, 1971).
Hospital	Pulmonary edema	Noted increased arterial blood gas determinations, intubations, and total charges for patients hospitalized during 1 year after opening of an intensive care unit compared with those hospitalized 1 year prior. Found that those hospitalized after had longer hospital stays but showed no difference in mortality (Griner, 1972).
Hospital	Myocardial infarction	Observed increased use of laboratory tests, bacteriologic exams, X-rays, ECGs, oxygen therapy, and sedatives over a 30-year period. Found no difference in length of hospital stay or mortality (Martin et al., 1974).
Outpatient Clinic	Hypertension	Found no correlation between patients' total annual charges for laboratory tests and blood pressure control (Daniels and Schroeder, 1977).
Hospital	Medicine (various diagnoses)	Examined physician attention to laboratory test results and found that both normal and abnormal results were often ignored by physicians (Griner and Liptzin, 1971; Williamson et al., 1967; Dixon and Laszlo, 1974).
Hospital	Medicine (various diagnoses)	Applied ordering criteria for serum lactic dehydrogenase and calcium determinations and found 50–75 percent of patients receiving multiple determinations in a 7-day period had received unnecessary tests (Eisenberg et al., 1977).
Outpatient Clinic	Various diagnoses	Applied definitions of appropriate prescribing to commonly used drugs and found 13 percent of prescriptions calling for excessive amounts (Maronde, 1971).

these shortcomings, the results of one study led to tougher criteria for admission to the intensive care unit at Strong Memorial Hospital in order to reduce excessive use of the unit (Griner, 1972).

Blood pressure control, a more proximal measure of treatment outcome, also has been used to test marginal effectiveness of care. When physician ordering of laboratory tests was matched to blood pressure control for a sample of similar ambulatory hypertensive patients, no relation was found between average annual laboratory costs per patient and patient outcome. Physicians who used more and costlier laboratory tests did not necessarily provide a better outcome for their hypertensive patients (Daniels and Schroeder, 1977).

One measure of excessive use of testing is the attention paid by physicians to results. Retrospective audits of medical records reveal that both normal and abnormal laboratory test results apparently are often ignored by physicians (Griner and Liptzin, 1971; Williamson et al., 1967; Dixon and Laszlo, 1974). This implies that the laboratory determinations were not needed in the first place. For example, in one study, reports of white blood cell differential counts were withheld to assess physicians' need for the test result (Griner and Liptzin, 1971). Two measures were used: 1) the number of phone calls to the laboratory requesting the test results; and 2) the frequency of tests reordered during the subsequent 48 hours. In none of the 37 test cases were phone calls placed to the laboratory requesting the test result. In 40 percent of the cases, the differentials were ordered daily before and after the withholding of results; of the remaining 23 cases, only 7 were reordered within 48 hours.

In another setting, a committee of physicians at a community hospital defined minimally acceptable physician responses to abnormal screening test results; e.g., did the physician mention the result in the chart or order follow-up tests? Applying these criteria to abnormal findings from urinalyses, fasting blood glucose tests, and hemoglobin studies, they found minimally acceptable physician responses for only 35 percent of the cases studied (Williamson et al., 1967). In another study, Dixon and Laszlo (1974) found that only 5 percent of chemistry panel tests yielded results that caused physicians to alter patient care. The latter two studies, however, were weakened by their definition of inattention to test results: ignoring test results was defined operationally as failing to acknowledge results in medical records or to follow up with additional testing. Although it may be considered essential for good care, chart notation may not be a valid measure of physician attention to test results. Especially in the case of normal or unchanged abnormal findings, the physician may respond to the test result, yet not note it in the chart. The degree to which excess ordering is thereby overestimated is unclear.

Eisenberg et al. (1977) developed ordering criteria for serum lactic dehydrogenase and calcium determinations and applied them to patients receiving multiple orders for these tests over a one-week period. Fifty to 75 percent of the patients were found to have undergone unnecessary tests. Observations of frequent unnecessary orders also have been made for blood cross-match, barium enema, upper gastrointestinal series, and nursing service orders (Devitt and Ironside, 1975; MacEwan et al., 1978; Vautrain and Griner, 1978; Marton et al., 1980). In these cases, overordering was judged by assessing the extent to which the ordered service either provided needed clinical information or changed therapy.

Maronde et al. (1971) studied outpatient drug prescribing at the Los Angeles County-University of Southern California Medical Center. Definitions of appropriate use of each drug in the medical center formulary were developed by a group of physicians and pharmacists at the center. Applying these definitions to prescriptions for 78 commonly used pharmaceuticals, they found that 13 percent of the prescriptions called for excessive amounts of drugs. Excessive prescriptions occurred most frequently for sedatives and barbiturates, ranging up to nearly 40 percent for some individual drugs and raising the prospect of potential disease.

The evidence on the marginal value of physicians' orders is preliminary and fragmentary, but it provides many examples that hospital services are overused. If this is the case, physicians may be able to help their patients more by ordering less, and physicians in hospitals may be able to reduce hospital expenditures without endangering quality of care.

Why Physicians Order Hospital Services

The principal goal of physicians is to ensure the health of their patients. There may be many alternative pathways to that goal, differing in both treatment and cost. Physicians vary considerably in the amounts and types of services that they order for their patients. For example, in an outpatient setting, internists have been found to differ as much as 17- to 20-fold in mean annual charges per patient for laboratory and X-ray services when caring for similar patients (Daniels and Schroeder, 1977; Schroeder et al., 1973). Physicians also vary in their ordering of numerous other services, including surgery, diagnostic procedures, and pharmaceuticals, as well as additional days of hospital stay (Schroeder et al., 1973; Heasman and Carstairs, 1971; Childs and Hunter, 1972; Lyle et al., 1976; Roos et al., 1977). Most of these studies tried to control for patient diagnosis and severity among physicians by selecting similar patients for comparison. Two of them, however, failed to control for patient characteristics, making it unclear how much variability in ordering actually could be attributed to physicians (Childs and Hunter, 1972; Roos et al., 1977).

One major setting contributing to greater use of hospital services by physicians is the teaching hospital. In 1978, hospitals affiliated with medical schools accounted for 36 percent of all acute-care hospital beds and 47 percent of total national hospital expenditures (American Hospital Association, 1979). In teaching hospitals, physicians use more resources for the same types of patients than do physicians practicing in community hospitals—greater use of consultations, laboratory tests, X-rays, and scans (Schroeder and O'Leary, 1977; Feigenson et al., 1978). Greater use of diagnostic tests per patient in a university hospital accounted for 56 percent of the differences in charges for similar patients between this hospital and a neighboring community hospital, even though patients were admitted by the same internists at both institutions (Schroeder and O'Leary, 1977). Use of specific blood tests, radiologic procedures, and consultations was significantly greater for patients in the teaching hospital. Greater use of services at teaching hospitals has been attributed, at least in part, to house staff inexperience. Results of a case simulation study of physician ordering behavior supports this reasoning: describing how they would care for a set of hypothetical patients, residents "ordered" more tests and procedures than did experienced physicians, who relied more on history and physical examination (Hardwick et al., 1975). The dual medical-educational purpose of teaching hospitals also may be responsible for greater resource use: ordering of tests or procedures can have both clinical benefits for patients and educational ones for residents and medical students. It should be noted, however, that the educational return on increasing levels of ordering probably also follows the pattern of diminishing returns.

A physician's clinical decisions may be influenced by any number of individual, organizational, and economic considerations, most of which promote the increased use of services (Eisenberg, 1979; Schroeder and Showstack, 1979). Below, we discuss three of the more important incentives for physicians to order more, rather than fewer, services. The potency of these three major reasons to order may also be influenced by many other characteristics of medical practice such as clinical specialty, organizational mode, perceived risk of malpractice litigation, and method of physician reimbursement.

Belief that Patient Care Will Be Improved

Physicians request services for patients principally to improve the quality of patient care. Thus, more diagnostic, monitoring, and therapeutic services are ordered in the belief that a condition will be diagnosed, that possible complications will be averted, that the patient's fears (or physician's anxieties) will be assuaged, and, finally, that the disease will be cured. With the dramatic increase in the number and type of services available, few physicians can be fully informed of the indications for and the appropriate use of all hospital resources (Zieve, 1966; Williams et al., 1979). At one hospital, for example, some physicians ordering graded treadmill tests were unaware of the appropriate indications, interpretation, and follow-up for the tests. As a result, they often ordered the procedure inappropriately and excessively while believing it to be in their patients' best interest (Abbott et al., 1977).

Clinical diagnosis and treatment are complex, and by nature entail uncertainty. In highly ambiguous situations, physicians order more services than in more clear-cut situations (Pineault, 1977). Physicians in training are particularly vulnerable to the fear of missing information, in part because attending physicians and senior house staff are more likely to criticize junior house staff for ordering too few rather than too many tests and procedures (Dans, 1978). Uncertainty about how to use hospital services, added to the ambiguity of clinical situations and the fear of missing vital clinical information, may account for much of the overuse observed in hospitals (Casscells et al., 1978).

Patient Demand

Patients influence physician ordering by requesting particular treatments or by reinforcing liberal ordering practices. Patients often associate advanced technological procedures and medications with good care. In a survey of patient attitudes toward testing in general and toward the upper gastrointestinal X-ray series in particular, Marton et al. (1978) found that nearly two-thirds of the patients believed that "the better a doctor is, the more tests he will order in evaluating a patient's problem." Moreover, these patients valued the upper gastrointestinal series highly even when it had little actual clinical value for diagnosis or treatment in their individual cases. With regard to prescriptions for medications, Maronde et al. (1972) attributed multiple and excessive prescriptions for psychoactive drugs to "prescription shoppers." Although the number of these patients was not large, they posed the potential problem of serious adverse drug interactions. Although it has been asserted that patient demand is partially responsible for increased drug prescribing, little empirical evidence exists to assess the magnitude of the effect on physician ordering (Hemminki, 1975).

Financial Incentives

Many financial incentives encourage physicians to order increasing amounts of services. Physicians may receive direct financial compensation for ordering or administering tests and procedures, depending on the organization of their practice. The financial incentive occurs most strikingly in private practice settings in which physicians own major pieces of equipment, such as X-ray and electrocardiogram machines, and have a financial stake in promoting use of this equipment (Schroeder and Showstack, 1978). These same financial incentives exist when physicians have part ownership of hospitals with accompanying laboratories, when they are members of group practices that include radiologists or other similar specialists, or when they invest in private clinical laboratories (Relman, 1980). Physicians also have financial incentives to treat patients in the hospital rather than in the office and to perform surgery when surgical procedures can be substituted for office visits (Burney et al., 1979). Most of the examples of financial incentives for physician ordering arise from outpatient settings. While hospital reimbursement patterns tend to create financial incentives as well (see below), their impact on physician ordering has not been documented.

These three major factors all encourage physicians to order more, not fewer, hospital services. Except for concurrent review of length of hospital stay and prospective review of admissions, there are no examples of incentives to order fewer. On the contrary, placing a standing order for tests is as easy as requesting a single test. Other factors also contribute to potential overuse of services. Physicians may be ignorant of the prices of services; in a number of hospitals, physicians have been quizzed on the charges for frequently ordered tests and procedures (Skipper et al., 1975, 1976; Kelly, 1978; Dresnick et al., 1979; Nagurney et al., 1979; Kirkland, 1979). In most instances the majority of estimates were clearly erroneous, usually on the side of underestimating the charges. Finally, since hospital care is paid largely by third-party payers, not by patients, there is no direct financial barrier to doing "the most" for the hospitalized patient.

Hospitals Encourage Physician Ordering of Services

Although we have focused primarily on physicians and the "demand" for hospital services, the "supplier," or the hospital, also encourages ordering of services. Like physicians, hospitals have powerful financial and organizational incentives to promote use of their services. Hospitals that successfully foster physician ordering are rewarded with solvency, perceived higher quality of care, and growth (Schulz and Rose, 1973). Hospitals may not intervene directly in physician decisions, but they set a climate favorable to increased ordering.

Before the widespread availability of medical insurance, use of hospital services was restricted by patients' ability to pay and hospitals' ability to finance charity care. These limitations effectively placed a ceiling on hospital prices and utilization; violating the ceiling risked insolvency. With present broad insurance coverage for the majority of patients (over 90 percent of hospital costs are reimbursed by third-party payers), hospitals can now be assured of increased income and, in some cases, profit, for each added patient day or service ordered (Gibson, 1980; Schulz and Rose, 1973). Since hospitals are paid largely on the basis of their costs, there is little incentive to reduce costs. Rather, at least in those states without reimbursement controls, the more hospitals expend, the more they are paid. Moreover, as the cost of providing care rises, cost-based third-party payment levels rise also. Thus, with income almost guaranteed for any clinical service ordered, it is to the hospital's financial advantage to promote hospitalization and the use of hospital services for patients.

Hospitals attract patients largely by encouraging physicians to use their facilities. Although the strength of the relation is unclear, physicians may be more likely to admit patients to hospitals that offer the most advanced services and technologies, such as computerized tomography. In fact, physicians may actively advise hospitals on equipment purchase decisions (Lewis, 1979). Both physicians and the general public perceive the availability of sophisticated equipment and services to mean better quality of care. Hospitals that grow by adding the latest technologies, special care units, and newest beds both increase their own prestige and business and enhance the reputations of their administrators.

Growth in number of beds and services also raises a hospital's fixed costs and reduces the proportion of costs controllable by management. To pay for new equipment, technical staffing, or beds, hospitals promote increased utilization. This may express itself indirectly: hospitals may make these services, which are generally well reimbursed, more attractive and convenient to use than others that are reimbursed poorly, if at all. Scheduling ease, availability of expert consultants, rapid turnaround for test results, and round-the-clock availability of tests or procedures can all be manipulated to encourage greater use of specific hospital services. Thus, the hospital's strong financial and organizational incentives provide a climate that encourages physicians to order more services for their patients.

Can Physician Ordering Patterns Be Changed?

In response to alarm at the growing physician-determined use of hospital services, the sometimes questionable value of these services, and the abundance of powerful incentives to maintain the growth in use of services, various means to intervene in the ordering process and to slow the rise in service ordering have been proposed and examined. Table 2 summarizes published reports concerning the four major strategies that have been assessed in hospital settings: education; audit with feedback; restrictions or rationing; and positive incentives. Most of the strategies have been tested only in teaching hospitals and on physicians in training, and in general the number of reports is small, although recently increasing.

Education

Attempts to educate physicians to modify their patterns of service use generally have focused either on appropriateness of care or on cost of tests and procedures. These efforts are based on the assumption that physicians would choose to change their ordering behavior if they understood better the costs and benefits of each service. Several programs have demonstrated an initial reduction in ordering, but long-term effects on individual physicians generally have not been assessed.

Educational programs to teach physicians the indications for ordering services have yielded mixed results. Physicians learning the appropriate indications for prothrombin time and thyroid function tests temporarily demonstrated lower use of these tests than physicians who received no such education (Eisenberg, 1977; Rhyne and Gelbach, 1979). In one case, however, a six-month follow-up of the same physicians revealed that they had resumed their previous patterns (Rhyne and Gelbach, 1979). Promulgating criteria for ordering determinations of serum lactic dehydrogenase had no effect on the rate of overuse of this test (Eisenberg et al., 1977). The failure in this instance was attributed to lack of incentives for the house staff to change their ordering patterns, lack of support from attending physicians, and the limited focus of the effort. An effort to teach appropriate therapy for urinary tract infections resulted in significantly improved prescribing behavior and a 40 percent reduction in cost of care compared with a concurrent control group who received no education (Klein et al., 1980). Guidelines for ordering blood for surgery patients have been associated with major long-term declines in blood use, as much as 50 percent over an eight-year period (McCoy, 1962; Mintz et al., 1978). Medical students' knowledge of indications for ordering seems to grow when they review actual patient records; moreover, the review process appears to improve their attitudes about

TABLE 2
Summary of Research on Intervention Strategies

Intervention	Settings	Findings
Education • in cost of services • in decision-making • in ordering protocols • in all of the above	Hospital, medical school, group practice clinic	Efforts focused on reducing or improving ordering of laboratory tests, X-rays, ECGs, blood and pharmaceuticals. When only one approach is employed, use may be reduced, but results are mixed. When a multidimensional approach is used, long-term effect is observed. Success may depend on senior faculty and departmental support and on continuous effort (e.g., Eisenberg et al., 1977; Rhyne and Gelbach, 1979; Klein et al., 1980; Griner, 1979).
Audit with Feedback	Hospital, outpatient clinic	Attempts made to reduce laboratory, pharmacy, and surgery service use and length of hospitalization were generally successful. "High-cost" and "high-use" physicians tend to reduce their ordering the most (e.g., Schroeder et al., 1973; Mitchell et al., 1975; Pozen and Gloger, 1976; Martin et al., 1980).
Restrictions or Rationing	Hospital	Efforts made to reduce ordering of laboratory tests only. Rationing reduces use and improves proportion of tests ordered appropriately (Dixon and Laszlo, 1974; Gray and Marion, 1973).
Positive Incentives	Hospital	One attempt to reduce laboratory test use. Positive incentive, in form of material reward, found to be relatively ineffective (Martin et al., 1980).

cost control although it is not clear that it changes their behavior (Garg et al., 1979; Zeleznik and Gonnella, 1979).

Educating physicians about the cost of medical services appears to be an effective cost-containment strategy, at least in the short run. Whether in real life or in simulated situations, teaching the cost of services reduces the ordering of laboratory tests, X-rays, electrocardiograms, electroencephalograms, and hospital charges per patient (Freeman, 1976; El Khatib et al., 1977; Henderson et al., 1979). Results of all of these studies were based on comparisons with control groups. In only one reported instance, a simulation study, were any physicians found to ignore costs (Lawrence, 1979).

The most impressive results of an educational program were reported from the Strong Memorial Hospital, where an extensive educational effort appeared to curtail the use of chemistry tests and chest X-rays and reduce the rate of growth in use of hematology determinations and microbiology cultures (Griner, 1979). Over a seven-year period, laboratory, EKG, and chest X-ray use was monitored and then compared for the years 1970 and 1977. Increases in use and costs at the Strong were lower than the national average; and, for the period 1975 to 1977, use at the Strong was lower than that at a nearby affiliated teaching hospital. The lack of a concurrent comparison group for the entire period, however, makes it difficult to attribute the cause of the lower use. Other changes at the hospital acknowledged by the author, such as change in patient or physician mix, increased use of chemistry panels over individual tests, decreased reliance on particular nonautomated tests, and the elimination of the chest X-ray from the admission screening battery, in addition to the educational program, could have affected use. Nevertheless, this educational effort was unique for its broad coverage of a variety of topics, including test specificity and sensitivity, probability theory, laboratory charges, and reimbursement mechanisms. The multifaceted and ongoing nature of this approach and the personal involvement of a respected senior clinician may have contributed to the long-term reductions in use of hospital services reported.

Audit with Feedback

In this intervention, physicians' use of services is reviewed by senior physicians, their performance compared with that of others, and the results of the comparison shared with each physician. This "audit and feedback" approach is successful in reducing the ordering of laboratory tests, especially among "high-cost" or "high-use" physicians (Schroeder et al., 1973; Lyle et al., 1979). After one such audit at the George Washington University Medical Clinic, overall mean annual laboratory charges declined by 29 percent. Moreover, the previous "high-cost" physicians lowered their laboratory charges by 42 percent. A study at the Peter Bent Brigham Hospital indicates that house staff who underwent audits of their laboratory use by senior physicians ordered significantly fewer tests than either house staff in a control group or those in a group offered material rewards to lower their laboratory use (Martin et al., 1980). Similar audits of surgery cases also were effective in reducing length of stay for patients undergoing cholecystectomy. After results of an audit were presented to surgeons at one hospital, average length of stay dropped by one day; again, it was the "longer-stay" physicians who most reduced hospitalization time (Mitchell et al., 1975). Pozen and Gloger (1976) reported to physicians monthly on their ordering of laboratory tests and of three major cardiovascular medications for outpatients. The feedback on prescribing included the calculation of an index to evaluate appropriateness of the quantities prescribed. The reporting had no effect on laboratory ordering when compared with a control group, but it substantially improved the ordering of medications in appropriate quantities.

Audit and feedback also can be effective on a broader scale. One audit that examined regional differences in the performance of tonsillectomies reported a 13-fold difference in the per capita rate of tonsillectomies across thirteen regions in Vermont. After feedback of these results to the regions, tonsillectomy rates declined by 46 percent over a five-year period; again, the region with the highest previous rate reduced its rate the most (Wennberg et al., 1977).

Restrictions or Rationing

Another means to reduce use of hospital services is to place limits on the number of tests or services that can be ordered or to encumber the process of ordering. Under a rationing program, medical house staff were limited to ordering a maximum of 8 chemistry and hematology tests per patient day, except in cases of emergency. They reduced their use of chemistry tests significantly from a mean of 6 to a mean of 2 per day primarily by eliminating unnecessary follow-up tests (Dixon and Laszlo, 1947). House staff who were required to consult a laboratory hematology resident before ordering thrombin, prothrombin, and partial thromboplastin tests also reduced their ordering of these tests markedly (Gray and Marion, 1973). A third reported attempt to ration services at a teaching hospital was abandoned as being too difficult to maintain (E. Amador, personal communication, 1978).

Positive Incentives

Comparisons of fee-for-service systems and health maintenance organizations certainly suggest that positive financial incentives can affect hospital utilization patterns in the aggregate (Luft, 1978). Little information exists, however, on the effectiveness of positive incentives in altering individual physicians' ordering behavior for hospitalized patients. The project at the Peter Bent Brigham Hospital created positive incentives, in the form of journal subscriptions and textbooks, for reducing use of specified laboratory tests. Results indicate that these incentives were not effective (Martin et al., 1980). Considering the strong effect that positive incentives exert on physicians in organized systems of medical care, it seems reasonable to assume that they could be powerful determinants of individual physician behavior in other settings as well. Results of research on the type, strength, and effect of such incentives will be eagerly received.

These four strategies for modifying physician patterns of ordering hospital services are all designed to inform or guide the physician into more clinically appropriate ordering patterns. Yet they represent strikingly different approaches to the problem and run the gamut from almost certain effectiveness (audit with feedback) to questionable feasibility (restrictions or rationing). For positive incentives especially, but also for restrictions and rationing, few published reports exist to aid in their evaluation. At some of the institutions where strategies have proved effective, a key determinant of success seems to be the participation of respected senior clinicians; the importance of this particular factor, however, has not been assessed.

Implications for Hospital Cost Containment

Clinical decision-making and policy decision-making share an important quality: a "treatment" often must be prescribed for a problem even when its effectiveness is uncertain. In both medicine and policy, "sure cures" are neither always available nor without their own potentially deleterious side effects. In selecting therapies, however, a clinician or policy maker can do much to maximize possible benefits and to minimize costs of the treatment plan.

Leaving aside the clinical example, hospital administrators, medical educators, and state and federal policy makers increasingly are encouraging their institutions to approach the problem of hospital cost increases by developing cost-containment programs that focus on physician ordering behavior. Their motivation for doing so may stem from fear of impending federal regulation of hospital expenditures, support for the Voluntary Effort, or personal belief in the importance of cost and appropriate ordering. It should be emphasized that hospital support for any cost-containment strategy cannot be expected unless adequate incentives exist for that support. As we have shown, a number of optional strategies are available to alter physician ordering of services. The primary criterion by which to assess these options is their relative effectiveness in improving physician ordering patterns, even though, as explained above, evaluative data are incomplete. Other factors, however, affect both the costs and benefits of each strategy; hence they also must be considered. We will discuss briefly each of the four strategies according to several other factors—ease and cost of implementation, permanence of effect, and the urgency of the need for change.

Current evidence suggests that the strategy most likely to reduce ordering appears to be audit with feedback. In each of the reported trials, this strategy has reduced physician ordering levels most reliably, and it has done so for a variety of hospital services and in a number of settings. Unfortunately, although audits seem to be effective, they are expensive because of the time and effort required of physicians to review patient charts and to communicate the results. Audits with feedback also may be difficult to implement; physicians may feel that their autonomy and personal responsibility for patient care are being threatened. The precedent of utilization review committees, however, may facilitate implementation of the audit mechanism.

Education follows audit as the next most effective strategy. As noted above, physicians tend to order fewer or less expensive services when made aware of their costs. It is not known, however, how long this effect lasts. Providing physicians with patients' bills or price lists is inexpensive and relatively easy to do. If a hospital's or medical school's purpose is to imbue physicians with the knowledge and the ability to make cost-effective clinical decisions, then education in decision-making and in the specificity, sensitivity, and indications for tests may be in order. This education may or may not have an effect and, if it does occur, may dissipate over time. Success of educational efforts depends on access to capable faculty, or, at the very least, to specific educational materials. Such efforts also require substantial preparatory work in developing curricula, in gathering resource materials, and in gaining consensus for ordering criteria.

The next most reliable strategy for changing physician behavior seems to be restricting ordering or rationing services, although very few evaluations of restrictions have been reported and none have used concurrent control groups to assess impact. Where restrictions have been tested, they appear to have had an effect on ordering of services. If effective, their impact would probably be immediate and enduring as long as the restrictive policies were enforced. None of the evaluations has examined possible compensatory behaviors, however, such as ordering chest physical therapy or chest X-rays when respiratory therapy treatments are restricted. Such substitutions seem more likely with restrictions, especially arbitrary restrictions, and point up the possibly limited utility of restrictions as a cost-containment strategy. Moreover, restrictions are often odious, difficult to implement, ethically questionable, and costly to maintain. They require the capability to monitor ordering, to flag disallowed orders, and to communicate directly back to the ordering physician so that patient care will not suffer.

Not enough is known yet about the effect of positive incentives on use of hospital services. Although the cost-reducing behavior of health maintenance organizations may be motivated by positive financial incentives, their savings are attributable largely to lower hospitalization rates (Luft, 1978). It is unclear how such incentives affect physician use of services for hospitalized patients. In the only good study of positive incentives in a fee-for-service setting, the offer of rewards to physicians was ineffectual in reducing their ordering (Martin et al., 1980). More studies are needed to measure the possible benefits of more attractive positive incentives in a range of fee-for-service hospital settings. Even if this strategy is shown to be effective, however, financial, ethical, and political considerations may hamper its implementation.

Conclusion

Our tremendously expanded capacity to diagnose, monitor, and treat illnesses has been accompanied by a growing tendency to overuse hospital services, many of which are costly. As detailed in a number of reports, only a portion of the many tests ordered for hospitalized patients is actually used for patient management. Overuse of services contributes neither to quality of care nor to patient outcome, may well be detrimental to care in some cases, and certainly raises the cost of hospital care. These findings strongly suggest that the ordering of hospital services and the cost of hospital care may be reduced selectively without adversely affecting patient care.

Numerous incentives confronting physicians and hospitals encourage increased ordering of hospital services even when, as in the practice of "defensive medicine," patient care will not be improved. There are no strong forces in fee-for-service medicine to balance these incentives and to moderate physician ordering. Nevertheless, several strategies for modifying physician ordering patterns have been tested and found to be relatively effective, at least in the short run. Some of them, however, are costly or difficult to implement.

Audit with feedback and education appear to be the most effective strategies to reduce physician ordering. Yet each requires considerable effort to implement. Data on the effectiveness of restrictions and, especially, of positive incentives are fragmentary and preliminary, making it difficult to predict how well they might change physician ordering. They are certainly the most controversial of the four strategies. Although more research on any of these strategies would clarify their impact and feasibility, efforts to understand the benefits of restrictions and positive incentives are needed the most.

If some of the strategies discussed successfully reduce physician ordering of hospital services, their application will significantly improve the chances of controlling hospital cost inflation, at least in the short run. On the other hand, if cost-effective means to reduce unnecessary use of hospital services are not found and then implemented, prospects for controlling hospital costs are poor. While hospital occupancy rates and length of stay may continue their present decline, ordering of ancillary and other hospital services will continue to increase, further raising the bill for a patient day as more services are administered during fewer patient days.

A successful cost-containment effort may also have a negative effect by putting some hospitals in a difficult position: their expected income will drop, and they may not be able to respond adequately by cutting costs because a large proportion of their costs will be fixed, the result of previous growth in beds and equipment. If reimbursement levels are not raised sufficiently to offset reduced volume, hospitals will feel the pinch, facing higher costs and lower revenues per patient day. For some financially weak hospitals, cost containment may spell hospital closure, a scenario that may be desired by advocates of "competition" as a solution to rising costs of ·medical care.

On the positive side, this situation may bring community hospitals and physicians together to decide the cost-effective allocation and use of hospital resources. Moreover, if hospital reimbursement mechanisms that limit the hospital's ability to increase reimbursement continue to spread (Biles et al., 1980), hospital administrators will have great need of strategies by which to change the pattern of physician use of services for hospitalized patients.

References

Abbot, J.A., Tedeschi, M.A., and Cheitlin, M.D. 1977. Graded Treadmill Stress Testing: Patterns of Physician Use and Abuse. *Western Journal of Medicine* 126:173–178.

American Hospital Association. 1979. *Hospital Statistics, 1979 Edition.* Chicago: American Hospital Association.

Barkin, J., Vining, D., Miale, A., Jr., Gottlieb, S., Redhammer, D.E., and Kalser, M.H. 1977. Computerized Tomography, Diagnostic Ultrasound and Radionuclide Scanning. Comparison of Efficacy in Diagnosis of Pancreatic Carcinoma. *Journal of the American Medical Association* 238:2040–2042.

Biles, B., Schramm, C.J., and Atkinson, J.G. 1980. Hospital Cost Inflation under State Rate-Setting Programs. *New England Journal of Medicine* 303:664–668.

Burney, I.L., Schieber, G.J., Blaxall, M.O., and Gabel, J.R. 1979.

Medicare and Medicaid Physician Payment Incentives. *Health Care Financing Review* 1:62–78.

Casscells, W., Schoenberger, A., and Graboys, T.B. 1978. Interpretation by Physicians of Clinical Laboratory Results. *New England Journal of Medicine* 299:990–1001.

Childs, A.W., and Hunter, E.D. 1972. Non-medical Factors Influencing Use of Diagnostic X-Ray by Physicians. *Medical Care* 10:323–335.

Daniels, M., and Schroeder, S.A. 1977. Variation among Physicians in Use of Laboratory Tests. II. Relation to Clinical Productivity and Outcomes of Care. *Medical Care* 15:482–487.

Dans, P.E. 1978. The Great Zebra Hunt: A View of Internal Medicine from the Walk-In Clinic. *Pharos,* July, 2–6.

Devitt, J.E., and Ironside, M.R. 1975. Can Patient Care Audit Change Doctor Performance? *Journal of Medical Education* 50:1122–1123.

Dixon, R.H., and Laszlo, J. 1974. Utilization of Clinical Chemistry Services by Medical House Staff. *Archives of Internal Medicine* 134:1064–1067.

Dresnick, S.J., Roth, W.I., Linn, B.S., Pratt, T.C., and Blum, A. 1979. The Physician's Role in the Cost-Containment Problem. *Journal of the American Medical Association* 241:1606–1609.

Eisenberg, J.M. 1977. An Educational Program to Modify Laboratory Use by House Staff. *Journal of Medical Education* 52:578–581.

————. 1979. Sociologic Influences on Decision-Making by Clinicians. *Annals of Internal Medicine* 90:957–964.

————, Williams, S.V., Garner, L., Viale, R., and Smits, H. 1977. Computer-based Audit to Detect and Correct Overutilization of Laboratory Tests. *Medical Care* 15:915–921.

El Khatib, M., Skipper, J.K., Gliebe, W., Garg, M.L., and McNamara, M. 1977. Physicians' Knowledge of Cost: Effects on Utilization Behavior. Abstract, American Public Health Association Meeting.

Enthoven, A.C. 1978. Shattuck Lecture: Cutting Cost Without Cutting the Quality of Care. *New England Journal of Medicine* 298:1229–1238.

Feigenson, J.S., Feigenson, W.D., Gitlow, H.S., McCarthy, M.L., and Greenberg, S.D. 1978. Outcome and Cost for Stroke Patients in Academic and Community Hospitals: Comparison of Two Groups Referred to a Regional Rehabilitation Center. *Journal of the American Medical Association* 240:1878–1880.

Freeman, R.A. 1976. Cost Containment. *Journal of Medical Education* 51:157–158.

Garg, M.L., Gliebe, W.A., and Kleinberg, W.M. 1979. Student

Peer Review of Diagnostic Tests at the Medical College of Ohio. *Journal of Medical Education* 54:852–855.

Gibson, R.M. 1980. National Health Expenditures. 1979. *Health Care Financing Review* 2:1–36.

Gray, G., and Marion, R. 1973. Utilization of a Hematology Laboratory in a Teaching Hospital. *American Journal of Clinical Pathology* 59:877–882.

Griner, P.F. 1972. Treatment of Acute Pulmonary Edema: Conventional or Intensive Care? *Annals of Internal Medicine* 77:501–506.

————. 1979. Use of Laboratory Tests in a Teaching Hospital: Long-Term Trends: Reductions in Use and Relative Cost. *Annals of Internal Medicine* 90:243–248.

————, and Liptzin, B. 1971. Use of the Laboratory in a Teaching Hospital: Implications for Patient Care, Education, and Hospital Costs. *Annals of Internal Medicine* 75:157–163.

Hardwick, D.F., Vertinsky, P., Barth, R.T., Mitchell, V.F., Bernstein, M., and Vertinsky, I. 1975. Clinical Styles and Motivation: A Study of Laboratory Test Use. *Medical Care* 13:397–408.

Heasman, M.A., and Carstairs, V. 1971. Inpatient Management: Variations in Some Aspects of Practice in Scotland. *British Medical Journal* 1:495–498.

Hemminki, E. 1975. Review of Literature on the Factors Affecting Drug Prescribing. *Social Science and Medicine* 9:111–115.

Henderson, D., D'Allessandri, R., Westfall, B., Moore, R., Smith, R., Scobbo, R., and Waldman, R. 1979. Hospital Cost Containment: A Little Knowledge Helps. *Clinical Research* 27:279A.

Hutter, A.M. Jr., Sidel, V.W., Shine, K.I., and DeSanctis, R.W. 1973. Early Hospital Discharge after Myocardial Infarction. *New England Journal of Medicine* 288:1141–1144.

Kelly, S.P. 1978. Physicians' Knowledge of Hospital Costs. *Journal of Family Practice* 6:171–172.

Kirkland, L.R. 1979. The Physician and Cost Containment. *Journal of the American Medical Association* 242:1032.

Klein, L., Charache, P., Johannes, R., and Lewis, C. 1980. Effect of Physician Tutorials on Prescribing Patterns and Drug Cost in Ambulatory Patients. *Clinical Research* 28:296A.

Knapp, D.A., Speedie, M.K., Yaeger, D.M., and Knapp, D.A. 1980. Drug Prescribing and Its Relation to Length of Hospital Stay. *Inquiry* 17:254–259.

Lawrence, R.S. 1979. The Role of Physician Education in Cost Containment. *Journal of Medical Education* 54:841–847.

Lewis, H.L. 1979. Who Makes Decisions about New Technology in Hospitals? *Hospitals* 53:114–121.

Luft, H.S. 1978. How Do Health-Maintenance Organizations Achieve Their "Savings"? *New England Journal of Medicine* 298:1336–1343.

Lyle, C.B., Applegate, W.B., Citron, D.S., and Williams, O.D. 1976. Practice Habits in a Group of Eight Internists. *Annals of Internal Medicine* 84:594–601.

————, Bianchi, R.F., Harris, J.H., and Wood, Z.L. 1979. Teaching Cost Containment to House Officers in Charlotte Memorial Hospital. *Journal of Medical Education* 54:856–862.

MacEwan, D.W., Kavanagh, S., Chow, P., and Tishler, J.M. 1978. Manitoba Barium Enema Efficacy Study. *Radiology* 126:39–44.

Maronde, R.F., Lee, P.V., McCarron, M.M., and Siebert, S. 1971. A Study of Prescribing Patterns. *Medical Care* 9:383–395.

————, Siebert, S., Katzoff, J., and Silverman, M. 1972. Prescription Data Processing: Its Role in the Control of Drug Abuse. *California Medicine* 117:22–28.

Martin, A.R., Wolf, M.A., Thibodeau, L.A., Dzau, V., and Braunwald, E. 1980. A Trial of Two Strategies to Modify the Test-Ordering Behavior of Medical Residents. *New England Journal of Medicine* 303:1330–1336.

Martin, S.P., Donaldson, M.C., London, C.D., Peterson, O.L., and Colton, T. 1974. Inputs into Coronary Care During 30 Years: A Cost Effectiveness Study. *Annals of Internal Medicine* 81:289–293.

Marton, K.I., Sox, H.C., and Wasson, J.H. 1978. The Clinical Utility of the Upper Gastrointestinal Series. *Clinical Research* 26:334A.

————, Sox, H.C., Wasson, J.H., and Duisenberg, C.E. 1980. The Clinical Value of the Upper Gastrointestinal Tract Roentgenogram Series. *Archives of Internal Medicine* 140:191–195.

McCoy, K.L. 1962. The Providence Hospital Blood Conservation Program. *Transfusion* 2:3–6.

McNerney, W.J. 1980. Control of Health-Care Costs in the 1980's. *New England Journal of Medicine* 303:1088–1095.

Mintz, P.D., Lauenstein, K., Hume, J., and Henry, J.B. 1978. Expected Hemotherapy in Elective Surgery: A Follow-Up. *Journal of the American Medical Association* 239:623–625.

Mitchell, J.H., Hardacre, J.M., Wenzel, F.J., and Lohrenz, F.N. 1975. Cholecystectomy Peer Review: Measurement of Four Variables. *Medical Care* 13:409–416.

Nagurney, J.T., Braham, R.L., and Reader, G.G. 1979. Physician Awareness of Economic Factors in Clinical Decision-Making. *Medical Care* 17:727–736.

Pineault, R. 1977. The Effect of Medical Training Factors on Physician Utilization Behavior. *Medical Care* 15:51–67.

Pozen, M.W., and Gloger, H. 1976. The Impact on House Officers of Educational and Administrative Interventions in an Outpatient Department. *Social Science and Medicine* 10:491–495.

Relman, A.S. 1980. The New Medical-Industrial Complex. *New England Journal of Medicine* 303:963–970.

Rhyne, R.L., and Gelbach, S.H. 1979. Effects of an Educational Feedback Strategy on Physician Utilization of Thyroid Function Panels. *Journal of Family Practice* 8:1003–1007.

Rogers, D.E. 1975. On Technologic Restraint. *Archives of Internal Medicine* 135:1393–1397.

Roos, N.P., Roos, L.L., and Henteleff, P.D. 1977. Elective Surgical Rates: Do High Rates Mean Lower Standards? Tonsillectomy and Adenoidectomy in Manitoba. *New England Journal of Medicine* 297:360–365.

Schimmel, E.M. 1964. The Hazards of Hospitalization. *Annals of Internal Medicine* 60:100–110.

Schroeder, S.A., Kenders, K., Cooper, J.K., and Piemme, T.E. 1973. Use of Laboratory Tests and Pharmaceuticals: Variation Among Physicians and Effect of Cost Audit on Subsequent Use. *Journal of the American Medical Association* 225:969–973.

————, Marton, K.I., and Strom, B.L. 1978. Frequency and Morbidity of Invasive Procedures. Report of a Pilot Study from Two Teaching Hospitals. *Archives of Internal Medicine* 138:1809–1811.

————, and O'Leary, D.S. 1977. Differences in Laboratory Use and Length of Stay between University and Community Hospitals. *Journal of Medical Education* 52:418–420.

————, and Showstack, J.A. 1978. Financial Incentives to Perform Medical Procedures and Laboratory Tests: Illustrative Models of Office Practice. *Medical Care* 16:289–298.

————, and Showstack, J.A. 1979. The Dynamics of Medical Technology Use: Analysis and Policy Options. In Altman, S.H., and Blendon, R., eds. *Medical Technology: The Culprit Behind Health Care Costs?* 178–212. DHEW Publication No. (PHS)79-3216. Washington, D.C.: U.S. Government Printing Office.

Schulz, R.I., and Rose, J. 1973. Can Hospitals Be Expected to Control Costs? *Inquiry* 10:3–8.

Scitovsky, A. 1979. Changes in the Use of Ancillary Services for "Common" Illness. In Altman, S.H., and Blendon, R., eds. *Medical Technology: The Culprit Behind Health Care Costs?* 39–56. DHEW Publication No. (PHS)79-3216. Washington, D.C.: U.S. Government Printing Office.

Seidl, L.G., Thornton, G.F., Smith, J.W., and Cluff, L.E. 1966. Studies on the Epidemiology of Adverse Drug Reactions. III.

Reactions in Patients on a General Medical Service. *Bulletin of the Johns Hopkins Hospital* 119:299–315.

Showstack, J.A., Schroeder, S.A., and Steinberg, H.R. 1981. Evaluating the Costs and Benefits of a Diagnostic Technology: The Case of Upper Gastrointestinal Endoscopy. *Medical Care* 19:498–509.

Skipper, J.K., Smith, G., Mulligan, J.L., and Garg, M.L. 1975. Medical Students' Unfamiliarity with the Cost of Diagnostic Tests. *Journal of Medical Education* 50:683–684.

———. 1976. Physicians' Knowledge of Cost: The Case of Diagnostic Tests. *Inquiry* 13:194–198.

Smith, D.M., Roberts, S.D., and Gross, T.L. 1979. Components of the Costs of Care for Medicine Patients at an Urban Care Center. *Clinical Research* 27:284A.

Vautrain, R.L., and Griner, P.F. 1978. Physician's Orders, Use of Nursing Resources, and Subsequent Clinical Events. *Journal of Medical Education* 53:125–128.

Wennberg, J.E., Blowers, L., Parker, R., and Gittelsohn, A.M. 1977. Changes in Tonsillectomy Rates Associated with Feedback and Review. *Pediatrics* 59:821–826.

Williams, S.V., Eisenberg, J.M., Pascale, L.A., and Kitz, D. 1979. Determining the Causes for Unnecessary Testing. *Clinical Research* 27:286A.

Williamson, J.W., Alexander, M., and Miller, G.E. 1967. Continuing Education and Patient Care Research: Physician Response to Screening Test Results. *Journal of the American Medical Association* 201:118–122.

Zeleznik, C., and Gonnella, J.S. 1979. Jefferson Medical College Student Model Utilization Review Committee. *Journal of Medical Education* 54:848–851.

Zieve, L. 1966. Misinterpretation and Abuse of Laboratory Tests by Clinicians. *New York Academy of Science Annals* 134:563–572.

Acknowledgments: This work was supported by grants from the California Medical Education and Research Foundation, the California Hospital Association, the Henry J. Kaiser Family Foundation, and the John A. Hartford Foundation.

We wish to thank Jonathan A. Showstack, Anne A. Scitovsky, Philip R. Lee, John Eisenberg, Albert R. Martin, Paul F. Griner, Keith I. Marton, Harold S. Luft, J.P. Myers, Elizabeth Afshari, and our colleagues at the Institute for Health Policy Studies for their assistance in the critical review and preparation of this paper.

Address correspondence to: Dr. Steven A. Schroeder, University of California, San Francisco, 1326 Third Avenue, San Francisco, CA 94143.

Physician Involvement

in Hospital Decision Making

MICHAEL A. REDISCH*

The focus of government health care policy over the past two decades has subtly changed from earlier commitments to provide health care to all who are in need. While assurance of access to care is, of course, still of great concern, the foremost policy issues of today revolve around ways to constrain future increases in health care costs. The major policy battleground is the hospital sector, where the most serious health care cost increases have occurred.

Governmental concern goes beyond the simple figures that show health expenditures rising from 5.2 percent of Gross National Product in 1960 to 8.6 percent of Gross National Product in fiscal 1976 (see Gibson and Mueller, 1977). A similar rise in relative expenditures in the consumer durable sector would traditionally be interpreted as the result of informed choices made in the economic marketplace by consumers of those products. However, medical care in general and hospital care in particular operate in markets so heavily underwritten by public programs and by private insurance that conventional market signals are weak or nonexistent. In 1975, 92 percent of hospital care was paid for by some form of third-party payer, a fact that tends to obscure the cost impact of hospital care on

*Any views expressed in this paper are those of the author and do not necessarily reflect the official position of the U.S. General Accounting Office.

The authors wishes to thank Jon Gabel for a number of comments that were helpful in the preparation of the paper.

In *Hospital Cost Containment: Selected Notes for Future Policy*, edited by Michael Zubkoff, Ira E. Raskin, and Ruth S. Hanft. New York: PRODIST, 1978.

the household budget. Furthermore, the individual seeking care is usually not fully informed of the potential outcomes of that care; instead, he must put his faith and trust in a physician who is allowed to commit the individual to utilize a bundle of scarce health resources. Among them is the physician's own time, and thus a potential conflict of interest is created.

The individual, therefore, typically does not purchase health care through the same mechanism or with the same attitudes as he does other goods and services. The result is governmental concern and intervention as the share of the nation's resources devoted to health care continues to rise.

A number of as yet untested proposals are being offered to combat inflation in the hospital without unduly limiting access to or quality of care. These suggestions include certificate-of-need laws, hospital rate review, various forms of prospective reimbursement, return to the direct wage and price controls of the Economic Stabilization era, or market strategies revolving around the growth of Health Maintenance Organizations.

However, too often in attempts to conceptualize the process by which the hospital sector will react to one or more of these control mechanisms, a central and overriding feature of the U.S. hospital system is omitted. The unique relationship between the hospital and the physician in the production of health care in this country is ignored by many of those attempting to understand or predict the reaction of hospitals to specific government policy. Instead, the hospital is typically viewed as an institution differing from ordinary firms only to the extent that a major portion of hospital care is provided in a not-for-profit setting.

An explanation for the lack of a strong physician figure in most models of hospital behavior can probably be traced to the payment mechanism for health care in the United States. The patient hospitalized here is typically subject to two separate billings; one for "hospital" services and one for "personal physician" services. This dual billing system has led to a conceptually false dichotomy whereby the hospital and physician are often erroneously viewed as independent entities selling services in functionally segmented health markets. Yet from the patient's point of view, "health care" in a hospital setting should be viewed as a single product jointly produced by the combined actions of hospitals and physicians. That patients in fact do take this view is suggested by Yett et al. (1971), who estimate that the demand for hospital care in a state aggregated cross-section is more responsive to changes in a physician surgical fee index than changes in the (more heavily insured) price of a bed day. Davis and Russell (1972) also estimate a demand equation for inpatient care that contains a significantly negative coefficient for the physician fee variable.

This paper will examine the hospital-physician relationship more from a' perspective of supply-side response to a set of social and economic incentives than from the perspective of consumer demand for hospital-based health care. It is in the area of modeling supply-side behavior that distortions and erroneous implications can be caused by an improper specification of the role of the physician in determining resource use in the hospital. As Jacobs (1974) has noted, many of the attempts to model hospital behavior either view the hospital as controlled completely by administrators' preferences or lump all decision-making groups into a heterogeneous whole, creating a fictional entity not related to reality. These "organism" models, viewing the "hospital" as the acting body, tend to obscure the way operational decisions are jointly arrived at through the individual actions of patients, trustees, physicians, administrators, and other hospital personnel.

Here we will attempt to delineate more specifically the roles that the physician may play in strategies aimed at controlling cost increases in hospitals. Any effective mechanism for containing the ongoing rapid rises in hospital costs must explicitly take into account the involvement of physicians in hospital decision making. Few administrators like to admit how limited is their control over the operation of their hospitals. They would like to believe that by their efforts alone, order and direction are distilled from anarchy. Yet it is the physician, operating as a separate entity outside the control of the Board of Trustees or the administrator, who directs most of the major resource decisions made in the hospital setting. The physician recommends admission, takes responsibility for ordering diagnostic procedures and therapeutic measures, and determines when the patient is fit to leave the hospital. In addition, it is the physician who typically engages in a lobbying effort with hopes of committing the administrator and trustees to invest in additional bed space, in personnel to help him provide more and better patient care, and in new and expensive technology.

A model of complete physician control, while admittedly an abstraction of reality, is still close enough to be considered a useful tool for analyzing various policy formulations (see Pauly and Redisch, 1973, for a rigorous statement of such a model). The two lines of internal authority in the hospital can lead to inevitable conflict between administrators and physicians. Yet the administrator has little stake in opposing physicians, particularly under a regime of unconstrained cost reimbursement. In fact, the administrator typically finds his own job security most closely tied to his ability to satisfy the demands of the medical staff. Viewed in this light, the administrator's role is simply to provide labor, supplies, and facilities to independent physicians. It is the physician who directs the actual provision of care in the hospital.

Trustees are also organizationally structured to exert external control on physician behavior. In a not-for-profit hospital there are no stockholders or owners of equity capital. The Board of Trustees presumably represents the public interest and bears some form of legal and moral responsibility for all activities, professional and otherwise, that occur within the institution. However, while each member of a typical board is a competent individual in his own field, he is unprepared for participation in the types of issues and decisions involved in the management of the hospital. Ordinarily he has limited knowledge of the medical profession, and his knowledge of the hospital is usually restricted to personal contact as a patient or as a relative of a patient.

A group of laymen without training in medicine thus may find it difficult to fulfill adequately responsibilities related in any way to quality of care, the practice of medicine, or the evaluation of medical staff. Almost all resource-related decisions in the hospital can be classified under one or more of these "medical" rubrics. It is therefore not surprising to see a tendency in most hospitals for the board to abjure direct responsibility and to delegate authority to some internal physician group. This tendency is, of course, actively supported by the American Medical Association, which suggests that "the responsibility of the hospital governing board is to provide the foundation for self-governance by the organized medical staff" (American Medical Association, 1974b:12). Once again de facto physician control over resource-related decisions is not hard to establish.

We will discuss in some detail the physician's role in the hospital cost inflation process and examine the impact of hypothesized physician behavior on the expected relative success of alternative policies for containing hospital costs. First, however, a description of the way inflation has taken place in the hospital will prove helpful.

The hospital cost inflation process will be examined with the patient day (or adjusted patient day, accounting for outpatient department care, American Hospital Association, 1969:466) as the reference unit of output. We feel that a specific illness incident treated as a case is a more meaningful measure of hospital "output" in the social welfare sense than the number of days of varying services devoted to patient care. However, use of the patient day is a more tractable measure and will allow us to explain relationships involving resource use (for example, factor input utilization decisions, a hospital investment function, the operational inflationary mechanism in the hospital environment) as well as or better than the case. This is particularly true since there is yet no precise, generally agreed upon way to measure the economic or medical aspects of "case mix."

The 10 to 20 percent annual increases in per diem hospital costs since 1965 are critically related to changes in the quantities, qualities, and sophistication of the services that are lumped together under the output designation of a patient day. Previous efforts to document the rise in cost per patient day have broken down these cost increases into four basic components: (1) rising wage levels of employees; (2) increased personnel per patient day; (3) rising cost of nonlabor inputs; and (4) increased use of nonlabor inputs per patient day. M. Feldstein (1971a), Davis and Foster (1972), and Waldman (1972) have all independently estimated that rising unit input costs and increased real input use have contributed approximately equal amounts to the rise in per diem costs in the late 1960s and early 1970s.

The American Hospital Association has claimed a recent change in the proportionate share of hospital cost increases related to rising unit input costs (Council on Wage and Price Stability, 1976:13). It estimates that pure factor price increases accounted for over 70 percent of hospital cost increases from January 1974 until June 1975. This reversal, if true, was due to expanded minimum wage laws and collective bargaining, increased malpractice insurance premiums, and higher energy costs. While hospital input prices may temporarily move faster than the general rate of inflation, it is still expected that increases in real inputs have led and will continue to lead, unless checked, to the growing share of hospital care in our national product accounts.

The origin of the rise in the volume of labor and nonlabor inputs utilized per patient day can be traced in part to the ability of the physician over time to reduce his own input or operating costs by transference of functions and costs to the hospital. Examples of this trend include the obstetrician who relies more and more on nursing staff and who rushes in at the last minute for the actual delivery, or the attending physician who utilizes house staff to care for his patients on Wednesdays and Saturdays. Johnson (1969) notes that nurses now perform many tasks that until two decades ago were limited to physicians, for example, the starting of blood transfusions, introduction of intravenous fluids, and injections. Such transference will continue into the future as attending physicians are relieved of suturing and many other responsibilities in surgery, coronary care, emergency room duties, and dialysis.

If this transference were done in an economically and socially efficient manner, then society could capture the potential gain generated by substitution of low-cost hospital inputs for high-cost physician time. While hospital costs would register increases, these would be more than compensated for by decreases in aggregate physician bills to patients. However, this does not appear to have happened. Instead, aided by the separation of bills for the costs of joint hospital-and-physician services, the physician has shown a great willingness to bill as much in his "supervisory" capacity over hospital inputs as when he performs services directly. Physicians are thus able to increase output (and incomes) without dramatic increases in fees. As an extreme example, the Medicare program often finds itself asked to pay under Part A (the hospital side of Title XVIII) its proportionate share of the salary of the resident who performs surgery while simultaneously being asked to cover under Part B (the physician side) the bill submitted by the supervising physician.

The physician's growing financial stake in the direction of resources other than his own labor may be seen by examining data from 1955 to 1971. Over this period physician incomes rose by around 7.2 percent per year while physician fees (as measured by the Consumer Price Index) rose by only 4.4 percent per year. Physician practice hours per week and practice weeks per year fell slightly (see Leveson and Rogers, 1976). The maintenance of this high rate of income growth under these conditions was accomplished by increasing physician productivity through dramatic increases in the nonphysician resource intensity of medical care.

Even if the physician did not continue to bill in part for services transferred to the hospital, the trend toward a greater and greater role for hospital inputs has still led to major inefficiencies in the production of health care. The physician and his patient are usually not even cognizant of the costs of basic hospital services. The hospital will typically tend to prorate the costs of all inputs (except those used to produce ancillary services) over all users of those inputs, through the use of room rates or daily service charges, which cover more than 50 percent of daily patient expense in most hospitals. Thus the utilization of increasing amounts of basic services by an individual patient will have a negligible impact on that patient's bill, since these costs are spread over all patients in the hospital. As the medical staff increases in size, each physician will tend to become less and less aware of the effects of his actions on others, since there are large numbers of patients of other physicians who share in the costs of these basic services. Unfortunately, the cumulative effect of this myopic behavior results in the rapid escalation of basic hospital services and of the hospital's room and board charge. The basic service increase is reflected in the time trend of the semiprivate room charge component of the Consumer Price Index, which almost tripled from 1965 to 1975.

The situation is exacerbated by the extent of insurance for

hospital services. Even when the hospital directly bills the patient for use of specific services, the physician is aware that the major burden of that bill will be borne not by the patient but by some third-party payer. To the extent that hospital care is more heavily insured than ambulatory physician care, the physician is likely to suggest a hospital stay for a patient who could be treated as well (and more efficiently) on an ambulatory basis. The practice of admitting patients into the hospital for an overnight stay to run a series of what are essentially diagnostic tests is the classic example of such behavior. But this specific practice has begun to die out as insurors have taken steps both to cover these tests when performed on an ambulatory patient and to reject payments for inpatient admissions whose sole justification is diagnostic testing.

Thus there appear to be three forces at work that mutually tend to reinforce the physician's incentive to utilize hospital services in an economically inefficient manner. The separation of physician and hospital bills for jointly produced health care, the proration of basic hospital service costs over all patients, and the pervasiveness of insurance for hospital services all make the apparent cost to the physician of additional hospital service very small relative to the true social costs of the inputs used to produce that service. Major incentives are created for the physician to oversubstitute hospital inputs for his own labor and to order the production of only marginally beneficial health and hotel services in the hospital.

At the same time, the physician seems reluctant to utilize health care inputs when he himself must bear the full costs and directorial burden of those inputs. For example, Reinhardt (1972) estimates that physicians could profitably employ in their offices more than twice as many physicians' assistants as they now do. Rather than take the risk and the added responsibility of a larger staff to supervise, physicians have chosen to pass up this potentially profitable option. Yet they seem to show no such compunction when it comes to ordering for their patients increasing amounts of hospital inputs, for which they bear no direct financial or managerial burden.

While the number of inputs used to produce basic hospital room and board services have increased over time, the really dramatic increases in hospital resource intensity seem to be largely related to increases in the availability and utilization levels of a set of diagnos-

TABLE 1   **Growth in Selected Hospital Series**[a]

	1968	*1969*	*1970*	*1971*	*Percent Change 1968-1971*
Operating cost	$55.51	$60.89	$69.60	$78.75	41.8
Operating room visits	.05456	.05071	.05223	.05373	-1.5
Pathology tests	.06327	.11652	.11504	.10914	72.5
Nuclear medicine procs.	.00252	.00705	.00690	.00965	282.9
Pharmacy line items	.35610	.79150	.91918	1.0449	193.4
In- & outpatient lab tests	2.2046	2.2964	2.5393	2.8588	29.7
In- & outpatient radiology procs.	.31753	.31604	.33519	.36378	14.6
Therapeutic radiology procs.	.00685	.01394	.01577	.01894	176.5
Blood bank units	.03759	.05881	.05333	.06333	68.5

[a]All figures are reported in whole units normalized on adjusted patient days. Thus in 1968 operating cost per adjusted patient day in the sample was $55.51 and the average number of pathology tests per adjusted patient day was .06327.

Sources: The data were provided by the Health Services Research Center (the Center) of Northwestern University and the American Hospital Association (AHA). They were obtained by the Center from the Hospital Administrative Services (HAS) Division of the AHA. Data are submitted to HAS on a monthly basis by several thousand voluntarily participating hospitals. These hospitals may then compare their performance in providing services with that of similarly situated institutions.

No payment for services is based on the completed HAS forms, and the data are not audited. HAS puts the raw monthly data onto a computer tape and runs some simple statistical checks that are meant to eliminate "order of magnitude" errors. The Center obtained a tape of this monthly data file for close to four hundred hospitals. The tape was than "annualized" on a calendar year basis for the years 1967 to 1971. Hospitals reporting less than nine months of data were eliminated from the sample, and it was assumed that hospitals reporting between nine and eleven months of data would have reported "average" figures (based on months they did report) for the missing months. In addition, statistical checks were performed to eliminate obviously erroneous outliers. There still appear to be some order-of-magnitude errors in the data, and certain hospitals and unreliable variables will have to be removed in later empirical work.

All identifying hospital characteristics (geographic area, teaching status, affiliations, services offered other than those reported on the HAS forms, etc.) were removed by either HAS or the Center. The data were then made available to the author.

It was quickly decided that the data for 1967 were too fragmented and erratic to be of much use. (HAS was just starting up and many hospitals were unfamiliar with the forms.) Also, those hospitals that did not appear in all years (1968 to 1971) were eliminated from the sample. The original sample consisted of 348 hospitals in 1968, 370 in 1969, 379 in 1970, and 375 in 1971. After removing those hospitals that did not appear in one or more years, we were left with a sample of 285 hospitals. These were fairly evenly spaced out over all hospital bed-size groups. The average bed size in the final sample varied slightly from year to year about an aggregate mean of 249 beds.

tic and therapeutic medical services provided in a hospital setting under the direction and control of physicians. The increases can be seen quite clearly in Table 1. Over a period of time (1968 through 1971) in which the number of operating room visits per adjusted patient day actually declined slightly in these sample hospitals, we can see explosive growth in the utilization levels per adjusted patient day of seven medical services (pathology tests, nuclear medicine

procedures, pharmacy line items, inpatient and outpatient laboratory tests, inpatient and outpatient radiology procedures, therapeu-
radiology procedures, and blood bank units). There is no break in
the general pattern when hospitals are grouped into separate bed-
size classes. In a separate paper by the author (Redisch, 1974),
hedonic cost indices are estimated that suggest that the growth of
these seven medical services accounts for more than one-third of the
increase in cost per adjusted patient day in the sample hospitals.
Since approximately one-half of the per diem cost rise is related to
rises in unit costs of basic inputs, these estimates imply that two-
thirds of the increase in real inputs per adjusted patient day in the
sample hospitals were related to increases in the per diem use of
these seven medical services.

Much of this increase can be traced to the growth of highly
specialized treatment centers within hospitals. Coronary care units,
intensive care units for adults and for newborns, burn units, and so
on, contribute to a highly structured form of patient care. (The ratio
of private, not-for-profit hospitals reporting intensive care units
jumped from 11 percent in 1960 to more than 70 percent today.)
There may be a tendency to establish routines in patient monitoring
in these units. Patterns of diagnostic ancillary service use can
develop that may bear little relation to the needs of the individual
patient (see Griner and Liptzen, 1971).

Growth in ancillary service use has also been encouraged by new
hospital technology, such as multiple channel autoanalyzers, that
lowers unit costs of individual tests when operating at a high
volume. However, these scale economies may soon be dissipated
through a "Xerox effect" (in many business offices, the surge in
volume after the introduction of duplicating machines may more
than make up for the drop in unit costs). Physicians who once
ordered a small number of lab tests to confirm their original clinical
diagnosis now order a full range of ten or twenty tests to "see what
comes up." This somewhat spurious demand for laboratory tests can
then be used to justify the purchase of still more automated lab
equipment.

Moreover, rapid growth in ancillary service use is stimulated by
a major new force in the practice of medicine. The rising number of

dissatisfied patients who choose to sue their physicians and hospitals for malpractice, the decreasing reluctance of physicians to testify against one another in the contest of such suits, and the growing propensity of the courts to award large sums of money to patients who are successful in pursuing these suits have all contributed to an increasing tendency for physicians and hospitals to practice "defensive medicine."

This ancillary service growth, contributing such a large share to the rise in per diem hospital costs, is under the direct control of the physician. Furthermore, it is not at all clear that this intensive use of a fairly common set of hospital services has positively contributed to the overall level of the "quality" of hospital care. Berki, for example (1972:31), notes that it is not known whether the more intensive use of laboratory procedures corresponds in fact to increases in the quality of care or to medically unjustified overuse of convenient, income-generating services. Ofttimes what may emerge from haphazard diagnostic testing is one or two false positives that lead to further testing or to inappropriate treatment. For example, Schimmel (1964) notes that 20 percent of the patients in Yale's Intensive Care Unit suffered complications from diagnostic tests, drugs, and various therapeutic measures.

Until now we have talked about hospital cost inflation primarily in terms of increases in costs per adjusted patient day. Yet government policy should be directed not just at these "unit" or daily costs, but at the aggregate level of hospital expenditures, as reflected in per capita hospital costs. Per capita costs are determined by the product of per diem costs and the number of patient days per capita. And the latter is determined by the per capita hospital admission rate and by the average length of stay for hospital care. Thus far we have examined the influence of the physician on per diem costs. We must now consider his degree of control over the admission decision and the discharge (or length of stay) decision.

Work by Wennberg et al. (1975), concerning several Maine communities at a single point in time, suggests that the admission decision is the most important explanation of variations in per capita hospital costs and expenditures. They find that average length of stay or cost per admission is less important than per capita admissions in explaining those variations. Physicians' uncertainty about the need for service or the value of alternative therapies is the likely cause of large observed differences in age- and sex-adjusted per capita hospital admission rates across what would be considered fairly homogeneous communities. Wennberg and his associates conclude that "the resource implications of differences in management within hospitals are less important than decisions to manage patients at the ambulatory or the institutional level of care" (Wennberg et al., 1975:305).

While growth in per diem costs plays a larger role than growth in per capita admissions in explaining increases in per capita hospital costs over time, it *is* true that the admission decision is a central one in initiating the hospital cost inflation process. The decision seems dominated by a group of socioeconomic incentives aimed at both the patient and the physician, and by the varying perceptions of individual physicians as to what constitutes medical need.

Perceptions of medical need do vary among physicians. In England, medical care is not rationed by the price mechanism and physicians face identical economic incentives across all of their patients. In a study of over three thousand normal deliveries in the Oxford Record Linkage Study area in 1962, M. Feldstein (1968) found that the most important single factor influencing any woman's expected hospital stay during delivery was the standard practice of the obstetrician in charge of the case. This was found to be more important in determining length of stay than the age of the woman, the number of previous children, her social class, or other characteristics.

Physicians have a great deal of discretion in deciding whether the "medical needs" of the patient include admission to a hospital. Their determination of this need may be influenced by a number of social and economic forces not directly related to the medical condition of the patient. For example, Rafferty (1971) has observed that in two Indiana hospitals increases in the general incidence of illness in the community, resulting in increases in the rate of bed occupancy, made physicians reluctant to hospitalize patients for less severe illnesses or for minor elective procedures. Similarly, Davis and Russell (1972) found that rises in occupancy rates lead to treatment of marginal patients in the outpatient department. When beds are relatively scarce, they are saved by physicians for the seriously ill.

The resource decisions that physicians implicitly make in response to perceived social needs do not have to be minor ones. Titmuss (1950) notes that in 1939 almost half the patients in English hospitals (some 140,000 individuals) were discharged in anticipation of war casualties, at a time when there were 200,000 people on hospital waiting lists. Major changes in the way health care is delivered can be accomplished if they are considered part of desirable public policy with a degree of universal public acceptance.

While it is clear that "medical need" is the major determinant of health care utilization, we have shown that various social forces and differences in the medical perceptions of individual physicians also influence the decision to utilize hospital services. In addition, economic incentives to the patient and to the physician produce nontrivial changes in the level and mix of care. Bishop (1973:29) notes that the simplification of an extended care facility (ECF) transfer form and, more important, an agreement by a third-party payer to cover physician services in the ECF led to net savings by the insuror and the ending of a hospital expansion plan.

New York City provides another example of how physicians' personal economic incentives can affect their behavior in a way that is particularly relevant for future health care policy decisions. In the late 1950s, Group Health Insurance (GHI) and the Health Insurance Plan of Greater New York (HIP) both provided a wide range of health services at a marginal out-of-pocket cost of approximately zero to similar sets of subscribers in New York City. GHI paid participating physicians a fee for each service performed, while HIP contracted with groups of physicians who agreed to provide care to HIP enrollees in return for payment on an annual capitation basis. The rates for nonsurgical, nonobstetrical physician visits were similar for each plan, but GHI enrollees had an average of 7.18 hospitalized surgical procedures per hundred persons per year, while the rate for HIP enrollees was only 4.18 (Monsma, 1970:151). It may be that "too many" appendectomies, hysterectomies, and tonsillectomies were performed by GHI surgeons, or it may be that "too few" were performed by HIP surgeons. The only statement that emerges with any clarity is that the financial incentive to the physician somehow seems to have heavy impact on definitions of "medical need" when elective surgery is considered.

The impact of personal economic incentives to the physician can be further viewed in the study by Gaus et al. (1976), which compared various aspects of HMO performance with those of the nonprepaid, fee-for-service system for the Medicaid population. It was found that Medicaid beneficiaries enrolled in two medical foundations exhibited no statistically significant differences in hospital use when compared with a matched sample of Medicaid beneficiaries utilizing the fee-for-service system. The foundations accepted capitation payment for their Medicaid enrollees but reimbursed affiliated physicians on a fee-for-service basis. In contrast, Medicaid beneficiaries enrolled in a group of HMOs with non-fee-for-service physicians were observed to have 356 days of hospital care per 1,000 persons per year. This was a remarkable 62 percent lower than the 934 days per 1,000 persons per year measured for the fee-for-service Medicaid control group.

The authors conclude that the fact that foundations show no major differences in hospital use, despite the financial incentives at the organization level to do so, indicates that the financial incentive of capitation payment to the HMO organization may by itself not have significant impact on the hospitalization practices of affiliated physicians. The major cost impact of HMOs appears to lie not simply in having an organization (the HMO) take the risk for total care of the beneficiary. Instead, it lies in having the physician limit his incentives to hospitalize patients by removing him from the fee-for-service setting, by separating to some extent resource control from the medical staff, and by reconstituting medical practice within the context of a salaried, multispecialty group.

These conclusions are partially confirmed at a wider level by Bunker (1970), who observes a much lower rate of surgical procedures per 1,000 persons in England than in the United States. Similarly, Adelstein (1973) shows that the per capita number of x-ray exams is much higher in this country than in other countries.

Surgery and radiology in England are performed by salaried specialists working full time as hospital staff members, while surgery and radiology in the United States are typically performed by independent physicians faced with the perverse incentives of a fee-for-service reimbursement system.

This documentation of the pervasive influence of physicians in determining resource allocations within the hospital implies that control measures to hold down the rate of inflation of hospital costs, if aimed solely at the hospital, will be disappointing. Certificates of need, rate review, or alternative forms of prospective reimbursement all *do* provide the administrator with an added rationale for confronting and standing up to the physician staff. Yet the benefits to the administrator of siding with the staff are usually so high that true confrontations are exceedingly unusual.

Most hospital administrators see themselves in competition with other hospitals for physicians, not for patients, since it is only through a physician that an individual may be admitted to a hospital. As long as there are other hospitals that will admit him to practice, a physician is not totally dependent on a particular hospital for his livelihood. But a hospital that cannot retain a satisfied medical staff will soon find its occupancy rate falling, its per diem costs rising, and its ability to function as a health care institution seriously impaired. Furthermore, if cost guidelines are given to a hospital on a per diem basis, many administrators may find themselves in the seemingly paradoxical situation of allowing certain marginal equipment and personnel decisions or capital projects to attract or keep physician staff so that the occupancy rate will be high enough to move the hospital within the per diem cost constraints.

It is not surprising that administrators will put off as long as possible the inclusion of medical staff into any negative budgetary decisions that must be made. Most physicians practicing in a group of Western Pennsylvania hospitals that were being reimbursed on a prospective basis by the local Blue Cross organization were not even aware of this fact (see Applied Management Sciences, 1975). Cost containment was considered an administrative issue, not a medical one.

If hospital budgetary controls are made so tight that they cannot be met by simply eliminating any administrative slack in the hospital, then affiliated physicians will have to become more directly involved in the hospital's budgetary process. However, even when the administrator is forced to confront his medical staff on cost issues, he is at a disadvantage. Physicians can argue persuasively and with a unique degree of authority about medical need and quality of care. It is difficult for the lay administrator to pick and choose among these arguments and make resource decisions that hurt one physician group but not another. Even when these negative decisions are chosen, they are most likely to be based on the degree of power of the various physician specialty groups within the hospital, rather than on criteria based on some nebulous concept of social efficiency norms. There has been a paucity of sophisticated evaluation relating medical care inputs to health outcomes, even for expensive pieces of equipment. Without such evaluation, hospital administrators have little with which to judge competently or counter physician arguments concerning quality of care.

A more effective control mechanism might make an impact on the physician directly, rather than through the administrator. Yet the costs of policing physicians through direct regulation on a case-by-case basis can be excessive. Medical cases are highly differentiated goods. No two patients are ever exactly the same, even if they exhibit the same general set of symptoms. If the decision to hospitalize were based solely on medical reasoning, the physician would be hospitalizing a disease rather than a person with a disease.

The current method of applying case-by-case regulation is through a form of professional peer review structured around local Professional Standards Review Organizations. Yet peer review in this form may prove more effective as a quality control measure than as a cost control device. Historically, peer review in the health care sector seems to have been oriented toward preventing abuse of patients and not toward preventing abuse of resources. Skeptics have claimed that this orientation will continue, and that hospital costs will rise as PSRO-mandated "resource ceilings" quickly become "quality floors."

A more effective form of case-by-case peer review may be simply to have third-party payers provide full funding on a prospective basis for a second opinion by an "impartial" board-certified surgeon whenever a physician feels that nonemergency surgery is indicated. One study in this area, with a one- to four-year follow-up of cases, showed that "in the voluntary programs, one out of four screened patients, and in the mandatory programs, one out of seven and a half screened patients, appear to be permanently 'deferred' from surgery" (McCarthy and Kamons, 1976:7).

However, peer review in any form should not be expected to play a dominant role in strategies aimed at containing health care costs. The history of peer review in fields other than health has been marginal at best, because of an unwillingness or lack of power to impose meaningful controls. The inability of peer review to function effectively as a cost control device in fee-for-service health care settings gains credence from empirical studies of fee-for-service group practices in California. Physicians in these practices share costs but either bill patients directly or share in the net receipts according to a weighting scheme based on volume of the individual physician's patients. Costs have been observed to be as high as or higher than those in similarly situated solo practices (Newhouse, 1973).

The potential economies of sharing paramedical personnel and office equipment have been dissipated by physician behavior. With a large number (N) of physicians in practice together, each physician knows that by prescribing extensive use of the groups' resources he bears the burden of only $1/N$th of the costs but gains a proportionately greater share of the revenues. Even though physicians have a direct economic stake in the actions of their colleagues, peer group pressures in this ambulatory setting have not been effective cost control devices as physician staff size becomes unwieldy.

And the future may be less bright. Noll (1972) has shown that the regulatory process in areas other than health care has quickly degenerated into a system of peer control. This occurs when the only groups competent to evaluate the regulated firms are themselves current or former members of the industry.

Direct government intervention through the regulatory or rate-review process also does not appear to be the panacea that will bring hospital cost inflation in line with price rises in the rest of the economy. Work by Salkever and Bice (1976) and by Hellinger (1976) in evaluating the early impact of certificate-of-need legislation, and the study by Gaus and Hellinger (1976) of prospective reimbursement systems show that even in those few cases where these regulatory devices evoke a statistically discernible effect in the desired direction, the magnitude of this effect, while large in dollar terms, is quite small relative to cost increases in the hospital sector.

The "co-option" of the regulatory process in health care seems to have already begun in some areas. For example, the Center for the Analysis of Public Issues (1974) makes charges relating to health care regulation in New Jersey. On a more inferential level, Cromwell et al. (1975:121) note that only one out of forty-one certificate-of-need applications was denied to hospitals in the Greater Boston area in 1973.

There is thus a real danger that health care regulation will be proposed and supported by members of the industry as a mechanism for supplanting whatever competitive elements remain with a legal, enforceable cartel. This view would allow for state hospital associations to petition their legislatures to put them under the protective umbrella of a state-mandated prospective reimbursement system that is meant to *guarantee* an "adequate" cash flow to each hospital. This view would also encompass the use of comprehensive health planning by local hospital groups as a vehicle for keeping Health Maintenance Organizations from encroaching on their territory.

Even if direct hospital regulation turns out to be a moderate success, its role will have to be strengthened by some basic structural changes in the way physicians are educated and reimbursed. Today the typical physician, acting in the interests of himself and his immediate patients, puts little weight on the larger issues of economic efficiency and social benefit. This attitude has been reinforced by the strong technological imperative instilled in physicians during their medical training programs (and is tacitly encouraged by the present cost-based system for financing hospital care).

The professional training of physicians has traditionally not emphasized the concept of the physician as a manager of health care resources confronted with complex issues of cost and efficiency. Instead, the physician emerges from his training period with a perception of the hospital as a rent-free workshop, a place where he feels justified in pressing administrators and trustees to add those medical care inputs that allow for full, modern treatment of patients while simultaneously enhancing the physician's income and prestige.

Individual physician and patient issues, not social issues, dominate the training process and are carried over into the medical practice. For example, physicians who specialize in treating patients with a given disease will not agree to the exclusion of facilities at hospital A, where they hold staff appointments, unless they are granted staff privileges at hospital B, where the planning agency would like to concentrate all facilities for diagnosis and treatment. The physician not only has a financial interest involved; there is also the matter of the preservation and employment of professional skills.

At times this type of behavior is costly not only to society but to the individual patient as well. The only one to gain is the physician. Rosenthal (1966:109) quotes, as a not so extreme example, the President's Commission on Heart, Cancer, and Stroke to show that in the early 1960s 30 percent of the 777 hospitals equipped to do closed-heart surgery had no such cases in the year under study, and 87 percent of the 548 hospitals that did have cases performed fewer than one operation per week. Furthermore, 77 percent of the hospitals equipped to do open-heart surgery averaged less than one operation per week, and 41 percent averaged less than one a month. Little of this sporadic surgery was of an emergency nature, and the mortality rate of both procedures when done infrequently was far higher than in institutions with a full work load.

This phenomenon is, of course, closely linked to the explosive growth in the opportunities for application of new and high-cost technology in health care. Recent innovations in medical care have been characterized by an emphasis upon complex diagnostic and therapeutic techniques usually requiring hospitalization and the physician-controlled application of complicated, expensive equipment. Examples include cancer radiation therapy and chemotherapy, renal dialysis, organ transplants, open-heart surgery, brain and body scanners, and intensive care units for burn, trauma, and heart patients. The overall cumulative effect of health care technology in this country, in combination with hospital-oriented, cost-based health insurance, has been to shift the focus of the health system from office-based, primary care medical practice toward hospital-based, specialist care medical practice.

Furthermore, this shift in focus is made more acute by the interaction of technological applications in health care and the current orientation of medical training programs. The new high-cost hospital technology necessitates specialization and fosters a narrow professionalism among new physicians. That is, for reasons relating to income, prestige, and the way that modern medicine is practiced, new physicians are drawn toward the practice of specialized medicine within an urban, institutionalized setting. This trend in turn creates ever greater demands from physicians to induce hospitals to adopt still more technology. Thus the cycle is completed and starts anew. And thus delivery of health care has shifted from general practitioners toward high-priced specialists operating in expensive settings. From 1963 to 1973 the overall number of physicians in the United States increased by 32.5 percent. There was a 53.5 percent increase in medical specialists, a 29.8 percent increase in surgical specialists, a 50.3 percent increase in all other specialists, and a 26.5 percent *decline* in the number of general practitioners (American Medical Association, 1967 and 1974b).

The massive movement toward specialization has helped fuel the hospital cost inflation process through the specialist-technology relationship described earlier. M. Feldstein (1971b:871), using a pooled cross-sectional time series for individual states for the period 1958–1967, estimates that the addition of one or more specialists in a state in that time interval would cause hospital costs to increase by $39,000 per year. Conversely, general practitioners were shown to be a substitute for hospital care. Feldstein estimates that the introduction of an additional GP into a state would cause hospital costs to decrease by $39,000 per year. Thus the true costs of producing ever-increasing numbers of specialists must include these induced hospital costs as well as any added educational costs (in part underwritten by public funds) and higher physician fees associated with specialization. These additional costs should be taken into account in any decisions impacting on the extent of public funding for the production (that is, education) of hospital-oriented physicians.

The greatest potential in utilizing the physician to contain hospital costs, however, may lie in the movement, whenever possible, away from fee-for-service as the method of reimbursing physicians and away from a system in which individual physicians control hospital inputs without bearing any responsibility for them. Such a movement, if feasible at all, would probably have to take place in piecemeal, incremental fashion. Capitation or salaried service may marginally increase in popularity, but it seems clear that, even with a major restructuring of the health care system through national health financing legislation, these two methods of reimbursing physicians will for some time appear only as options to physicians who desire alternatives to fee-for-service. Any new system, to be politically feasible, must meet with at least grudging acceptance by physicians. While most physicians see the hospital as an adjunct to their practice and an extension of their office, a vocal minority visualizes the hospital as a threat to the private practice of medicine. The AMA and individual physicians have fought long and hard to maintain de facto control of resource decisions in hospitals to keep this fear from becoming a reality. The AMA (1974b:20) suggests that "a physician should not bargain or enter into a contract whereby any hospital, corporation, or lay body may offer for sale or sell for a fee the physician's professional services." The only exceptions to this stated AMA principle are salaried "educational" staff appointments. The AMA's position has been that hospitals are "exploiting" salaried physicians by making shadow profits on their activities to support other departments (American Medical Association, 1959).

However, physician groups can no longer severely punish individual physicians who are induced to defect from traditional fee-for-service reimbursement. The courts have ruled that hospitals may not deny staff privileges to a physician simply because he is a member of a group practice or is not a member of the local county medical society.

The amount of money society can afford to spend to induce defections may prove to be quite large. From July 1975 to June 1976 hospital costs increased by $7.2 billion (Gibson and Mueller, 1977). This represents 27 percent of the total cost of physician services in that period, or around $23,000 per U.S. physician, and a much higher figure when divided only by fee-for-service physicians.

We have suggested that a large part of these annual hospital cost increases is related to the growing intensity of care caused partly by the method by which physicians are reimbursed and partly by the way they are free from responsibility for hospital inputs. Movement away from the perverse incentives of fee-for-service, in combination with the separation to some extent of resource control from the medical staff, could produce the dramatic drops in per capita hospital utilization similar to the ones associated with HMOs. It is these anticipated savings that society could decide to use to encourage defections from fee-for-service practice.

Adoption of a European-style health care system, with hospitals primarily the domain of salaried specialists, and with general practitioners operating independently in office-based settings, might be a step in this direction. Many physicians are already practicing in hospitals on a straight salary, such as interns and residents (who comprise more than 20 percent of active physicians in many states), full-time salaried chiefs of staff, and other physicians serving educational functions. Still other physicians could be induced to practice on a salaried basis if the salary were high enough. (While many physicians are ideologically opposed to anything but fee-for-service reimbursement, others are concerned not about ideology but about levels of income and hours of work today and in the future.)

However, adoption of a European-style system for the United States would present many problems. The level of physician salaries and of payment responsibilities would have to be determined. State laws against the corporate practice of medicine would have to be redesigned (they are currently being rewritten in many states to allow for the functioning of HMOs). A way would have to be found to gradually allow new staff privileges only to salaried specialists. And more important, while this system removes many of the perverse incentives individual physicians face with respect to the utilization of hospital resources, it does nothing by itself to provide incentives to the hospital to contain costs.

A more practical approach that should be viewed as a movement in this general direction would be to push for salaried status for three specific hospital-based physicians. Anesthesiologists, pathologists, and radiologists often control small fiefdoms within the hospital. They practice under reimbursement methods that are financially very favorable to them (fee-for-service or some percentage of their departments' gross or net revenues). It is suggested that these reimbursement methods contribute simultaneously to their high average income level and to rising levels of hospital costs resulting from the inordinate growth of their departments' services.

There are, of course, other alternatives to full-scale fee-for-service in addition to the European model. New concepts deserve encouragement, such as variants of the reimbursement plan being developed by the Blue Shield organization in Wisconsin. Individuals or groups of primary care physicians can elect capitation for a number of their patients. That is, they agree to provide a basic set of primary care services "on demand" in return for a fixed monthly fee. (The monthly fee and the set of primary care services can vary from physician to physician.) A pool is set up to pay for referrals to specialists and for hospitalization costs of patients. If the pool is not depleted by year end, the remainder is distributed back to the participating physicians.

Other new methods might be tried that attempt to make the physician responsible for the level of hospital costs. Monetary disbursements could be made to all physicians in an area where hospital costs are below projections, and also for residents or other full-time staff in a specific hospital. While this might create some incentives for the physician peer review process to focus in on some financial criteria, there would be many complications inherent in determining both a projected level of costs and a disbursement method. When variants of this reimbursement method have been tried (as in medical foundations), the evidence appears to show that fee-for-service incentives to the individual physician are stronger than peer group pressure (see Gaus et al., 1975).

The major physician-related impetus to cost containment in hospitals may come from the growth and encouragement of nonfoundation-type HMOs. It has already been suggested that these HMOs keep hospital costs in check not by the organization as an entity going at risk to provide medical care, but from the actions of staff physicians who are removed from fee-for-service reimbursement, who practice in multispecialty groups, and who do not operate with complete autonomy in regard to resource control. Encouragement of HMOs could take many forms. For example, a major insurance plan with deductibles for hospital and physician care and a 20 percent copayment provision for physician services (such as Medicare) could offer to drop all deductibles and co-insurance payments for beneficiaries who joined HMOs that agreed to provide care at a cost to the program of 80 percent of the average beneficiary cost in the area.

In the end it must be remembered that the search for a single panacea to contain hospital and other health care costs is likely to be a futile one. There are major forces at work in the health care arena. They are related to the interaction of physician incentives, patient passivity (induced in part by high levels of insurance), new technology, and cost-related hospital reimbursement. These forces are not unique to the American health care system. Costs of hospital care and other forms of health care can be observed to be rising rapidly in many societies operating under a wide range of regulatory activity and financing arrangements. The lesson to be learned is that there does not appear to be a single, simple solution to the health care cost crisis. Instead, the problem is one that will have to be solved (or at least partially alleviated) through a number of small, discrete steps. Utilizing the physician as a lever to help contain hospital costs is one of those steps.

References

Adelstein, S.
    1973   "The risk-benefit ratio in nuclear medicine." Hospital Practice 8 (January).

American Hospital Association
    1969   Hospitals, Journal of the American Hospital Association (August, Guide Issue).

American Medical Association
    1959   "AMA/Acts on hospital-physician relations." Hospitals, Journal of the American Hospital Association (December): 17–19.
    1967   Distribution of Physicians in the U.S., 1963. Chicago: AMA Managerial Services Division.

1974a   Distribution of Physicians in the U.S., 1973. Chicago: AMA Center for Health Services Research and Development.

1974b   Physician-Hospital Relations. Chicago, Ill.

Applied Management Sciences

1975   Analysis of Prospective Reimbursement Systems: Western Pennsylvania. Prepared for the Office of Research and Statistics, Social Security Administration, U.S. DHEW, under Contract No. HEW-OS-74-226.

Berki, S.E.

1972   Hospital Economics. Lexington, Mass.: Lexington Books, D.C. Heath & Co.

Bishop, C.

1973   Public Regulation of Hospitals: Summary of a Conference. Health Care Policy Discussion Paper No. 4, Harvard Center for Community Health and Medical Care (March).

Bunker, J.

1970   "Surgical manpower: A comparison of operations and surgeons in the United States and in England and Wales." The New England Journal of Medicine 282 (January): 135–143.

Center for the Analysis of Public Issues

1974   Bureaucratic Malpractice. Princeton, N.J.

Council on Wage and Price Stability

1976   The Problem of Rising Health Care Costs. Staff Report, Washington, D.C. (April).

Cromwell, J., P.B. Ginsburg, D. Hamilton, and M. Sumner

1975   Incentives and Decisions Underlying Hospitals' Adoption and Utilization of Major Capital Equipment. Prepared by Abt Associates, Inc., for National Center for Health Services Research and Development. Contract No. (HSM) 110-73-513 (September).

Davis, K., and R. Foster

1972   Community Hospitals: Inflation in the Pre-Medicare Period. Social Security Administration, Research Report No. 41. Washington, D.C.: Government Printing Office.

Davis, K., and L.B. Russell

1972   "The substitution of hospital outpatient care for inpatient care." Review of Economics and Statistics 54 (May): 109–120.

Feldstein, M.S.

1968   Economic Analysis for Health Service Efficiency. Amsterdam: North-Holland Publishing Company.

1971a   The Rising Cost of Hospital Care. Washington, D.C.: Information Resources Press.

1971b   "Hospital cost inflation: A study of nonprofit price dynamics." American Economic Review 61 (December): 853–872.

Gaus, C.R., B.S. Cooper, and C.G. Hirschman
1975   "Contrasts in HMO and fee-for-service performance." Social Security Bulletin 39 (May): 3–14.

Gaus, C.R., and F.J. Hellinger
1976   Results of Hospital Prospective Reimbursement in the United States. Paper presented to the International Conference on Policies for the Containment of Health Care Costs and Expenditures. Fogarty International Center (June).

Gibson, R.M., and M.S. Mueller
1977   "National health expenditures, fiscal year 1976." Social Security Bulletin 40 (April): 3–22.

Griner, P., and B. Liptzen
1971   "Use of the laboratory in a teaching hospital: Implications for patient care, education, and hospital costs." Annals of Internal Medicine 75 (August).

Hellinger, F.J.
1976   "The effect of certificate-of-need legislation on hospital investment." Inquiry 13 (June): 187–193.

Jacobs, P.
1974   "A survey of economic models of hospitals." Inquiry 11 (June): 83–97.

Johnson, E.
1969   "Physician productivity and the hospital: A hospital administrator's view." Inquiry 6 (September): 59–69.

Leveson, I., and E. Rogers
1976   "Hospital cost inflation and physician payment." American Journal of Economics and Sociology 35 (April): 161–174.

McCarthy, E., and A. Kamons
1976   Voluntary and Mandatory Presurgical Screening Programs: An Analysis of Their Implications. Presented at American Federation for Clinical Research, Atlantic City (May 2).

Monsma, G.
1970   "Marginal revenue and the demand for physicians' services." In H.E. Klarman, ed., Empirical Studies in Health Economics. Baltimore: John Hopkins Press.

Newhouse, J.P.
1973   "The economics of group practice." Journal of Human Resources (Winter): 37–56.

Noll, R.C.
1971   Reforming Regulation. Washington, D.C.: The Brookings Institution.
Pauly, M., and M.A. Redisch
1973   "The not-for-profit hospital as a physicians' cooperative." American Economic Review 63 (March): 87–99.
Rafferty, J.
1971   "Patterns of hospital use: An analysis of short-run variations." Journal of Political Economy 79 (January–February): 154–165.
Redisch, M.A.
1974   Hospital Inflationary Mechanisms. Presented at Western Economic Association Meetings, Las Vegas, Nev. (June).
Reinhardt, U.
1972   "A production function for physician services." Review of Economics and Statistics 54 (February): 55–66.
Rosenthal, G.
1966   "The public pays the bill." Atlantic 218 (July): 107–110.
Salkever, D.S., and T.W. Bice
1976   The Impact of Certificate-of-Need Controls on Hospital Investment, Costs, and Utilization. Final report to the National Center for Health Services Research, DHEW, Contract No. HRA-106-74-57 (August).
Schimmel, E.
1964   "The hazards of hospitalization." Annals of Internal Medicine 60 (January): 100–116.
Titmuss, R.
1950   Problems of Social Policy. London: HMS Office and Longmans, Green.
Waldman, S.
1972   The Effect of Changing Technology on Hospital Costs. Research and Statistics Note No. 4, DHEW Publication No. (SSA) 72-11701 (February 28).
Wennberg, J., A. Gitteljohn, and N. Shapiro
1975   "Health care delivery in Maine III: Evaluating the level of hospital performance." Journal of the Maine Medical Association 66 (November).
Yett, D., L. Drabek, M. Intriligator, and L. Kimball
1971   A Macroeconomic Model for Regional Health Planning. Presented at the 46th Annual Conference of the Western Economic Association (August).

II Hospitals and Technology

Medical Technology

and Hospital Costs

JUDITH L. WAGNER
AND MICHAEL ZUBKOFF

Introduction

Medical technology, particularly the kind found in hospitals, has undergone a curious shift in public acceptability over the past five years. Those who influence and shape national health policy have shown increasing alarm over the way in which new technologies are developed and introduced into the health care system. With few exceptions, the present concern is with the proliferation of new technologies in hospitals.[1] New equipment, procedures, or systems appear to be introduced by hospital decision makers often without knowledge of or concern for their relative effectiveness or efficiency. Technology purportedly follows its own imperative, eluding effective control by regulatory or financing agencies (Rabkin and Melin, 1976). Most important, new hospital technologies have allegedly raised health care costs, and herein lies the major source of

---

[1] The exceptions are important. Some observers have noted the low development or implementation of technologies for use in primary care that would allow the substitution of low-cost for high-cost manpower (see White, Murnaghan, and Gaus, 1972). Barriers to development and diffusion of technologies that would be very useful to the handicapped have been noted in a recent report by the National Research Council (1976).

In *Hospital Cost Containment: Selected Notes for Future Policy*, edited by Michael Zubkoff, Ira E. Raskin, and Ruth S. Hanft. New York: PRODIST, 1978.

alarm. Clifton Gaus of the Social Security Administration recently stated:

> The long-term cumulative effect of adopting new health care technologies is a major cause of the large yearly increases in national health expenditures and in total Medicare and Medicaid benefit levels [Gaus, 1975:12–13].

Technology has clearly acquired a bad name; increasingly, policies to assess, evaluate, or control the introduction of new technologies on the federal and state levels have been suggested as cost-containment strategies (see, for example, Russell, 1976; Rabkin and Melin, 1976; Gaus and Cooper, 1976; Weiner, 1976). Debates over the nation's ability to continue to pay for new technologies as it has in the past have flourished (DeBakey and Hiatt, 1976).

The obvious question arises as to why technology, and particularly hospital technology, has been singled out at this time as a particular problem of hospital behavior. The answer lies in the convergence of three lines of criticism of the health care system.

First, recent studies decomposing hospital cost inflation into its constituent parts have provided some circumstantial evidence linking technology to increased hospital costs. In 1972, Waldman estimated that increases in real inputs accounted for 50 percent of the annual changes in per diem hospital costs between 1951 and 1970. Similar findings by Worthington (1975) and, most recently, Feldstein and Taylor (1977) have demonstrated the changing nature of the hospital product. Feldstein and Taylor found that about 75 percent of the rise in hospital costs relative to the general economy can be attributed to increases in labor and nonlabor inputs per patient day. Although there is no one-to-one correspondence between the increasing level of intensity of care (as measured by increasing inputs) and the rate of technological change, a clear implication of these studies is that the introduction of new technologies is responsible for much of the trend.

The second factor leading to the assault on hospital technology is the mounting evidence that many health services, indeed perhaps *all* medical care, have made little difference in health outcomes. Nonmedical factors appear to have been more important in reducing mortality and morbidity rates over the past fifty years than has medical care. The works of Cochrane (1972) and McKeown (1976) have raised considerable doubt about the efficacy of many medical procedures. It has become increasingly clear that clinical research is not organized to provide definitive information on the effectiveness of existing or new medical procedures. In the absence of hard scientific proof, several observers have suggested that we should avoid heavy investments in technologies that enhance the delivery of dubious services (see, for example, White, Murnaghan, and Gaus, 1972; Banta and McNeil, 1977). Arguments for redistribution of health dollars to areas of health promotion and prevention are based on an acceptance of this thesis (Lalonde, 1972).

A third source of concern lies in the disappointing record of programs designed to control hospital capital expenditures. State certificate-of-need laws and state programs for approval of large capital expenditures under Section 1122 of the 1972 Social Security Amendments have been in existence long enough for some evidence to be accumulated about their effectiveness in controlling the proliferation of expensive pieces of capital equipment. The record has been dismal. Not only have health planning agencies proved to be unprepared to make appropriate judgments about new technologies, but certificate of need appears to have shifted the composition of capital spending from investments in new beds to investment in sophisticated equipment (Salkever and Bice, 1976). Capital equipment expenditures should not be unequivocally equated with adoption of new technologies, but the lack of effective control over this aspect of hospital expenditure has raised the question whether any control over decisions of hospitals to adopt new and expensive technologies exists.

The convergence of these three separate types of evidence has created an environment of cynicism about the value of new technologies to the delivery of health care. If health care services make so little difference to the community's health level, then investments in an increasing level of sophistication embodied in new technology become especially suspect. As the major repository of the visible symbols of sophisticated technology, the hospital is a natural target for criticism. Sensitive to this emerging anti-technology trend, the authors of DHEW's 1976 *Forward Plan for Health* defended technology's contribution to the well-being of the nation:

During the past 30 years, national investment in biomedical and behavioral research has been enormously productive and has revolutionized clinical care. It is true that it is not yet possible to prevent many of our most frequent and costly illnesses, but that is not because such "high technology" (in Lewis Thomas' concept) is not a goal of research; rather, it is that research progress has not yet permitted the kind of definitive interventions that antibiotics brought for many infectious diseases. . . . Nevertheless, 30 years and billions of dollars of public funds have been invested in this progress against disease, and the public believes it has a right to the benefits of its investment whether such benefits are "half way" or not [pp. 93–94].

Because the issue of technology is so visible at present and the policies that have been suggested to deal with problems of technology are so varied and in some cases extreme,[2] it is important to differentiate among the kinds of "technology problems" that have been identified. As the previous discussion indicates, inferences about the improper use of technology by the health care system have been drawn from very different kinds of evidence, including the volume of inputs devoted to the production of hospital services and the level of capital expenditures undertaken by hospitals. For the most part, critics have not distinguished among the particular problems that they address. Confusion stems partially from the broad scope of hardware and software activities that are often thought of as technology. According to the definition offered by the U.S. Congressional Office of Technology Assessment (OTA), medical technologies include techniques, drugs, procedures, or systems combining these elements, used in the practice of medical care (U.S. Congress, OTA, 1976a). The very comprehensiveness of this definition blurs some of the critical policy problems currently under consideration. More important, however, is a general failure to

[2]See, for example, Bogue and Wolfe (1976), calling for the establishment of a moratorium on the purchase of CAT scanners.

distinguish between problems associated with the improper use of existing technologies and the process by which new technologies are developed, introduced, and diffused into the medical care system. Often, the two problems are lumped together, as in a recent article by Banta and McNeil (1977), focusing on problems associated with new and existing diagnostic technologies. Policy recommendations often involve combined strategies to control both the use of existing capabilities and the introduction of new technology. As a result, exactly which problems specific policies address and how these policies will affect different aspects of the "technology problem" are often unclear.

For the purpose of this chapter, the technology problem can be divided into two subproblems, each with its own policy implications. The first is the problem of the way in which the health care system allocates resources to and uses existing technologies. The second is the problem of technical change involving the introduction of new equipment, systems, or procedures into the health care system. Each of these problems must be defined separately, although it is obvious that the way in which existing technologies are used has immense impact on the direction and speed of technical change in the health care system.

Problems Involving Existing Technology

If we accept the OTA definition of medical technology, the problem of existing technology becomes synonymous with the more general problems of resource allocation and use of health care services. And if, as Perrow has claimed (1965), the hospital itself is the technological instrument of the medical profession, then all problems of utilization of hospital services and allocation of resources to hospitals are inherently problems of the inappropriate use of existing technologies. Most frequently, critics of "existing technology" focus on particular elements of hospital behavior or resources that are "technological" by nature, such as equipment (U.S. Congress, OTA, 1976b), capital-intensive facilities (Russell and Burke, 1975), diagnostic tests (Rushmer, 1976; and Banta and McNeil, 1977), or surgical procedures (Orloff, 1976). These particular elements are identified as sources of abuse of existing technology because they represent the "sophisticated" element of medical care. The tendency of the health care system to bias the allocation and use of resources toward these more sophisticated elements is often referred to as the "technological imperative" (Rushmer, 1976). To the extent that the tendency to overinvest in and overuse sophisticated services is just part of a larger tendency to overuse health services or to invest too many labor or nonlabor resources in the production of hospital services, the problem is not related to technology itself and should not be singled out as one of technology. The impact of present reimbursement and regulatory policies on hospital resource allocation, particularly on decisions to overinvest in capital assets and overuse services, should be viewed as a problem of cost control and not of technology per se.

However, insofar as decisions to invest in or use certain equipment, procedures, or drugs are made on the basis of their level of technical sophistication, the existence of the "technological imperative" must be accepted. A number of arguments have been put forth to justify the view that technology is a problem in its own right. Changes in medical education have purportedly placed increasing emphasis on objective tests and precise measurement when less technologically advanced methods might still be adequate for diagnosis and treatment (Gellman, 1971). Medical students and residents, trained in the most sophisticated institutions, expect and depend upon the availability of diagnostic and therapeutic assists in the form of instrumentation and facilities. Thus, clinical decision makers may be functionaries of the technological imperative.

Several economists have theorized that patient demand for medical care is, among other things, a function of the perceived quality of care (Feldstein, 1976). Others postulate that the objective of the hospital is to maximize a weighted function of the quality and quantity of the services it produces (Newhouse, 1970). How quality is perceived by patients and hospital decision makers thus has a major influence on the behavior of the health care system with respect to technologically sophisticated procedures and services. Feldstein (1976) hypothesizes that hospital decision makers' perceptions of quality depend on the amount of labor and nonlabor inputs devoted to the production of medical care. However, perceived quality may be correlated as much with the level of sophistication of those inputs as with their absolute amounts.[3] If, too, patients perceive quality in terms of high levels of sophistication in the delivery of services, including the application of many and frequent diagnostic tests, performance of equipment-bound procedures (such as respiratory therapy), and increases in the number and training level of health care personnel, then physicians and hospitals will respond by emphasizing those inputs. Similarly, if an important element of the patient's perception of hospital quality were the efficiency of its billing procedures, then the hospital would invest capital and labor resources to improve these. Thus, to the extent that it does exist, the source of the technological imperative rests largely on the value that patients and hospital decision makers place on technological sophistication for its own sake.

Newhouse (1970) has posited that under a predominantly charge- or cost-based system of third-party payment, the hospital decision maker could conceivably push both quality and quantity to the point where the additional utility to the hospital is zero. If quality is equated with the availability and use of sophisticated services, then this hypothesis implies a level of sophistication much beyond that which would result were marginal utility equated with the marginal cost of these services.

The problem of existing technology can thus be related to three factors: structural changes in the nature of medical education, which stresses dependence on scientific instrumentation; patient demands for technological sophistication as a surrogate for high "quality" care; and the failure of the cost-reimbursement system to constrain hospitals from increasing their investment in expensive and sophisticated technological capabilities. On balance, these factors create powerful incentives for the hospital to invest in the showpieces of technological sophistication, including clinical instrumentation, special care units, specialized facilities for complex procedures (for example, cardiac catheterization and cardiac surgery), and automated clinical laboratory systems.

[3] See for example, Grimes and Moseley (1976), relating hospital characteristics with indices of their performance.

The implications for public policy to deal with these sources of abuse of the existing armamentarium of equipment and procedures available to hospitals and physicians are fairly clear. First, the present reimbursement system as it is currently structured needs a major overhaul. Either detailed regulation of the investment decisions of hospitals and health care facilities must be undertaken, or reimbursement systems must be so structured as to provide different incentives to hospitals and health care facilities. Certificate-of-need programs represent one regulatory approach, but these laws generally fail to require the approval of capital purchases under some threshold level or to apply to all health care settings. Furthermore, the separation of the responsibility for regulation of health care expenditures from the responsibility for paying for the services produced creates an institutional weakness in the certificate-of-need arrangements.

Rate setting on a prospective basis is also a potential solution for the bias toward the use of sophisticated technology, but as Bauer's paper in this book points out, rate setting may not lead to the cost control results that many expect of it. Rate setting does not apply to decisions to use sophisticated services. These decisions remain for the most part the exclusive domain of physicians. Thus, rate setting may keep unit costs low, but it cannot be expected to control the utilization of services effectively. Also, hospital rate setting would not alter the internal bias within the hospital decision-making structure toward technologically advanced services. Because the hospital administrator views quality as related to sophistication, the tendency to invest in these services will still remain.

Ellwood (1975) has suggested that a system of competing prepaid group practices would provide the incentives to health care providers to make resource allocation decisions in the light of the relative cost effectiveness of each decision. With appropriate information on measures of performance of such prepaid plans, patients could trade off quality against cost in a fashion that would approach a more conventional market decision.

A second policy implication arising from the tendency to equate technological sophistication with quality of care is the need for a reexamination of the efficacy of medical practices, particularly those involving the use of expensive equipment, facilities, or personnel. Furthermore, the results of this reexamination must be transmitted or communicated to physicians and patients so that a more informed set of demands can be made for quality. Indeed, the results could also be used to control utilization of sophisticated services.

The organization of such deliberate and ongoing research into efficacy requires the delegation of a new set of responsibilities to some federal agency or the establishment of an agency to perform this role. At present, no federal health agency has the specific charge of evaluating the efficacy of existing medical practices.

The third policy implication argues for changes in methods of medical education, including incorporation into the educational process the information on efficacy produced through research efforts. Some critics of the medical education system have noted that medical schools do not provide any training in statistical decision theory to enable medical students to evaluate the relative information content of diagnostic tests (Schwartz, 1976). Of course, if the reimbursement system were altered so that hospitals and physicians had to choose among alternative uses of limited economic resources and if appropriate information on efficacy were produced by a research organization, medical education would be likely to reflect the new incentives and knowledge.

The Problem of Technical Change

Technical change refers to the complex and not well understood process by which new capability is developed and brought into use. New technical capability in health care refers to the ability to produce new products or services that did not previously exist or to produce existing products or services in a new way, with greater reliability or less cost. Because the nature of the hospital product is so poorly defined, these two kinds of capability are often difficult to distinguish from one another. For example, was gastric freezing a new service, or was it a "better" way to perform an old service—the treatment of ulcers? The most important distinction for policy purposes is between changes that at least theoretically enhance the quality of care and changes that lower the cost of providing care. Gastric freezing was clearly intended to fall into the former category.

Technical change implies that the new capability has resulted from scientific progress, not from changes in the hospital's economic environment. For example, if the hospital reorganizes previously scattered services into a separate respiratory therapy unit for economic reasons, it has not introduced a new technology, as some would claim (see, for example, Russell, 1976), but has merely adjusted methods of providing services. However, the introduction of intermittent positive pressure breathing (IPPB) as a new service clearly represents the adoption of a new technical capability, as would the replacement of existing laboratory methods with new automated laboratory equipment.

Technical change is a dynamic process that involves several identifiable but somewhat overlapping phases. The process has been classified in a number of ways (U.S. Congress, OTA, 1976a), but it can be summarized in terms of four major phases: (1) generation of clinically useful knowledge; (2) prototype development; (3) testing; and (4) diffusion. The first phase can be equated with scientific and biomedical research, or in some cases with technological development outside of health care. The development phase may occur as part of the first or may involve a significant time lap (President's Biomedical Research Panel, 1976a). Testing in the clinical environment is likely to be concurrent with development activities to some extent. Diffusion represents the final phase in which a technology is adopted for nonexperimental use by individual or organizational decision makers.

The dependence of diffusion of new technology on the outcome of scientific and biomedical research has complicated the policy problems associated with the process. Two major strains of criticism appear to be in direct conflict with each other. The first is that the process of technological change has raised health care costs too high; the second is that the pitfalls in each step of the process of technical change render it extremely delicate and in need of assists at critical points, particularly in the research and development phase. The first criticism implies that too much technology is emerging from the process; the second that too little results.

The result of this schism is a spate of policy recommendations that on their face appear contradictory. Those whose focus and experience lie in the early phases of the process are extremely sensitive to the obstacles that must be overcome to reach the testing and diffusion phases and the high mortality rate of ideas and inventions along the way (see, for example, Anderson, 1976). Among the obstacles cited are biomedical research funding policies that bias the kinds of clinically useful knowledge that develop (RAND Corp., 1976); property rights policies that provide inadequate incentives to developers of new technologies (U.S. Federal Council for Science and Technology, 1975); the small size and disaggregated nature of the potential markets (National Research Council, 1976); inadequate networks for communicating the results of clinically useful research to the health care community (U.S. DHEW, 1977) and the host of regulatory processes required before new technologies can reach their markets (Noll, 1975).

Those whose primary concern is the cost of new technologies cite the failure of those who test new technologies to consider the important concepts of efficacy and effectiveness in a complete or consistent fashion (Hiatt, 1975); the willingness of hospital decision makers to serve as an easy market since they bear no risk if the technology proves to be inadequate or quickly outmoded (Brown, 1972); the apparent bias in the system toward the development of hospital technologies instead of ambulatory or home setting (Hiatt, 1975); and the lack of any responsibility for early assessment of the impact of new technologies on costs or effectiveness (Arnstein, 1976).

The first set of arguments would call for public policy to facilitate the development and diffusion of new technologies and the elimination of bureaucratic and regulatory barriers. The second set would imply the intensification of public efforts to shape and control the process through research funding and regulatory avenues. The recent passage of the medical device amendments, which will require significantly new devices to obtain clearance prior to entry in the market is an interesting example of the conflict. Critics cite the impact that new drug regulation has had on both the rate of introduction of these new technologies and the structure of the drug industry (U.S. Congress, 1973). Supporters point to the need for

171

intervention in a field that poses ever increasing safety and efficacy questions, and to the savings that have resulted from the inability of unsafe or ineffective new drugs to reach the market.

The source of the conflict expressed in this context arises from the paucity of information now available about several critical aspects of the process of technical change. First, the empirical evidence on the impact that new technology has had on medical and social costs and effectiveness is fragmentary and inconclusive. We need to know the extent to which the process has worked inefficiently and whether new technologies have indeed raised costs as so many claim. Some recent research efforts have been devoted to this question. The results of that research are summarized in a subsequent section of this paper.

Second, we know very little about the way in which new medical technologies are developed. We do not even have a clear picture of who the developers are and what environments produce what kinds of technologies. The impact of government funding of biomedical research on the development of different kinds of technology is also unclear. The settings for development of different kinds of technology unquestionably vary. Considering the many different procedures, techniques, equipment, and systems that have come into being in the past ten years, it is reasonable to assume that the patterns of development among these will be highly varied. Research and development can occur in universities, hospitals, medical schools, large or small research and development laboratories, manufacturing firms, and even in physicians' offices; frequently, the process involves a combination of these settings. Although it is easy to theorize about the motivations of various kinds of participants in the development process, there is very little evidence to support a model to explain the determinants of technology development. The background studies commissioned by the President's Biomedical Research Panel (1976b) made a start in this direction, but they did not focus on the different kinds of developers and the differences among them. A frequently described model is the "advocacy" theory (Anderson, 1976). The individual scientist, engineer, or clinician has a strong personal faith in the value of his idea and mothers it through the paths of development. The success of a technology at least to the prototype state is said to be a function of the degree of advocacy it engenders as well as its usefulness. But we know so little about who actually does research and development and how they interact, that it is virtually impossible to diagnose failures in the development process.

Third, the evidence on how hospital decision makers adopt new medical technologies is scattered among several research disciplines with different approaches; consequently, the results are somewhat equivocal. It is important to identify not only the early adopters of new technologies and the time and spatial patterns of diffusion, but also how these factors differ among different classes of medical technologies. Unfortunately, the research has not looked directly at these questions; rather, individual studies have focused on a single technology or a specific type of hospital behavior, such as capital equipment purchases. Nevertheless, some tentative conclusions can be drawn from this literature. Indeed, there appears to be more systematic analysis of the process of medical technology diffusion than of any other important policy-related question in the area. The major findings of the literature on this question are summarized in a subsequent section.

The Economic Costs of New Technology

A number of studies have attempted to estimate the economic impacts of new technology. These studies measure different concepts of cost, including hospital costs, total costs of medical care, and net social costs. They also vary in the operational definition of technological change. These variations render objective comparison difficult; nevertheless, the results do provide some insight into the relation between technology and health care costs.

In a study of the impact of new technology on the cost of hospital care, Davis (1974) used data from approximately 200 non-profit hospitals for the period 1962 to 1968. Using time as a proxy for technological change, Davis found that when demand and supply variables had been taken into account, hospital expenses per admission rise about 2 percent annually. The time trend variable is an imperfect proxy since it also includes effects due to gradual changes that influence demand, including changing attitudes about hospital care, improved methods of ambulatory care, or other changes in behavior over time that are not accounted for by explicit variables in her model. Davis suggests that the time estimate provides an upper limit for an estimate of the effect of technological change on hospital costs, but the other influences represented by the time variable could have had a negative effect, leading to an understatement of technology's effect on hospital costs.

Several researchers have studied the impact of technical change on total medical care costs. Mushkin et al. (1976) analyzed the total impact of biomedical research on health expenditures from 1930 to 1975. Using a time residual as a proxy for biomedical advances, they found that this factor was responsible for an annual reduction in total health expenditures of 0.5 percent. This result compared favorably with a twenty-year study by Fuchs (1972), which found that technology and biomedical change had a positive residual effect on total health care expenditures in the amount of 0.6 percent annually. The difference in these studies may be attributable to differences in the study periods (Fuchs' study compared the years 1947 to 1967) and to other effects included in the studies. These longitudinal studies include the effects on medical care costs of the significant advances in the treatment of communicable diseases during the period under study. They also include the net effect of shifting disease patterns of the population. Thus, the relatively favorable outcome with respect to the role of technology and biomedical research over the entire study period obscures some of the changes in the health of Americans. The pattern of cost changes in the recent past may not be consistent with long-run trends.

Scitovsky and McCall (1975) have analyzed the changes in cost of medical care associated with selected illnesses. Between 1964 and 1971, the net increase in the average cost of treatment of an episode of illness was calculated for eight conditions: otitis media; forearm fractures; appendicitis; maternity care; cancer of the breast; pneumonia; duodenal ulcer; and myocardial infarction. In almost every instance, there were cost-raising and cost-saving changes in treatment. However, Scitovsky and McCall noted that "the costs of treatment of conditions requiring hospitalization rose at a considerably faster rate than those of conditions treated on an ambulatory basis" (p. 15). Cost-raising sources were found to include shifts to more expensive drugs, an increase in the number of laboratory tests per case, and an increase in the number of miscellaneous inpatient and outpatient services. However, the most dramatic cost increases occurred in the treatment of myocardial infarction; these changes were traced principally to the increasing use of intensive care units. Thus, we see that sources of medical cost increases reflect an epidemiological shift from diseases requiring outpatient to those requiring inpatient care, and a shift of setting of care within the hospital from less specialized services to more specialized units. Unfortunately, the analysis does not permit any comparison of cost-increasing conditions with cost-decreasing conditions because of the selected nature of the conditions considered. Combined with Mushkin's results, these findings show that the ultimate impact of technological change on medical care costs is not clearly cost-increasing. A more selective approach to analysis is required. Cooper (1976) has observed that the important policy issues lie not in the total impact of technological change across all diagnoses and settings of care but in the misallocation of resources in whatever settings they occur. However, if the overall effect of the introduction of technology does not clearly lead to inordinate increases in the cost of medical care, then the impact of an elaborate system to control the introduction of new technologies may not be worth the administrative costs involved.

Although the application of benefit-cost analysis to health programs has a long history (see Klarman, 1974), only one study has attempted to measure the "social" costs of a broad class of technological developments. This study, by Orloff (1976), estimated the net contribution to medical and nonmedical social costs of research in surgery over the study period. Using the life-cycle earnings approach to valuation of changes in morbidity and mortality, this study found that the most significant research contributions had resulted in a net saving of $2.8 billion for the year 1970. The study suffers from the bias of dealing only with selected surgical advances, but there was some attempt to consider the leading advances in the period under study as identified by a panel of surgeons. It is possible that the surgical advances not considered would have shown systematic increases in hospitalization and total social costs.

Although the studies described here represent significant advances in the economics of technological change in medical care, they fall short of providing policy guidance. New technologies appear to be raising hospital costs, but it is not altogether clear that these increases are not offset by savings in other sectors of the health care delivery system or by nonmedical benefits to society.

A major problem with these analyses is the lack of a normative base for comparison. The real question is not how much total health care costs increased or decreased, but how far that change differed from what would be possible under an ideal system of technical change, that is, a system in which development and adoption decisions were made with full information and with the maximization of social benefits as the objective.

The Diffusion of New Hospital Technologies

In order to devise good policies to control the introduction of new technologies, it is necessary to know a great deal about how they find their way into hospitals and into the practice of medicine. What factors determine whether and when a hospital adopts a new technology? How do these factors differ among classes of hospital technologies? What are the characteristics of early adopters and of late adopters? How do they differ? What determines the speed with which new technologies are introduced? And, most important, how does the process diverge from patterns of diffusion that would occur in an ideal situation?

The literature offers answers to some of these questions but leaves the central question of the ultimate effectiveness of the diffusion process unanswered. What we do know must be synthesized from several independent bodies of research, representing different disciplines. Economists have studied the economic characteristics of the adopting unit and the new technology; sociologists have studied the attributes of organizations and individuals determining their propensity to adopt new technologies; political scientists have considered the political environment in which change takes place.

Definitional problems pose significant barriers to comparison of research studies. Not only do operational definitions vary because of constraints on data available to various researchers, but there are also basic conceptual differences in various approaches. In order to avoid confusion, we must define some terms commonly used in this literature. First, the adoption of a new technology refers to a decision by an adopting unit (defined as an individual or organization) to make use of the technology's capability. Adoption is often confused with utilization of a new technology. For many hospital technologies, adoption is synonymous with the purchase or lease of equipment, construction of a facility, or decision to offer a new service. When, however, the adopting unit is likely to be the physician (as is the case with new drugs or surgical procedures not requiring extraordinary equipment), then adoption cannot be easily distinguished from the first use of the technology. Because so many hospital technologies require a decision to make capital expenditures, the determination of whether and when a hospital has adopted a new technology is often based on the time of the commitment of capital resources.

Diffusion refers to the pattern of adoption decisions over time and sometimes space. The diffusion process is often expressed as the number of units adopting a new technology as a function of the time or distance from its first availability on the market. Diffusion studies often differentiate early adopters from late adopters and attempt to characterize them. The time path of adoption of new medical technologies may be either too fast or too slow depending on the real social value of the change.

Many studies focus on the determinants of "innovation" by individuals or organizations. Innovation is defined as the first use of a product or program by a given adoption unit.[4] The adoption of a new technology is, then, one kind of innovation possible within the hospital. Innovations can include program or organizational changes

---

[4]See Mohr (1969) for a discussion of alternative definitions of innovation.

as well. Much of the literature on innovation in health care organizations has involved the study of these nontechnological innovations. Using these studies to make inferences about the determinants of technological innovations may be dangerous, as the external validity of such studies across innovation types has not been demonstrated in the literature.

Economic studies of technological diffusion outside of health care have provided empirical support for the hypothesis that the rate of innovation is a function of the profitability of the innovation and the resources required for adoption relative to the size of the firms in the industry (see Mansfield, 1961, 1968). To apply these findings to technological innovation in health care, it would be necessary to redefine "profitability" to be more consistent with the objectives of hospitals. In fact, it is the generalization of this concept that most studies of the diffusion of medical technologies address. Substitutes for profitability must be found to explain differences in the way that particular technologies are adopted by hospitals. As discussed above, these substitutes are most often postulated to be some combination of quantity and quality of services provided by the hospital, where quality may be perceived in different ways by hospital decision makers. Economic studies of diffusion of hospital technologies relate adoption of specific technologies to variables believed to be related to these objectives and to the resources available to the hospital.

In a recent study of nuclear medicine facilities, Rapoport (1976) used statewide data to regress the speed of diffusion over different time periods against a number of factors, including the ratio of the state's population in urban centers, state income, availability of physicians, hospital size, percent of hospitals affiliated with medical schools, and the variation in size among hospitals. Depending on the time period under study, these variables explained between 50 and 75 percent of the total variation in diffusion rates across states. The most interesting result was the strong negative relationship between the medical school affiliation variable and the diffusion rate in all time periods. Rapoport offers the explanation that in areas with many affiliated hospitals, which acquired nuclear medicine early, the nonaffiliated groups may not have considered themselves capable of competing in this arena and thus did not adopt this new technology as rapidly as hospitals in states with few such medical school affiliations. Thus, regionalization of this service may have occurred by default.

Cromwell et al. (1975) have studied the relationship between the existence of particular high technology facilities in a state and a number of explanatory variables. Their results show that the diffusion of equipment-intensive hospital services such as intensive care units, open heart surgery, x-ray therapy, cobalt therapy, radium therapy, diagnostic radioisotope, and therapeutic radioisotope services is significantly and positively related to per capita income, age, total per capita number of physicians in the state, the ratio of specialists to total physicians, and for certain facilities, the existence of a certificate-of-need law.

Studies of innovation in health care organizations have related adoption of innovations to factors such as organizational size, wealth, or access to resources; organizational structure; the nature of the environment facing the organization; and attributes or attitudes of individual decision makers within the organization. In a study of respiratory therapy technologies, Gordon et al. (1974) showed that innovation in hospitals is a function of several structural characteristics of the organization, including the degree of decentralization of decision making, the visibility of consequences of medical care within the organization, and the complexity of the medical staff resources of the hospital. This study looked only at respiratory therapy services which were judged by an expert panel to be elements of "good" medical care. Whether these factors would remain important as determinants of adoption of technologies of questionable efficacy is uncertain; the study also failed to include any technologies requiring substantial capital resources.

Resource availability has surfaced as the leading determinant of innovation in health departments and other public health agencies (see Gordon and Fisher, 1975). Studies of innovations in these agencies have concentrated on program changes rather than on the adoption of new medical technologies; therefore, their external validity for the adoption of medical technology in hospitals is suspect. However, evidence from the economics literature tends to support this finding. In a study of capital expenditure decisions by hospitals, Ginsburg (1972) showed that the availability of capital funds and hospital size were important determinants of the overall level of capital investment, whereas composition of investment depended on demand factors. In a more recent study of capital equipment expenditure decisions by fifteen hospitals, in the greater Boston area, Cromwell et al. (1975) found that larger hospitals spend proportionately more on capital equipment than smaller hospitals, but the relationship between capital expenditures and the availability of financial resources was found to be insignificant.

Taken together, these studies show that hospitals are likely to adopt new technologies when they are large, complex, and wealthy institutions. Medical centers and teaching hospitals can be expected to be the early adopters of new technologies, although there is no information on how well these early adopters differentiate between "good" and "bad" technologies.

The diffusion literature has provided virtually no information on the channels of communication responsible for the dissemination of information on new technologies. What role early adopters such as medical schools play compared with suppliers in communicating information on new technologies has not been studied. Nor have researchers studied at what stage in the process of diffusion new technologies become standards of medical practice, virtually guaranteeing their ultimate penetration of the health care system. The impact of the emergence of health planning and concepts of regionalization on different patterns has also not been assessed.

If, as one might expect, medical centers offering a full array of services and training are the early adopters of new medical technologies, followed by the rest of the hospitals, then it would be useful to focus policy development on these units. The impact of recent experimental reimbursement policies on adoption decisions may be perverse. Many hospital prospective reimbursement systems group hospitals according to certain characteristics for the purposes of rate setting. Often these include teaching status, bed size, case mix, or "service intensity." By so doing, these formulas are likely to compare the costs of early adopters with one another and thus ensure the continued resource availability to future adoption of new technologies by these hospitals. As other groups of hospitals respond to the new standards of medical practice developed in these centers, their costs get pulled upward as well.

Conclusion

The one clear implication of this discussion is that there are major gaps in what we know about the real impact of hospital technologies, new or existing, on social costs and benefits. We do not fully understand the nature of the development process, nor do we know how sensitive that process is to changes in the health care delivery or financing system.

This lack of knowledge does reveal that there needs to be increasing federal attention paid to the generation of valid information on the efficacy of medical procedures, particularly those involving the use of new and existing "sophisticated" services (that is, capital-intensive, equipment-oriented, requiring a high level of staff capabilities). That such information is not currently generated is reflected in our inability to determine the extent to which the hospital industry makes appropriate adoption decisions. We do not even know to what extent we are wasting our health care dollars on relatively ineffective but technically sophisticated services.

In the long run, the problem facing policy makers will be where on the trade-off curve between health care costs and benefits we should be and how to ration the availability of expensive technologies whose benefits are clear. To date, we have shown that the health care system as it works today cannot ration such technologies effectively (witness the renal dialysis program). Up to now we may have wasted resources, but we have been able to offer the benefits of new technologies to an ever wider class of beneficiaries. In the future, we may not be able to do so.

Refernces

Anderson, N.
   1976   "Critical steps in the development of new health technology."
           Paper prepared for the Conference on Health Care Technology

and Quality of Care, Boston University, November 19–20, 1976. Boston: Boston University, Program on Public Policy for Quality Health Care.

Arnstein, S.
1976   Statement by Sherry Arnstein, Senior Fellow, Intramural Research Section, National Center for Health Services Research, U.S. DHEW, at the Conference on Health Care Technology and Quality of Care, Boston University, November 19–20, 1976. Boston: Boston University Program on Public Policy for Quality Health Care.

Banta, H.D., and B.J. McNeil
1977   "The costs of medical diagnosis: The case of the CT scanner." Photocopy. Washington, D.C., Office of Technology Assessment.

Bogue, T., and S.M. Wolfe
1976   "CAT scanners: Is fancier technology worth a billion dollars of health consumers' money?" Washington, D.C.: Health Research Group.

Brown, R.E.
1972   "Managing the mushrooming growth of America's hospital system." In Regulating the Hospital, a report of the 1972 National Forum on Hospital and Health Affairs. Durham, N.C.: Department of Health Administration of Duke University.

Cochrane, A.L.
1972   Effectiveness and Efficiency: Random Reflections on Health Services. London: The Nuffield Provincial Hospitals Trust.

Cooper, B.
1976   Statement by Barbara Cooper, Office of Research and Statistics, Social Security Administration, at the Conference on Health Care Technology and Quality of Care, Boston University, November 19–20, 1976. Boston: Boston University Program on Public Policy for Quality Health Care.

Cromwell, J., et al.
1975   Incentives and Decisions Underlying Hospitals; Adoption and Utilization of Major Capital Equipment. Cambridge, Mass.: Abt Associates.

Davis, K.
1974   "The role of technology, demand and labor markets in the determination of hospital costs." In Mark Perlman, ed., The Economics of Health and Medical Care. New York: John Wiley & Sons.

DeBakey, M.E., and H.W. Hiatt
1976   "Medical technology: How much is enough?" In Proceedings of the National Leadership Conference on America's Health Policy. Washington, D.C.: National Journal.

Ellwood, P.M., Jr.
1975   "Alternatives to regulation: Improving the market." In Institute of Medicine, Controls on Health Care. Washington, D.C.: National Academy of Sciences.

Feldstein, M.S.
1976   Quality Change and the Demand for Hospital Care. Discussion Paper No. 475, Harvard Institute of Economic Research, Cambridge, Mass.

Feldstein, M.S., and A. Taylor
1977   "The rapid rise of hospital costs." Discussion Paper No. 531, Harvard Institute of Economic Research, Cambridge, Mass.

Fuchs, V.
1972   Essays on the Economics of Health and Medical Care. New York: Columbia University Press.

Gaus, C.R.
1975   "What goes into technology must come out in costs." Excerpt from testimony of the Social Security Administration before the President's Biomedical Research Panel, September 29, 1975, in The National Leadership Conference on America's Health Policy. Washington, D.C.: National Journal.

Gaus, C.R., and B.S. Cooper
1976   "Technology and Medicare: Alternatives for change." Paper prepared for the Conference on Health Care Technology and Quality of Care, Boston University, November 19-20, 1976. Boston: Boston University, Program on Public Policy for Quality Health Care.

Gellman, D.D.
1971   "The price of progress: Technology and the cost of medical care." Canadian Medical Association Journal 104 (March 6): 401-406.

Ginsburg, P.B.
1972   "Resource allocation in the hospital industry: The role of capital financing." Social Security Bulletin 35 (August): 20-30.

Gordon, G., and G.L. Fisher, eds.
1975   The Diffusion of Medical Technology. Cambridge, Mass.: Ballinger Publishing Co.

Gordon, G., et al.
  1974   "Organizational structure, environmental diversity and hospital adoption of medical innovations." In A.D. Kaluzny, J.T. Gentry, and J.E. Veney, eds., Innovations in Health Care Organizations: An Issue in Organizational Change. Chapel Hill, N.C.: School of Public Health, University of North Carolina.

Grimes, R.M., and S.K. Moseley
  1976   "An approach to an index of hospital performance." Health Services Research 11 (Fall): 294.

Hiatt, H.H.
  1975   "Protecting the medical 'commons'—who has the responsibility?" The New England Journal of Medicine 293 (July): 235–241.

Klarman, H.E.
  1974   "Application of cost-benefit analysis to health systems technology." In Morris F. Collen, ed., Technology and Health Care Systems in the 1980's. DHEW Publication No. HRA-74-3016. Rockville, Md.: National Center for Health Services Research and Development.

Lalonde, M.
  1972   A New Perspective on the Health of Canadians: A Working Document. Ottawa: Government of Canada.

McKeown, T.
  1976   The Role of Medicine. London: The Nuffield Provincial Hospitals Trust.

Mansfield, E.
  1961   "Technical change and the rate of imitation." Econometrica 29 (October): 741–766.
  1968   Industrial Research and Technological Innovation: An Econometric Analysis. New York: W.W. Norton & Co., Inc.

Mohr, L.B.
  1969   "Determinants of innovation in organizations." American Political Science Review 63 (March): 111–126.

Mushkin, S.J., L.C. Paringer, and M.M. Chen
  1976   "Returns to biomedical research 1900–1975: An initial assessment of impacts on health expenditures." Photocopy. Washington, D.C.: Georgetown University, Public Services Laboratory.

National Research Council
  1976   Science and Technology in the Service of the Physically Handicapped. National Research Council, Assembly of Life Sciences, Division of Medical Sciences, Committee on National Needs for

the Rehabilitation of the Physically Handicapped. Washington, D.C.: National Academy of Sciences.

Newhouse, J.P.
1970   "Toward a theory of nonprofit institutions: An Economic Model of a hospital." American Economic Review 60 (March): 64–74.

Noll, R.G.
1975   "The consequences of public utility regulation of hospitals." In Institute of Medicine, Controls on Health Care. Washington, D.C.: National Academy of Sciences.

Orloff, M.J.
1976   "Contributions of research in surgical technology to health care." Paper prepared for the Conference on Health Care Technology and Quality of Care, Boston University, November 19–20, 1976. Boston: Boston University, Program on Public Policy for Quality Health Care.

Perrow, C.
1965   "Hospitals: Technology, structure, and goals." In J.G. March, ed., Handbook of Organizations. Chicago: Rand McNally.

President's Biomedical Research Panel
1976a   Report of the President's Biomedical Research Panel, Appendix B: Approaches to Policy Development for Biomedical Research: Strategy for Budgeting and Movement from Invention to Clinical Application. DHEW Publication No. (OS) 76-502. Washington, D.C.: Government Printing Office.

1976b   Report of the President's Biomedical Research Panel, Supplement 1: Analysis of Selected Biomedical Research Programs: Case Histories. DHEW Publication No. (OS) 76-506. Washington, D.C.: Government Printing Office.

Rabkin, M.T., and C.N. Melin
1976   "The impact of technology upon the cost and quality of hospital care, and a proposal for control of new and expensive technology." Background paper prepared for the Conference on Health Care Technology and Quality of Care, Boston University, November 19–20, 1976. Boston: Boston University, Program on Public Policy for Quality Health Care.

RAND Corporation
1976   "Policy Analysis for Federal biomedical research." In President's Biomedical Research Panel, Appendix B: Approaches to Policy Development for Biomedical Research: Strategy for Budgeting and Movement from Invention to Clinical Application. Washington, D.C.: Government Printing Office.

Rapoport, J.
1976   "Diffusion of technological innovation in hospitals: A case study of nuclear medicine." Photocopy. South Hadley, Mass.: Mount Holyoke College.
Rushmer, R.F.
1976   "The technological imperative." Editorial, American Journal of Roentgenology 127 (August): 356-357.
Russell, L.B.
1976   "Making rational decisions about medical technology." Paper presented at the National Commission on the Cost of Medical Care, November 23, 1976, Chicago, Ill. Photocopy. Washington, D.C.: L.B. Russell.
Russell, L.B., and C.S. Burke
1975   Technological Diffusion in the Hospital Sector. Washington, D.C.: National Planning Association.
Salkever, D.S., and T.W. Bice
1976   "The impact of certificate-of-need controls on hospital investment." Milbank Memorial Fund Quarterly/Health and Society 54 (Spring): 185-214.
Schwartz, William
1976   Statement by William Schwartz, Vannevar Bush University Professor, Tufts University School of Medicine, at the Conference on Health Care Technology and Quality of Care, Boston University, November 19-20, 1976. Boston: Boston University, Program on Public Policy for Quality Health Care.
Scitovsky, A.A., and N. McCall
1975   Changes in the Costs of Treatment of Selected Illnesses 1951-1964-1971. San Francisco: Health Policy Program, University of California School of Medicine.
U.S. Congress
1973   Senate, Select Committee on Small Business, Subcommittee on Monopoly, Present Status of Competition in the Pharmaceutical Industry: Hearings. 93d Congress, 1st Session, February 5-8 and March 14, 1972. Washington, D.C.: Government Printing Office.
U.S. Congress, Office of Technology Assessment
1976a   Development of Medical Technology: Opportunities for Assessment. Washington, D.C.: Government Printing Office.
1976b   The Computerized Tomography (CT or CAT) Scanner and Its Implications for Health Policy. Draft. Washington, D.C.

U.S. Department of Health, Education, and Welfare
  1976   Public Health Service, Forward Plan for Health: FT 1978–82.
          DHEW Publication No. (OS) 76-50046. Washington, D.C.:
          Government Printing Office.
  1977   National Institute of Health, "The responsibilities of NIH at the
          Health Research/Health Care interface." Draft. Bethesda, Md.:
          National Institute of Health.
U.S. Federal Council for Science and Technology
  1975   Executive Subcommittee of the Committee on Government
          Patent Policy, University Patent Policy Ad Hoc Subcommittee,
          Report. Photocopy.
Waldman, S.
  1972   The Effect of Changing Technology on Hospital Costs. Research
          and Statistics Note No. 4, DHEW Publication No. (SSA) 72-
          11701 (February 28).
Weiner, S.M.
  1976   "State regulation and health technology." Paper prepared for the
          Conference on Health Care Technology and Quality of Care,
          Boston University, November 19–20, 1976. Boston: Boston Uni-
          versity, Program on Public Policy for Quality Health Care.
White, K.L., J.H. Murnaghan, and C.R. Gaus
  1972   "Technology and health care." The New England Journal of
          Medicine 287 (December): 1223–1227.
Worthington, N.L.
  1975   "Expenditures for hospital care and physicians' services: Factors
          affecting annual changes." Social Security Bulletin 38 (Novem-
          ber): 3–15.

Innovation of Health Services:
A Comparative Study of Hospitals
and Health Departments

ARNOLD D. KALUZNY

JAMES E. VENEY

JOHN T. GENTRY

This paper investigates the differential contribution of various organizational variables affecting the innovation of high-risk versus low-risk health service programs in two types of health care organizations: hospitals and health departments. It was found that variables are differentially related to both the type of program and the type of organization. Organizational size was a critical factor in program innovation as it relates to high-risk services in hospitals and low-risk services in health departments. Excluding size, characteristics of the staff, such as cosmopolitan orientation and training, were prime predictors for both high- and low-risk programs in health departments and low-risk programs in hospitals. The degree of formalization was the primary predictor of innovation of high-risk programs in hospitals. Cosmplitan orientation of the administrator was a critical factor in the innovation of high-risk programs in both hospitals and health departments.

The assessment of change in health care organizations, and particularly program innovation, has received increasing attention by social scientists. Using a wide range of explanatory variables, research, with few exceptions, has tended to concentrate on explaining variation in the innovation of a single program or that of aggregate change. For a review of these studies see Kaluzny (1972). While this represents progress, it is important to consider two underlying problem areas. First, it is necessary to inquire into the general area of programmatic change and whether factors associated with program innovation differ by type of program innovated. Essentially, this exploration involves assessment of a set of services and activities that have common characteristics, making possible generalization from known determinants of innovation of one program to other programs with similar characteristics. Secondly, explanation of differences by type of organization is necessary to provide insight into the specific organizational setting under which various factors are most appropriate. Thus, the introduction of a comparative study of organizational innovation permits an assessment of the generalizability of findings and provides an evaluation of the impact of organizational variables on concrete operational programs. Insight into these aspects is critical to the development of effective intervention strategies that may be used systematically to administer organizational innovation.

In an attempt to address these problems, the present study will provide a comparative analysis of organizational factors affecting the innovation of selected health services with a specific set of characteristics in two types of health care organizations: hospitals and health departments. The objective is to assess the differential contribution of organizational variables relating to the innovation of selected health services with specific characteristics as implemented within and between hospitals and health departments. To meet this objective, two specific questions are examined. First, is there a difference in organizational variables which accounts for innovation of services having different characteristics? Second, are there differences between organizational variables for hospitals as one type of health care organization and those for health departments as a distinctively different type of health care organization?

Method

Data for the study are based on questionnaires and interviews conducted in all organized county and city health departments in New York State excluding New York City ($n = 23$) and a sample of general acute hospitals ($n = 59$) located in the respective health department jurisdictions. Within each health department jurisdiction at least two hospitals were selected, unless only one hospital was available. The selection of hospitals was based on their innovative status and number of beds. Hospitals with three or more of the six program areas under study were considered innovative; all other hospitals were considered low innovators. Hospitals in each of the two innovation groups were further classified into those with more than 500 beds and those with 500 or fewer beds. Final selection of hospitals included all high-innovation hospitals regardless of number of beds and all hospitals of over 500 beds regardless of innovative status. One-fourth of the low-innovator hospitals with 500 or fewer beds were randomly selected. These hospitals were evenly divided on the basis of whether they had more or fewer than 300 beds.

Within sample organizations, four sets of respondents were selected. For hospitals, the list included (a) the administrator, (b) assistant-associate administrators and all department heads, (c) executive directors of the boards of trustees and a randomly selected sample of trustees, (d) chairmen of medical staff and a sample of physicians on the staff of the respective hospitals. For health departments, the respondents included (a) the director of the health department, (b) deputy and all department heads, (c) executive officers of the board of health and a sample of board members, and (d) a sample of staff public health nurses. Non-professionals and non-supervisory personnel were excluded because they were less directly involved in decision-making processes within the organization.

Administrators of both organizations were interviewed. In addition, questionnaires were sent to all personnel including the administrator. For hospitals, responses were received from 48 administrators (81 percent), 343 associate and assistant administrators and department heads (85 percent), 529 physicians (61 percent), and 366 hospital trustees (70 percent). In health departments, responses were received from 23 health officers (100 percent), 112 department heads (89 percent), 96 members of boards of health (61 percent), and 176 public health nurses (82 percent). Analysis of data from hospitals and health departments excluded from this analysis and non-respondents from within participating organizations indicates that the non-participants are not significantly different from organizations and respondents that did participate in the study.

Within participating organizations, attention focuses on the innovation of selected health services and activities associated with six program areas: home health, family planning, rehabilitation, mental health, medical social work, and chronic-disease screening. The specific services within each program area are shown in Table 1. These services were selected because of their association with the comprehensiveness and continuity of community health services. As the table indicates, the most commonly provided service for hospitals is physical therapy within a rehabilitation program, and, for health departments, home nursing within home health programs. Less commonly provided services for both hospitals and health de-

TABLE 1

Proportion of Hospitals and Health Departments
Implementing Services and Activities

Services and Activities	Proportion of Hospitals Implementing	Proportion of Health Departments Implementing
Home health		
Social services	11.7	20.9
Home nursing	9.6	66.3
Physician services (for coordination and planning of patient care)	7.7	28.8
Homemaker or health aide	5.4	43.4
Home-delivered food	2.3	1.5
Transportation	5.4	7.3
Patient care conferences	7.1	43.4
Physical therapy	11.9	51.7
Speech therapy	5.2	25.4
Family planning		
Provision as separate entity	11.7	41.5
Provision in conjunction with other services	20.2	43.4
Case-finding activities	14.2	26.3
Systematic follow-up procedures	13.3	49.8
Community case-finding activities using indigenous workers	4.6	28.8
Rehabilitation		
Routine evaluation of all patients	20.8	23.9
Standard nursing procedures	38.3	42.4
Physical therapy	67.9	41.5
Occupational therapy	31.7	16.6
Speech and hearing therapy	27.5	32.2
Mental health		
Outpatient diagnostic and treatment	26.3	23.4
Inpatient diagnostic and treatment	40.6	7.3
Use of indigenous workers for case-finding and information dissemination	8.5	8.8
Integration with other health services	20.8	36.7
Follow-up care after hospitalization	20.0	44.9
Medical social work		
Psychological and social consultation	29.6	22.9
Information and referral	42.7	29.3
Predischarge planning (hospitals)	40.0	
Assist families with legal problems (health departments)		7.3
Chronic disease screening		
Cervical cytology	36.3	53.7
Ocular tonometry for glaucoma	18.9	26.8
EKG cardiac anomaly	17.3	11.7
Multiple blood chemistry	36.0	19.5
Self-administered health questionnaire	4.8	5.9

partments are generally within the home care programs, with home-delivered food the least commonly provided.

Organizational Innovation

In using the concept of innovation, a number of alternatives have been considered for the classification of the dependent variable, i.e., degree of innovativeness of the organizations under study. Most of the classification schemes have various shortcomings. The least complex score which has been used with these data is classification of organizations on a scale of innovativeness using a simple sum of the 32 study services provided by each organization while controlling for the date of innovation. If innovation is considered as the simple adoption of services, the more services adopted the more innovative is the organization.

However, the gross services-provided score has several drawbacks. First is the fact that an organization providing a large number of services may have implemented them at some point in the fairly distant past but may not currently be undergoing substantial change. In essence, an organization, innovative in the past and hence receiving a high innovation score, may no longer be innovative. Another related problem is the difficulty of relating explanatory organizational variables based on cross-sectional data to retrospective data on innovation.

A partial solution to these problems has been to consider only programs implemented within the five-year period prior to the study in developing a score of innovation. This tends to limit the effect of extensive early adoption of services and also the possibility that early innovators may no longer be innovative. The use of data for the last five years does, however, produce one conceptual problem. Because a finite number of services are under consideration, some highly innovative organizations may have implemented all or most of the services prior to the five-year period and then moved off into other even more innovative areas which our data do not tap. A partial control for this possibility can be developed using the number of services provided at the beginning of the five-year period.

A second major difficulty in developing an index of innovation based on the 32 services under study is the diversity of the services. As Table 1 shows, a score based on the total 32 services combines a large number of fairly diverse activities. On the face of it, no logical reason exists to assume that homemaker services are comparable to routine cervical cytology, or that speech and hearing rehabilitation are comparable to family-planning case finding. A logical procedure for assuring a greater degree of consistency within an innovation score using the 32 services is to generate a score for each of the six program areas. Such scores, however, seem unsatisfactory for two reasons. On the one hand, services such as family-planning case finding and mental-health case finding may have more in common with one another than with other family-planning or mental-health services. Speech therapy within the home and in-hospital speech therapy, family-planning case finding and mental-health case finding, or integration of either family-planning services or mental-health services with other routine activities of the institution represent similar examples. Consequently, it is difficult even to evaluate the meaning of specific program scores.

At the same time, the services under study do not represent an exhaustive list of activities or services a health establishment might provide. Despite the fact that a real effort has been made to include all services considered to be critical to the successful operation of the six program areas, a legitimate case might be made for other services, or, indeed, for other programs as the focus of study in innovation. Because specific services analyzed leave little potential for generalization to other unstudied services and little potential for discussing the attributes or underlying commonalities of services rather than the services themselves, a means must be found to classify services on some logical basis relative to the nature or effect on the organization.

Fliegel and Kivlin (1966), in a study of the adoption of innovative practices among farmers in the state of Pennsylvania, discuss a number of attributes of practices such as cost, payoff, social approval, and divisibility which may be used to describe such practices. Using judgments by various experts about the attributes of farm practices, they are able to find high correlations between the attributes of a particular practice and the degree of adoption of that practice.

Drawing on the work of Fliegel and Kivlin, a set of potential attribute categories was devised. To arrive at a rating for each of these attributes, a group of judges, all having relevant administrative experience, was asked to rate each of the 32 health care services under study on a set of 10 nine-point scales. The 10 attributes, their definition, the overall mean rating and standard error for both hospitals and health departments are shown in Table 2. While the specifics are discussed in a previous paper (Kaluzny and Veney, 1973), Table 2 shows that the ratings for both hospitals and health departments are quite similar for all attributes. The two possible exceptions are rate of cost recovery where the mean differs by as much as the standard error of the hospital measure, and association with the major activities of the enterprise where the mean differs by half of the standard error. The standard errors of the ratings for both hospitals and health departments are also relatively similar with the exceptions being in initial cost, continuing cost, and social approval where there was slightly more variation among the services for health departments than for hospitals.

For the purposes of this paper the question is whether attribute judgments for each service can be used to classify services into logically related categories. A factor analysis, carried out for each of the 32 services and the mean value of all judgments on the ten attributes, produced two major factors for both hospitals and health departments. The respective factor loadings for the 32 services are shown in Table 3 along with the proportion of variance accounted for by both factors.

Analysis of the two separate factors for hospitals and health departments reveals some interesting characteristics. When the mean attribute score for services with high factor loadings on each factor was compared to the mean attribute score for services with low factor loadings, a pattern emerged. The mean attribute judgment appears in Table 4. Those services which generate high factor loadings in factor 1 for hospitals tend to be judged low in initial and continuing costs and high in payoff, social approval, complexity, clarity of results, association with major activities, and pervasiveness. Those services which generate high factor loadings for factor 1 in health departments tend to be the same types of services as appeared for hospitals. At the same time, the attributes tend to remain quite similar. This includes low initial and continuing cost and high payoff, clarity of results, and association with major activities of the enterprise.

The comparison of mean attribute judgments of those services with high loadings on factor 2 in both hospitals and health departments produces almost a mirror image of factor 1, except for the fact that certain services load high on both factors and certain ones

TABLE 2

Mean and Standard Error of Attribute Ratings
for Hospitals and Health Departments

Attributes	Hospitals		Health Departments	
	$\bar{X}$	*S.E.*	$\bar{X}$	*S.E.*
Initial cost: cost to initiate the use of this particular service or activity in a hospital (health department)	4.96	1.00	4.80	1.40
Continuing cost: cost to provide this service or activity on a continuing basis within a hospital (health department)	5.48	0.87	5.39	1.10
Rate of cost recovery: length of time it takes to return the investment cost of implementing this service or activity in a hospital (health department)	4.68	0.52	5.20	0.65
Payoff: impact the service or activity has in terms of improving the quality and/or continuity-comprehensiveness of overall services or activities provided in a hospital (health department)	7.11	0.71	7.00	0.71
Social approval: amount of increased community recognition gained by the hospital (health department) in providing this service or activity	6.30	0.71	6.45	1.01
Divisibility: feasibility of implementing part of the service or activity on a trial basis in a hospital (health department)	6.04	0.70	6.65	0.93
Complexity: ease with which the objectives of the service or activity can be explained or understood	6.55	0.62	6.58	0.74
Clarity of results: visibility of the implemented service or activity relative to objectives	6.34	0.83	6.46	0.79
Association with major enterprise of hospital (health department): degree to which service or activity has to do with direct patient care of the hospital/preventive services of health departments	6.71	1.00	7.18	1.00
Pervasiveness: degree to which the provision of this service or activity requires other changes in the hospital (health department)	5.98	0.74	5.58	0.64
Percentage which have service	20.46	15.14	28.95	16.17

TABLE 3
Factor Loadings for Each Study Service or Activity

SERVICE AND ACTIVITIES	HOSPITALS		HEALTH DEPARTMENTS	
	Column 1 Low Risk	Column 2 High Risk	Column 3 Low Risk	Column 4 High Risk
Home health				
Social services	.6924	.6117	*.6036	.5449
Home nursing	*.8747	.4560	*.9161	−.3048
Physician services (for coordination and planning of patient care)	*.8892	.3768	*.7632	.3571
Homemaker or health aide	.5922	*.7348	*.7341	.5235
Home-delivered food	.6230	.6401	.6313	.7259
Transportation	.7328	.6187	.6366	.7207
Patient care conferences	.2675	*.8741	−.0373	*.6466
Physical therapy	*.8229	.4714	*.9448	−.0312
Speech therapy	*.7629	.5629	*.8482	.4679
Family planning				
Provision as separate entity	*.8673	.4709	*.9201	−.0538
Provision in conjunction with other services	.5454	*.7770	*.6473	.4622
Case-finding activities	.3098	*.9123	.1274	*.8243
Systematic follow-up procedures	.2133	*.9580	.0015	.4164
Community case-finding activities using indigenous workers	.2616	*.8968	.0582	*.9100
Rehabilitation				
Routine evaluation of all patients	*.7374	.4794	.6837	.6179
Standard nursing procedures	.4674	.4555	.4772	.5733
Physical therapy	*.6320	−.4443	*.9673	.1100
Occupational therapy	*.8795	.2161	*.8429	.5136
Speech and hearing therapy	*.8564	.2660	*.9416	.3004
Mental health				
Outpatient diagnostic and treatment	*.9352	.1727	*.9287	.2581
Inpatient diagnostic and treatment	*.9261	.0122	*.8722	.3197
Use of indigenous workers for case-finding and information dissemination	.2895	*.8964	.1793	*.9646
Integration with other health services	.5597	*.7027	.5779	*.6697
Follow-up care after hospitalization	*.8355	.4388	*.8614	.3323
Medical social work				
Psychological and social consultation	*.8072	.3703	*.7862	.4376
Information and referral	4553	.4441	.3179	*.8265
Predischarge planning (hospitals)	.3702	.5295		
Assist families with legal problems (health departments)			.3549	*.8853
Chronic disease screening				
Cervical cytology	*.6957	.3589	*.8561	.0448
Ocular tonometry for glaucoma	*.7437	.5197	*.6413	.6110
EKG cardiac anomaly	*.8063	.4433	*.8670	.4751
Multiple blood chemistry	*.8466	.1661	*.8108	.5178
Self-administered health questionnaire	.0781	*.9538	−.0437	*.9375
Pct. Variance explained	82.0	13.7	73.5	18.9

* Indicates those services used in computation of high- and low-risk scores.

TABLE 4

Mean Attribute Ratings by Factor: High versus Low Loading

	HOSPITALS				HEALTH DEPARTMENTS			
	Factor 1		Factor 2		Factor 1		Factor 2	
	Loading		*Loading*		*Loading*		*Loading*	
	High	*Low*	*High*	*Low*	*High*	*Low*	*High*	*Low*
Initial cost	4.3 <	6.0	5.7 >	4.5	4.3 <	6.1	5.8 >	4.2
Continuing cost	4.9 <	6.3	6.2 >	5.0	5.0 <	6.5	6.3 >	4.9
Rate cost recovery	4.8	4.4	4.6	4.7	5.1	5.6	5.5	5.0
Payoff	7.4 >	6.7	6.5 <	7.5	7.0	7.0	6.9	7.1
Social approval	6.6 >	5.8	6.0	6.4	6.8 >	5.3	5.8 <	6.9
Divisibility	6.0	6.1	6.0	6.0	6.5	7.0	6.5	6.8
Complexity	6.8 >	6.2	6.1 <	6.8	6.7	6.3	6.4	6.7
Clarity of results	6.7 >	5.7	5.8 <	6.7	6.7 >	5.9	6.3	6.6
Association with major enterprise of hospital (health department)	7.2 >	5.8	5.8 <	7.2	7.4 >	6.5	6.5 <	7.6
Pervasiveness	6.3 >	5.4	5.4 <	6.3	5.6 ,	5.5	5.3	5.7

load high on neither. In general, however, those programs which load high on factor 2 in hospitals are characterized by judgments of high initial and continuing cost, low payoff, low complexity, low clarity of results, low association with the major activities of the enterprise, and low pervasiveness; while in health departments, they are high on judgments of initial and continuing cost and low on social approval and association with the major activities of the enterprise.

Except for the fact that separate factors in this type of analysis are conceptually and statistically assumed to reflect different underlying dimensions, one is tempted to view the services with high loadings on the first factor as primarily low-risk services and those with high loadings on the second factor as high-risk services. Because a substantial proportion of the total variance is contained in factor 1, both for hospitals and health departments, this course takes on additional appeal. While any number of names could be devised to differentiate between factor 1 and factor 2 in each case, it was decided to consider the critical underlying dimension to be the judges' assessment of risk involved in attempting to provide the services. On the basis of this information, two separate measures of innovation were devised for hospitals and health departments.

The first measure for hospitals, the level of implementation of low-risk services (those services marked by asterisks in column 1, Table 3) is a summation of all such services, i.e., home nursing, home physician services, physical therapy, and so on, implemented by each hospital. The second measure for hospitals, the level of implementation of high-risk services (those marked by asterisks in column 2, Table 3) is a summation of all such services, i.e., homemaker, patient care conferences, implemented by each hospital. Similar measures were constructed for health departments using data from columns 3 and 4 of Table 3. Those services with high loadings on both factors were eliminated from consideration as well as those with low loadings, in order to avoid confounding the results.

In accepting these measures of organizational innovation, there is some concern that organizations which had implemented numerous services prior to the last five years would be limited in the amount of innovation they would be able to record in the last five-year period simply because of the limit on the number of programs under study. If, for example, the organization had innovated most of the study services prior to the last five-year period, it would not be able to obtain a high innovation score by the measure being used no matter how innovative the organization actually was during the more recent period. By the same token, an organization having done nothing prior to the last five-year period could potentially implement a number of services during the last five-year period and be classified as highly innovative.

Consequently, before accepting the services implemented in the last five years as a measure of innovation, it was desirable to examine the relationship between that score and both an overall measure of innovation and a measure of the services provided by the organization prior to the last five years. An examination of these data, however, indicates that the measure of services implemented in the last five years as the innovation score is not artificially reduced by the finite limit to the number of services under study.

Table 5 shows the relationship between those services provided in the last five years and the total number of services provided as well as those services provided in the last five years as compared to those provided prior to the last five years. Only with

TABLE 5

Relationship of High- and Low-Risk Services of Hospitals and Health
Departments by Overall Innovation and Innovation Prior to the
Five-Year Study Period

| | INNOVATION WITHIN LAST FIVE YEARS | | | |
| | Health Departments | | Hospitals | |
	Low-risk	*High-risk*	*Low-risk*	*High-risk*
Overall innovation				
Low-risk	.717	—	.756	—
High-risk	—	.848	—	.901
Innovation prior to last five years				
Low-risk	0.48[a]	—	.138[a]	—
High-risk	—	.415 (.05)	—	.226[a]

[a] Not Significant

high-risk programs in health departments is there a significant correlation between those services provided in the last five years and
those provided prior to the last five-year period. This correlation,
moreover, is positive, which indicates that the more high-risk services provided prior to the last five years, the more such services an
organization is likely to innovate within the most recent five-year
period. This finding eliminates our initial concern that the finite
number of services would reduce the number any organization
could innovate over a five-year period relative to those begun prior
to that period. Moreover, the relatively high correlations between
total scores and the scores for the last five years, ranging from .901
for high-risk services within hospitals to .717 for low-risk services
within health departments, lead to the conclusion that the finite
number of services under study will not artificially decrease the innovation score assigned to any one organization. Thus, the number
of services innovated in the last five years in each of these areas is
the operating definition of innovation in this study.

Factors Influencing Organizational Innovation

Selection of the set of explanatory variables used in the analysis was
guided by the Pugh et al. (1963) scheme of conceptually distinct

levels of analysis in the behavior of organizations: (1) context within which the organization is found, (2) organizational structure and function, (3) organizational composition, (4) individual personality and behavior. The last level for our purposes was specified as selected personality and behavioral aspects of the administrator of the hospital or the director of the local health department.

The findings of the major studies of organizational innovation were a second important influence in designating specific factors that might account for variation in the innovation of the respective programs in the two types of organizations. In fact, the empirical analysis reported in this paper was primarily oriented toward considering variables within the conceptual levels of analysis for which some theoretical and/or empirical evidence had alreay been elaborated.[1] Thus, the major emphasis is not only to replicate and test relationships where possible, but, more important, to assess the generalizability of these propositions and/or empirical evidence to the innovation of high- versus low-risk programs in hospitals and health departments.

Organizational Context. Pugh et al. (1963) posit that the socioeconomic context of the organization has primary influence on its structure and function and thus on its innovative activity. Two contextual variables are considered. Size of organization is important to any analysis of organizational innovation simply because it connotes a summary of factors that constitute various organizational resources, complexities, etc. However, there is less agreement as to which aspects of size are related to program innovation and to the differential relationships between type of organization and type of program. Mytinger (1968) finds various indices of health department size, e.g., number of staff, size of budget, and characteristics of the jurisdiction, strongly influencing the innovation of various types of health care programs. Contrariwise, Mohr (1969), in a similar assessment of program innovation in health departments, notes that resources available as a consequence of size have no impact on the proportion of total increase of resources devoted to instituting or expanding innovative health care services. In this

---

[1] Variables already eliminated because of the minimal contribution and/or high correlation with other variables include rule observation, hierarchy of authority, organizational member's values toward change, and professional activism and professional training of the administrator.

analysis, organizational size for hospitals was defined simply as the number of beds within the organization. For health departments, size was defined as the population within the department's jurisdiction. In both cases, we expect organizational size to be positively related to program innovation.[2]

Other contextual variables considered relevant and obviously part of the general composite of variables involved with size are resources and specifically organizational slack. The latter is defined as the existence of uncommitted money or manpower available to the organization (March and Simon, 1964). Although this variable has received limited empirical documentation within health care organizations (Mohr, 1969), the notion as presented by March and Simon suggests that if slack resources exist, various specializations arise with respect to commitment to new programs or program elaboration. Thus, to the extent that variation exists between organizations, the availability of slack resources may differentially influence the amount and type of program innovation.

Two different measures of slack are utilized relative to the type of organization. For hospitals, slack is measured by the ratio involving the number of assistant-associate administrators per bed. It is inferred that the larger the ratio the greater the slack. A comparable measure was not available for health departments; however, as an approximation for this type of organization, slack was measured by the ratio of dollars to population coverage.

Organizational Structure and Function. Organizational structure and function in this analysis include three variables: (a) centralization as defined by the degree of participation in organizational decision making;[3] (b) formalization as defined by the degree to which

[2] Data for hospitals were obtained from the 1969 Hospital Guide Issue. The size of health department jurisdiction was based on data available in the City-County Data Book (1968).

[3] The index of participation in decision making was based on the extent to which individuals indicated participation in decisions concerning the following items: (a) allocation of total organizational income, (b) adoption and implementation of new organization-wide programs and services, (c) development of formal affiliation with other organizations, (d) appointment and promotion of administrative personnel, (e) appointment of medical staff members, and (f) long-range planning for new hospital-wide programs and services. Response categories involved (a) considerable participation, (b) some participation, and (c) no participation. The data were obtained from all respondent groups in both types of organizations.

rules define the person's activity within the organization;[4] (c) perceived performance as defined by the membership's satisfaction with the ability of the organization to meet community health needs and with the organization's reputation in the community.[5]

Although no available data exist on a comparative assessment of these variables in different types of health care organizations or as they relate to programs having different characteristics, there is a fair amount of agreement that both centralization and formalization are negatively related to innovation. Hage and Aiken (1967), in their study of sixteen health and welfare organizations, find that a high degree of participation and low formalization are highly associated with a high rate of program change. Palumbo (1969), in his assessment of health departments, presents similar findings. In a study of a single innovation, i.e., adoption of new drugs in hospitals, Rosner (1968), using a measure comparable to formalization, finds a negative relationship between the degree to which members of the organization follow procedures specified by superiors and that of innovation.

There has been no empirical attention given to performance satisfaction as a factor in organizational innovation. However, following March and Simon (1964), performance satisfaction refers to the amount of satisfaction with the organization's achievement relative to its changing environment. The underlying theory is that the lower the satisfaction with the organization's performance, the

[4] Formalization was based on scales developed by Hall (1963) and was measured by the individual's response to two questions: (1) Are how things are done here left up to the person doing the job? (2) Do most people here make their rules on the job? Response categories involved (a) basically true, (b) basically false, and (c) no opinion. Data were obtained from the administrators, assistant/associate administrators, and all department heads in hospitals and from the director, deputy, all department heads, and a sample of staff public health nurses in health departments.

[5] Organizational reputation was measured by a single question with five response categories: "To the best of your knowledge, what kind of reputation does this hospital (health department) have in the community?" (1) excellent; (2) very good; (3) good; (4) fair; (5) poor. Perceived need was similarly measured: "On the whole, how well do you feel this hospital (health department) is meeting the needs of the community as compared to similar hospitals (health departments) in this area of the country?" (1) extremely well; (2) very well; (3) adequately; (4) not well enough; (5) poorly. For both questions responses were received for all respondent groups within the organization.

greater the probability that programs will be innovated in an attempt to increase the level of satisfaction.

Organizational Composition.[6] Two variables are presented under this category: cosmopolitan-local nature of the staff[7] and the degree of training.[8] Both of these may be considered as a measure of organizational complexity and as such present a direct relationship with the rate of program change (Hage and Aiken, 1967). Empirical data on both health departments and general health and welfare organizations suggest that both these measures have a positive association with program innovation (Mytinger, 1968; Mohr, 1969).

Characteristics of the Administrator. Two basic characteristics of the administrator are considered. The first involves his values toward change and in this sense represents an index of his ability to

[6] Organizational composition variables are what Lazarsfeld and Menzel (1961) term analytical properties of collectivities, i.e., properties of collectives which are obtained by performing some mathematical operation upon some property of each single member.

[7] Index of cosmopolitanism-localism was based on the extent to which individuals within respective respondent groups participated in various professional activities. In hospitals, trustees and administrative staff responded to the degree to which they participated in (a) American College of Hospital Administrators and (b) American Hospital Association. Physicians responded as to their activities in the American Medical Association. In health departments, the members of the board of health, department heads, and staff nurses responded as to their participation in the (a) American Public Health Association and (b) the New York State Public Health Association. Response categories involved (1) attend meetings regularly; (2) have presented paper at meetings; and (3) currently hold or have held office.

[8] We used an organizational complexity scale developed by Hage and Aiken (1967). The index was scored as follows: (a) an absence of training beyond a college degree and the absence of other professional training received a score of 0; (b) an absence of training beyond a college degree and the presence of other professional training received a score of 1; (c) a presence of training beyond a college degree and the absence of other professional training received a score of 2; (d) a presence of training beyond a college degree and the presence of other professional training received a score of 3. Data were obtained for all assistant-associate administrators including department heads in both hospitals and health departments.

accept new concepts and ideas.[9] The second variable is the extent to which the administrator is cosmopolitan in his orientation.[10] Studies which have included the administrator as a unit of analysis strongly support the inclusion of both these variables in any consideration of innovation. Becker (1970), for example, notes that more cosmopolitan administrators tend to be early adopters of programs classified as having high adaptive potential. Similarly, Kaplan (1967), in an assessment of aggregate change, notes that administrators who manifest psychological flexibility have a higher proportion of program innovation. Finally, Mytinger (1968), in his study of health departments, finds the cosmopolitan orientation of the administrator strongly associated with program innovation.

Data Analysis and Findings

Before launching into the analysis of the data, it is necessary to give special attention to organizational size as one of the major variables under study. Organizational size, which has been discussed previously, was measured in hospitals by the number of beds the hospital reported in our interview. The measure of size for health departments was considered to be the number of people within the geographical area served by the health department. In a number of previous analyses of data from a national survey of hospitals and

[9] Index of values toward change was based on scales developed by McClosky (1958). Four questions from the original nine-item scale were selected: (1) I prefer a practical man any time to a man with ideas; (2) if something has existed a long time, there is very likely much wisdom in it; (3) I'd want to know that something would really work before I would be willing to take a chance on it; (4) groups can live in harmony in this country without changing the system in any way. Respondents were asked to "agree" or "disagree" with each of these four items. An "agree" response is a conservative response.

[10] The administrator's cosmopolitan orientation was based on the degree to which he was involved in professional groups. For hospital administrators this involved the American Hospital Association and the American College of Hospital Administrators. For health department directors, this involved the Public Health Association and the New York State Public Health Association. The response categories were the same as those presented in footnote 7.

health departments (Veney et al., 1971) and the New York data, size, either as measured by beds or by population served, has shown itself to be an influential variable. However, some question exists as to whether size per se is a causal variable. Size by its very nature stands as a proxy for a number of other characteristics of the organization. Examining national data, it was found that size of the organization was highly correlated with such things as population density, region of the country, urban/rural locations, and even with mean income and education of the population.

In a simple stepwise multiple regression in which these types of variables are permitted to enter the equation in order of explained variance, size generally serves to eliminate most of the variance which may be attributed to the characteristics of the region in which the organization is located. At the other end of the spectrum, we also found size to be highly correlated with the characteristics of the organization's structure and characteristics of the personnel of that organization. In the data under study, size correlates more highly with overall innovation for both high- and low-risk services and for both organizations than does any other variable with the exception of staff training within the high-risk programs in health departments (refer to Tables 6–9).

Because we believe that size is essentially a proxy for other characteristics of the organization, there are two ways in which size might be viewed. Size can be considered first as essentially a prior causal variable which is in part largely a characteristic of the region of the country in which the organization is located. Thus, densely populated urban areas tend to produce larger hospitals and larger health departments, which in turn attract more capable administrators and more capable staff, and produce a structure which is more favorable and amenable to change. This view of size suggests that the effect of the other variables under study could not be evaluated until the variance attributable to size had been eliminated from the innovation score. Under this assumption, size is an essentially uncontrollable external constraint.

The alternative view of size is as an emergent variable. From this view, growth is a part of the whole host of organizational characteristics, some of which can be manipulated and some of which cannot. Even from this view, size may be in part an uncontrollable external constraint, particularly as it is a function of location. However, size can also be seen as a characteristic of the structure and organization of the hospital, including the characteristics of the administrator.[11]

Given these two alternative views of size, the analysis was carried out both with size included, in which case it is considered to be a prior variable, and with size eliminated from the analysis. In the latter case, size itself is considered to be partly a function of the independent variables under study. Interestingly enough, as may be seen from the column marked R^2 in Tables 6–9, there appears to be an interaction effect between type of service, i.e., high- or low-risk, the organization which is doing the innovating, and the variable size. Table 6 shows that size is independently important to the innovation of low-risk services within health departments, and Table 9 shows that, alternatively, size is important to the innovation of high-risk services within hospitals. In health departments, as shown in Table 6, the over-all significant regression equation allows the prediction of 55 percent of the variance in low-risk innovation score with size included, but only 42 percent of the innovation score with size eliminated. By the same token, in Table 9, the significant regression equation allows a prediction of approximately 31 percent of the innovation score for high-risk services within hospitals, but, with size eliminated, the overall significant regression equation allows only the prediction of 21 percent of the variance in the innovation score for high-risk services.

However, as Tables 7 and 8 show, size is not a critical variable in the prediction of high-risk services within health departments or prediction of low-risk services within hospitals. Fifty-nine percent of the variance in the innovation score for low-risk services can be predicted using size within health departments and about 57 percent can be predicted without size. Similarly, as Table 8 shows, 31 percent of the variance in the low-risk innovation score can be

---

[11] This view of size as an emergent variable does gain some support from the data of the study itself. Thirty-nine of the 59 hospitals under study indicated that they had increased their number of beds in the five years prior to the study date. Twenty of these hospitals indicated that they had changed their size as much as 60 beds or more. At the same time 11 of the 23 health departments under study indicated that they had merged with another health department in the previous five years. These findings lead to an interesting direction for further research—the extent to which the set of independent variables under study here can predict change in size of health organizations over time. This examination remains for further analysis, however.

TABLE 6

Multiple Regression of Health Department Factors in Innovation of Low-Risk Services

Variable	*Multiple R*	R^2	*Simple R*	*B*	*Std. B*	*Beta*
Organizational size	.6273	.3935	.6273	.0053	.0024	.6939
Staff—professional training	.6962	.4847	.3928	.4231	.1856	.4349
Org—cosmopolitanism	.7075	.5005	.4543	.5712	.4425	.2891
Administrator—cosmopolitanism	.7301	.5331	.3817	-.0514	.0431	-.3076
Formalization	.7380	.5446	-.3812	.6813	.8622	.1682
Centralization	.7417	.5501	.1804	-.1990	.3506	-.1202
Slack Resources	.7436	.5529	.1134	-.1548	.4467	-.0619
Administrator—change values	.7442	.5538	.3249	.0739	.4121	.0384
(Constant)				-.5401		

Variable [a]	*Multiple R*	R^2	*Simple R*	*B*	*Std. B*	*Beta*
Org—cosmopolitanism	.4543	.2064	.4543	.8381	.3510	.4242
Staff—professional training	.6038	.3645	.3928	.4690	.1944	.4821
Administrator—change values	.6284	.3941	.3249	.5657	.4147	.2938
Centralization	.6458	.4171	.1804	.3372	.3522	.2036
Organizational performance	.6485	.4205	.2878	-.2392	.6828	-.0707
(Constant)				-16.1713		

[a] Organizational size excluded.

TABLE 7

Multiple Regression of Health Department Factors in Innovation of High-Risk Services

Variable	Multiple R	R²	Simple R	B	Std. B	Beta
Organizational size	.5518	.3045	.5518	.0012	.0008	.3554
Staff—professional training	.7591	.5763	.5984	.2259	.0735	.5041
Slack resources	.7659	.5866	-.0634	.1817	.1846	.1578
Administrator—cosmopolitanism	.7719	.5946	.4656	.0102	.0162	.1331
Centralization	.7732	.5978	.3263	.0580	.1277	.0760
Formalization	.7742	.5994	-.4601	-.1008	.3561	-.0540
(Constant)				-2.6349		

Variable [a]	Multiple R	R²	Simple R	B	Std. B	Beta
Staff—professional training	.5984	.3581	.5984	.2343	.0894	.5225
Administrator—cosmopolitanism	.6066	.4852	.4656	.0210	.0179	.2723
Formalization	.7191	.5171	-.4601	-.3141	.3454	-.1687
Slack resources	.7378	.5443	-.0634	.2014	.2127	.1749
Administrator—change values	.7503	.5630	.3020	.1230	.1865	.1396
Org—cosmopolitanism	.7526	.5664	.3176	.0687	.1948	.0755
Organizational performance	.7536	.5680	.3286	-.0634	.3311	-.0407
Centralization	.7539	.5684	.3263	-.0223	.1691	.0293
(Constant)				-4.1420		

[a] Organizational size excluded.

TABLE 8

Multiple Regression of Hospital Factors in Innovation of Low-Risk Services

Variable	*Multiple R*	*R²*	*Simple R*	*B*	*Std. B*	*Beta*
Organizational size	.3426	.1173	.3426	.0016	.0021	.1174
Staff—Professional training	.4212	.1774	.3165	.3038	.1820	.2211
Org—cosmopolitanism	.4624	.2139	.3403	.4562	.2377	.2906
Administrator—change values	.4893	.2394	.2330	.2757	.1768	.1929
Organizational performance	.5091	.2592	.0893	.5506	.3601	.1989
Centralization	.5363	.2876	−.0034	−.2922	.2184	−.1729
Administrator—cosmopolitanism	.5519	.3046	−.0050	−.0246	.0262	−.1152
Slack resources	.5554	.3085	.1779	.0015	.0023	.0910
Formalization	.5586	.3120	.3018	−.3991	.7784	−.0758
(Constant)				−5.1151		

Variable [a]	*Multiple R*	*R²*	*Simple R*	*B*	*Std. B*	*Beta*
Org—cosmopolitanism	.3403	.1158	.3403	.4905	.2319	.3131
Staff—professional training	.4129	.1705	.3165	.3089	.1811	.2248
Organizational performance	.4497	.2023	.0893	.6365	.3397	.2299
Administrator—change values	.4865	.2367	.2230	.2846	.1757	.1998
Centralization	.5179	.2682	.0036	.2945	.2174	.1743
Slack resources	.5339	.2851	.1779	.0024	.0020	.1423
Formalization	.5442	.2962	−.3018	−.5851	.7342	−.1111
Administrator—cosmopolitanism	.5518	.3045	−.0050	−.0201	.0255	−.0945
(Constant)				−4.3318		

[a] Organizational size excluded.

TABLE 9

Multiple Regression of Hospital Factors in Innovation of High-Risk Services

Variable	Multiple R	R²	Simple R	B	Std. B	Beta
Organizational size	.4851	.2353	.4851	.0037	.0014	.4241
Formalization	.5111	.2613	-.3159	-.4271	.5062	-.1244
Slack resources	.5247	.2754	.0709	.0014	.0015	.1335
Staff—professional training	.5356	.2868	.2006	.1344	.1184	.1500
Centralization	.5430	.2949	.0225	.1361	.1420	.1235
Organizational performance	.5516	.3042	.1481	.2132	.2342	.1181
Administrator—cosmopolitanism	.5574	.3107	.1865	.0117	.0171	.0837
Administrator—change values	.5598	.3134	.0442	-.0458	.1150	-.0491
Org—cosmopolitanism	.5616	.3154	.2472	.0607	.1546	.0594
(Constant)				-.9499		

Variable [a]	Multiple R	R²	Simple R	B	Std. B	Beta
Formalization	.3159	.0998	-.3159	-.8204	.4897	-.2390
Administrator—cosmopolitanism	.3702	.1371	.1865	.0211	.0172	.1520
Organizational performance	.4136	.1711	-.1481	.4286	.2289	.2374
Staff—professional training	.4392	.1929	.2097	.1497	.1177	.1670
Org—cosmopolitanism	.4484	.2011	.2472	.1544	.1560	.1512
Centralization	.4629	.2143	.0225	.1408	.1478	.1278
(Constant)				.6468		

[a] Organizational size excluded.

predicted using size in hospitals and 30 percent can be predicted without size.

These data, then, do not give us a firm mandate for eliminating size as a predictive variable. However, because we wish to examine those characteristics of the organiaztion which may be subject to change and their predictive power in determining organizational innovation, the remaining discussion will be limited primarily to that analysis in which size is not included.

Low-Risk Services

Tables 6 and 8 show the predictive equations for low-risk services within health departments and hospitals, respectively. Forty-two percent of the variance in innovation score for low-risk services within health departments may be attributed to the cosmopolitan orientation of organizational members, training of the staff, values of the administrator toward change, participation of organizational members in decision making, and their perceived performance of the organization. At the same time, 30 percent of the variance in innovation scores for low-risk services within hospitals can be accounted for by the cosmopolitanism of organiaztional members, training of the staff, perceived performance of the hospital, the values of the administrator toward change, participation of organizational members in decision making, available slack in the organization, formalization, and the cosmopolitanism of the administrator. Within both these organizations, the innovation score in low-risk services can best be accounted for, once size is removed, by the degree of cosmopolitanism on the part of organizational members. This variable accounts for 20 percent of the variance within health departments and 11 percent of the variance within hospitals.

The second most important variable in each case is staff training, which accounts for an additional 16 percent of the variance in health departments and an additional 6 percent of the variance in hospitals. Within both organizations, these two variables entered the equations in one-two order. In the ultimate prediction equation, cosmopolitanism of organizational members and training of the staff have the largest beta weights in each instance except within hospitals where performance satisfaction of the organization has a beta weight slightly stronger than the ultimate beta weight of training. The administrator's values toward change, with a beta weight of .29 in health departments and .20 in hospitals, is also important to over-all prediction. However, the perceived performance of the health department, with a beta weight of $-.07$, is not an important variable in predicting innovation of low-risk services, whereas perceived performance recorded a strong beta weight in hospitals.

Nevertheless, the conclusion might be safely reached from Tables 6 and 8 that the innovation of low-risk services, both within hospitals and health departments, may be attributed substantially to the same basic set of characteristics. Thirty-nine percent of the variance in the innovation of low-risk services may be accounted for in health departments by the cosmopolitanism of organizational members, training of the staff, and administrator's values toward change, in that order. The ultimate significant prediction is 42 percent. Twenty-four percent of the variance in innovation score for low-risk services within hospitals can be predicted by cosmopolitanism of organizational members, training of the staff, preceived performance of the organization, and administrator's values toward change, in that order. The significant overall prediction is 30 percent.

High-Risk Services

Within the scores for innovation of high-risk services, there is less obvious consistency than appeared in the case of low-risk services. The predictor equations for high-risk services are shown in Tables 7 and 9. As Table 7 shows, training of the staff is again critical to innovation of high-risk services in health departments. Training entered the equation first and accounts for about 36 percent of the variance explained. The second variable to enter the equation was cosmopolitanism again—in this case not the cosmopolitanism of organizational members but the cosmopolitanism of the administrator himself.

Examining the predictor equation for hospitals in Table 9, one finds a similar result. While formalization, reflecting the extent to which rules do not define individual activity within the organization, is the first and most important variable in the innovation of high-risk services in hospitals, accounting for about 10 percent of the variance, the cosmopolitanism of the administrator again comes in as the second most important variable in the equation and accounts for an additional approximate 4 percent. In this latter case the proportion of variance accounted for is fairly small, and it may be safe to suggest that while it is sufficient to have a highly sophisticated staff for the innovation of low-risk services either within hospitals or health departments, the sophisticated administrator is the critical element in the innovation of high-risk services. Though considerable agreement exists that low-risk services should be provided and that the structure of the organization itself may be sufficient to promote this provision of services, the highly sophisticated administrator essentially provides leadership in regard to the high-risk services if these are to be innovated. This conclusion based on the data at hand may be overly strong but certainly suggests an area for further study.

Further examination of Tables 7 and 9 shows that formalization enters the predictor equation third for health departments, reflecting the same variable in hospitals, whereas the third variable into the equation for prediction of high-risk services in hospitals is again the perceived performance of the organization. Training of the staff and cosmopolitanism of the administrator are the two most critical variables in predicting overall innovation of high-risk services in health departments as indicated by their beta weights, .52 and .27, respectively. In the final overall significant equation, formalization and perceived performance of the organization are the most important in predicting the R^2 for hospitals as reflected by their beta weights, $-.239$ and $.237$, respectively.

One conclusion that might be drawn from these data is that while there are definite commonalities between hospitals and health departments in the characteristics which lead them to innovate either low-risk or high-risk services, it is at the same time important to hospitals that they maintain a high degree of perceived performance. It is possible, of course, to view performance as a dependent variable itself and a function of the number of services provided. However, if one assumes that an organization perceiving itself as having high performance will strive to maintain this performance by continuing to be innovative in the area of health services, performance can be seen as a causal variable. In that sense, performance appears to be much more important to hospitals than to health departments.

The two most critical variables in predicting the overall R^2 for health departments in the high-risk area are training of the staff and the cosmopolitanism of the administrator. Together these account for about 49 percent of a total 56 percent predicted variance. Formalization, cosmopolitanism of organizational members, and the perceived performance of the organization account for 17 percent of an overall predicted 21 percent of the variance and are the three most important predictor variables in hospitals.

Discussion and Conclusions

What can be said about program innovation in a comparative set of hospitals and health departments? Were there differences between the types of organizational variables that affect the innovation of high-risk versus low-risk programs? Were differences in innovation largely a function of the fact that the organization was a hospital or a health department?

The results indicate that organizational size is a critical variable in program innovation as it relates to high-risk services in hospitals and low-risk services in health departments. However, surprisingly enough, size was not a critical factor in the innovation of high-risk services in health departments and low-risk services within hospitals.

While the role of organizational size is not well understood, the above would suggest that the very nature of the two organizations is different vis-à-vis the community. Health departments implement high-risk programs such as patient care conferences, case finding, and information and referral services regardless of department size because their traditional role is to provide services only where such services are not already provided by other community resources. Since these high-risk services are usually not provided by other health agencies, it thus becomes the responsibility of even small health departments to provide such services. In contrast, these high-risk activities are not traditional hospital functions. It is therefore only the large hospitals, where sufficient resources are available, that undertake high-risk types of activities.

The designation of such programs as occupational therapy, speech and learning therapy, and mental-health inpatient services as low-risk reverses this pattern. Hospitals, for example, are more likely than health departments to have such services regardless of size. It is with this type of services that health department size is important because size tends to provide the necessary economies of scale for implementation. For example, only a large health department can justify the inclusion of an occupational therapist in its staff.

In a sense, health departments, by implementing high-risk programs independent of size, suggest a more community-focused organization responding to the particular health needs and demands of the community. Hospitals, on the other hand, take the opposite position and develop a floor of low-risk services that are provided independent of organizational size and implement high-risk programs only in large-scale organizations where sufficient resources are available to support such activities. These findings are consistent with other findings (Kaluzny et al., 1971) in which it is shown that, unlike those of hospitals, the health care programs implemented by health departments do not demonstrate any systematic pattern of implementation, but tend to reflect individual community circumstances.

When we focus on variables within organizations (excluding size), composition variables represented by cosmopolitanism and training of the staff are critical to the innovation of low-risk services in both hospitals and health departments. This variable set is again important to the innovation of high-risk programs in health departments; however, personal variables of the administrator as measured by his own cosmopolitan orientation are an added ingredient to program innovation. A similar pattern is presented for hospitals, except that structure as reflected by less formalized rules defining individual activity within the organization replaces the composition variables, and satisfaction with organizational performance is added as the significant variable.

Thus, it would appear that a pattern emerges for both types of organizations and for both types of innovative services. Composition variables are central to innovation in both hospitals and health departments for low-risk services. These variables are also important to the innovation of high-risk services in health departments except that the personal variables of the administrator become critical for this type of service. On the other hand, structural variables replace composition variables as the primary factor in innovation of high-risk programs in hospitals while again the personal characteristics of the administrator present themselves as a critical variable.

These findings add to the growing body of literature that assesses factors affecting organizational innovation. However, as with most research, more questions are raised than are answered. Several are suggested here as implications for further research. First, empirical attention needs to be given to the concept of innovation as a process. It is quite likely that the process will be influenced by a number of variables on a differential basis. For example, as Wilson (1966) suggests, organizational complexity may positively affect the degree to which innovative concepts are conceived and proposed, but it may have a negative influence on actual implementation. Thus, the nature of the causality must be explicitly introduced, making necessary the conduct of longitudinal studies on a number of organizations.

Second, the study of innovation needs to be broadened to include other predicting variables outside the organization as well as the consequences of such innovation. While this analysis has focused primarily on the organization as the unit of analysis, it is important to consider in greater detail the context of that organization. This research would focus on community and interorganizational variables such as political climate, community decision-making patterns, and the nature and number of interorganizational programs. With regard to the implications of program innovation, consideration also needs to be given to their effect on organizational structure and function. For example, does innovation affect the perception of organizational performance? Do the rate and kind of innovation affect the structure of decision making within the organization?

Third, the study of attributes needs further attention. Although the current data point out the utility of such study in analyzing innovation, attention needs to be given to further methodological refinement in measurement procedures and in the consideration of relevant attributes (Zaltman and Lin, 1971). Moreover, the perception of attributes by organizational participants and how it affects organizational innovation at various points in time is also in need of research.

Finally, while we have been primarily concerned with assessing variables that relate to different types of program innovation and various types of organizations, our findings have obvious bearing on the development and application of change strategies in health care organizations. The results strongly argue against any view of organizational change and/or innovation as a relatively homogeneous phenomenon. The data presented here seem to indicate that factors tend to have a differential effect for different types of programs and for various types of organizations. Any efforts to intervene in an attempt to introduce new programs must take into account these variations.

Arnold D. Kaluzny, PH.D.
Department of Health Administration
School of Public Health
University of North Carolina
Chapel Hill, North Carolina 27514

James E. Veney, PH.D.
Department of Health Administration
School of Public Health
University of North Carolina
Chapel Hill, North Carolina 27514

John T. Gentry, PH.D.
Department of Health Administration
School of Public Health
University of North Carolina
Chapel Hill, North Carolina 27514

This research was supported by Health Services Research Center of the University of North Carolina through Research Grant HS–00239 from the National Center for Health Services Research and Development, Department of Health, Education, and Welfare.

References

Becker, M.
  1970   "Sociometric location and innovativeness: reformulation and extension of the diffusion model." American Sociological Review 35 (April): 267–282.

Fliegel, F. C., and J. E. Kivlin
  1966   "Attributes of innovations as factors in diffusion." American Journal of Sociology 72 (March): 503–519.

Hage, J., and M. Aiken
  1967   "Program change and organizational properties." American Journal of Sociology 72 (March): 503–519.

Hall, R. B.
1963   "The concept of bureaucracy: an empirical assessment." American Journal of Sociology 69 (July): 32–40.

Kaluzny, A. D.
1972   "Innovation in the health system: a selective review of system characteristics and empirical research." Paper prepared for the National Institutes of Health Conference on Medical Innovation, Cornell University, Ithaca, New York.

Kaluzny, A. D., and J. E. Veney
1973   "Attributes of health services as factors in implementation." Journal of Health and Social Behavior (June): 124–133.

Kaluzny, A. D., J. E. Veney, J. T. Gentry, and J. B. Sprague
1971   "Scalability of health services: an empirical test." Health Services Research (Fall): 214–223.

Kaplan, H. B.
1967   "Implementation of program change in community agencies." Milbank Memorial Fund Quarterly 45:3 (July): 321–331.

Lazarsfeld, P. F., and H. Menzel
1961   "On the relation between individual and collective properties." Pp. 422–440 in A. Etzioni (ed.), Complex Organizations: A Sociological Reader. New York: Holt, Rinehart & Winston.

March, J. G., and H. A. Simon
1964   Organizations. New York: John Wiley & Sons.

McClosky, H.
1958   "Conservatism and personality." American Political Science Review 52 (March): 27–45.

Mohr, L. B.
1969   "Determinants of innovation in organizations." American Political Science Review (March): 111–126.

Mytinger, R. E.
1968   Innovation in Local Health Services. Washington, D.C.: Government Printing Office, Public Health Service Publication No. 1664–2.

Palumbo, D. J.
1969   "Power and role specificity in organizational theory." Public Administration Review XXIX:3 (May-June): 237–248.

Pugh, D. S., D. J. Hickson, C. R. Hinings, K. N. MacDonald,
C. Turner, T. Lupton
   1963   "A conceptual scheme for organizational analysis." Administrative Science Quarterly VIII: 289–319.

Rogers, E., and F. F. Shoemaker
   1971   Communications of Innovation: A Cross-Cultural Approach. New York: Free Press.

Rosner, M. M.
   1968   "Administrative controls and innovation." Behavioral Science 13: 36–43.

Veney, J. E., A. D. Kaluzny, J. T. Gentry, J. B. Sprague, and
D. P. Duncan
   1971   "Implementation of health programs in hospitals." Health Services Research 6:4 (Winter): 350–361.

Wilson, J. Q.
   1966   "Innovation in organizations: notes toward a theory." Pp. 195–218 in J. D. Thompson (ed.), Approaches to Organizational Design. Pittsburgh: University of Pittsburgh Press.

Zaltman, G., and N. Lin
   1971   "On the nature of innovations." American Behavioral Scientist: 651–673.

III Hospitals and Health Care Costs

Hospital Rate Setting—
This Way to Salvation?

KATHARINE G. BAUER

Harvard Center for Community Health and Medical Care

Hospital rate setting is a new type of regulatory activity rapidly spreading in the United States. Between 1970 and 1975 the number of rate setting programs grew from two to twenty-seven. These programs, most of which are administered by Blue Cross plans or state governments, now control the hospital rates or charges to one or more major type of payer in twenty-three states, and affect to some degree more than 25 percent of the nation's acute care hospitals (U.S. Dept. HEW, 1975).

The federal government's involvement in hospital rate setting has up to now been minimal. Both Congress and the executive branch have been moving cautiously, made sensitive, perhaps, by the misfortunes that attended the massive switch to cost-based reimbursement when the Medicare program was introduced in 1966. This time, the federal government is closely scrutinizing experience in the states before adopting new methods of hospital reimbursement for Medicare or in plans for the administration of national health insurance.

Congress has, however, offered positive inducements to the states to develop rate regulation. Both the 1972 Amendments to the Social Security Act and the 1974 National Health Resources Planning and Development Act provide for federal support of new state and regional experiments in hospital rate setting and for the evaluation of results of programs in current operation. So far there is no conclusive evidence that rate-setting programs constitute an important means of containing hospital costs.

This paper reviews highlights in the state and regional experience as of 1975. After outlining the nature of rate setting and the impetus behind the movement, it examines some of the major issues that implementation has brought to the fore. In particular, we will

M M F Q / Health and Society / *Winter 1977*
© Milbank Memorial Fund 1977

note the kinds of assumptions on which this new and highly demanding form of regulation was premised, the sometimes contradictory expectations held for it, the strengths and weaknesses of various types of structures for its administration, and certain problems of methodology and information that handicap efforts of rate-setting bodies to accomplish their intended purposes. The final section deals with the kinds of risks and incentives that rate-setting programs introduce to the hospital industry, sometimes by intention, sometimes by inadvertence, and often because of the still limited state of their art.

Case studies of major rate-setting programs conducted or supervised by the author between 1973 and 1975 under contracts with the Social Security Administration provide the material for most of the descriptions and discussions of issues (Bauer and Clark, 1974a, b, c, d; Bauer, 1974a; Arthur D. Little, 1974a, b, c, d, e, f).

The What and Why of Hospital Rate Setting

Controls on the amounts of future reimbursement to which hospitals will be entitled take many forms. "Rate setting," by the purest definition, is only one of these forms. For purposes of convenience, however, we will use the term here in the broadest sense to include any means for determining the financial remuneration of hospitals whereby the amounts to be paid for specified units of service are established by some external authority prior to the period in which the services are to be given.[1]

The rate-setting programs in operation at the end of 1975 are extraordinarily heterogeneous. They operate under different types of auspices and organizational structures, cover different kinds of payers, use different types of methodologies, and present varied degrees of risks and sometimes conflicting incentives. While they pursue a common goal of trying to contain rates of increase in hospital costs, their specific objectives often differ considerably. Some emphasize controls on new spending for facility and program expansions, some stress improved hospital management, and some

[1]One could argue persuasively that this definition should be broadened to include the imposition of ceiling limits beyond which hospital price increases would not be reimbursed, such as under the federal wage-price control program, and under the regulations implementing Section 223 of the Social Security Act Amendments of 1972. For purposes of this paper, however, the narrower definition of rate setting has been used.

simply try to keep hospital cost increases in line with the movement of the general economic indicators. The approaches they use to achieve these objectives range from education, jawboning, and public disclosure to formula-derived rate projections. Their means for resolving conflicts may take the form of negotiation, mediation, and arbitration or of formal hearings, administrative case law precedents, and court decisions.

This diversity among the programs is stressed at the outset to warn the reader against summary statements about rate setting that will inevitably appear in the pages to follow. In fact, as will be seen, there is considerably more commonality in the activities rate-setting agencies *fail* to pursue than in the ones they do pursue. As a major example, no program aims its reimbursement risks and incentives at the physician members of hospital staffs, although all fully recognize that the day-by-day decisions such physicians make in hospitals are by far the most cost-consequential ones. Similarly, no program yet takes into systematic account the considerable differences among hospitals in respect to case mix, patient characteristics, and types of surgical procedures performed, although cost function analyses show these to be highly explanatory factors (Lave and Lave, 1971; Feldstein and Schuttinga, 1975). The most comprehensive study to date, analyzing the experience of all hospitals in two Canadian provinces, showed that diagnostic and age variables together accounted for more than 80 percent of the variation in costs among hospitals (Evans and Walker, 1972).

Finally, although hospitals and rate-setting bodies alike give considerable lip service to the quality issue, no program has tried to use the results of medical audits or other systematic quality of care measures as factors in rate-setting decisions.

Before describing the rate-setting programs in further detail, we will review the reasons behind their development.

The Rationale for Rate Setting as a Cost Control Measure

The current trend toward prospective rate setting rests on the premise that a major reason for the recent rise in hospital costs was the adoption by Medicare and Medicaid of retroactive cost-based reimbursement. By agreeing to reimburse hospitals for the actual "reasonable costs" incurred in providing services to patients, plus a share of depreciation and interest, it is argued, the third-party payers have encouraged these hospitals to spend freely—secure in the knowledge that they will get back whatever dollars they put out.

Former HEW Secretary Caspar W. Weinberger summed up this position when he told the Subcommittee on Health of the House Ways and Means Committee in hearings on June 12, 1975:

> I . . . firmly believe that the faulty design of Medicare and Medicaid is the principal culprit responsible for this super inflation in health care costs. The guaranteed government payment of health care costs in virtually any amount submitted by the provider, and with normal market factors absent in the health care area, inflation was bound to happen, and it did.

The third-party payers adopted one type of defense by the provisions of laws or contracts that excluded certain classes of hospital costs, such as bad debts and research, from the allowable cost-reimbursement obligation. Besides the federal wage-price control program and the Section 223 ceiling limits on Medicare payments, the next major attempt to contain costs through reimbursement has been the move to rate setting. The advantages seemed obvious: if a hospital could know its payment rate before it rendered its services, it would have the highest possible motivation to see that these services were produced in the most efficient manner, since its solvency would depend on keeping its spending within the limits of its anticipated revenues. The hospital would have positive incentives for efficiency as well, since if it could produce its services more cheaply than the predetermined rate had allowed, it could pocket the difference (Feldstein, 1968; Waldman, 1968).

Cost saving through improved hospital efficiency was to be the key: the public statements of theoreticians and program designers alike always stress that cost containment from rate setting will never be at the expense of access or quality.

Thus the rationale for cost containment through rate setting rests on several basic assumptions:

- rising costs are importantly associated with inefficiencies in the delivery of hospital services;
- these inefficiencies can be identified, and are amenable to control by hospital trustees and managers, were they to be so motivated;
- a more public and visible process of rate determination, with external review of institutional practices, can provide such motivation;
- those who establish prospective rates will have the skills and infor-

mation required to calculate rates that will neither underpay nor overpay each individual hospital for the particular mix and quality of products it provides;

the point at which these rates are set will be sufficiently exact to motivate each hospital to overcome the particular inefficiencies in its own production process and to avoid future actions leading to new inefficiencies, but without affecting patient access or quality of care.

None of these somewhat heroic assumptions appears to have been based on empirical observation of the experience of existing hospital rate regulation programs, such as the Canadian experience during the 1960s, nor the accomplishments of rate setting in improving production efficiency in other industries, such as railroads and public utilities. On the contrary, the rush to hospital rate setting appears to have been almost entirely reactive. To state legislators with their feet to the fire of hospital cost inflation, moving away from retrospective cost-based reimbursement seemed only logical; problems of implementing an alternative system of prospective reimbursement could be dealt with as they arose.

To be sure, most Blue Cross plans, already sensitive to the complexity of the issues surrounding hospital reimbursement, entered the arena more pragmatically. Rate setting seemed an approach worth trying; they would learn how to do it as they went along. But whoever the sponsor, little or no systematic analysis was made to project the magnitude of the benefits to be expected from rate setting, nor were doubts expressed as to the ability of rate setters, first, to define the "efficient production" of hospital care, second, to measure efficiency in relation to the quality of the product, and, finally, to fashion incentive and risk structures that would induce behavior changes in the actors responsible for creating the inefficiencies. Nor was the possibility of creating perverse, cost-increasing incentives considered.

The Impetus Behind Rate Setting

While many of the forces that moved Blue Cross plans and state governments to adopt hospital rate setting were unique to each locality, some were widely shared. They are important to understand, since they shaped the objectives of the ensuing programs.

In regions where hospital cost rises were the most precipitous, they forced corresponding rises in Blue Cross premiums that the plans feared might price them out of their markets. State insurance commissions joined them in anticipating insolvencies if the trend could not be halted. Similarly, governors and legislators in a number of states began to fear that rising hospital costs in Medicaid and other state programs if continued unchecked would bankrupt state treasuries. Meanwhile, constituents concerned about their taxes were pressing for controls, while constituents who paid their own hospital bills or were insufficiently protected by indemnity-type hospital insurance were pressing for relief.

Hospitals, too, were early backers of the rate-setting concept; their associations were usually active participants in program design. They saw several types of advantages. First, many hospital leaders believed that most of the rises in operating costs were stemming from a multiplicity of conditions genuinely beyond the hospital administrators' control. They believed that the external reviewing authorities would discover these facts for themselves once they began to scrutinize the details of operating costs. In the face of the public's concern and resentment, the arguments that hospitals mounted in their own defense appeared self-serving. Were the same arguments to be presented by independent rate-setting bodies, the credibility of hospitals would be enhanced.

The hospitals perceived a second advantage, namely in cash flow. Cost-based reimbursement is characterized by long-delayed retroactive adjustments by third-party payers that often plunge hospitals into fiscal crises; rate setting would allow hospital managers to predict their revenues for future periods and keep payments current with expenditures.

Most important, however, hospital leadership saw rate setting as a possible answer to the problem of cost shifting by major third-party payers. As over the years each payer tried to define ever more narrowly the particular hospital costs it would consider "allowable," expenses for items such as free care and losses from emergency room and outpatient care were falling between the cracks, becoming no one's responsibility. Hospitals were increasingly having to load such expenses on the bills of self-pay patients. The American Hospital Association's 1969 *Statement on the Financial Requirements of Health Care Institutions and Services*, a policy statement advocating elimination of such inequalities, proposed changes in reimbursement methods so that all legitimate hospital costs would be covered fairly by all payers. In subsequent guide-lines (AHA, 1972) the association formally accepted the principle that hospital rates be reviewed and set by independent state hospital commissions.

Thus, although the phenomenon of rising costs clearly sparked the move toward rate setting in the 1970s, we find that the major proponents, Blue Cross plans, insurance commissioners, taxpayers, state governments, and hospitals, often had quite different expecta-tions of what rate-setting programs should accomplish. In sum-mary, these diverse objectives included:

- curbing the rate of increase in the *unit price* of services (per diem, billed charges, etc.) for which hospitals would be reimbursed by some *particular class of payer*, such as Blue Cross, Medicaid, self-pay patients;
- curbing the rate of increase in *overall expenditures for hospitaliza-tion*, i.e., unit price times volume of service, for which the taxpaying public and insurance subscribers must eventually foot the bill;
- curbing the *shifts of legitimate hospital costs* from one type of payer to another.

Certain national commissions had even broader expectations, seeing rate setting as one component of a broad armamentarium of measures to bring about system changes that would increase not only the cost effectiveness of hospital care but of total health care expenditures (National Advisory Commission on Health Man-power, 1968).

Unfortunately, the methods employed to accomplish any one of these objectives can well block the attainment of other objectives. For example, the hospital's classic answer to criticism of high unit costs is to stimulate more admissions and increased volumes of ser-vices. Yet increased volumes (unless accompanied by bed reduc-tions) can easily translate to higher total expenditures for hospital care. Further, if volume increases are obtained by rendering types of care that patients do not in fact need, or could obtain less expensive-ly on an ambulatory basis, the level of cost effectiveness will decline.

Again, to the extent that any single class of payer is successful in minimizing his own share of hospital cost increase, the tendency to shift costs to other payers is encouraged. Conversely, successful fair share efforts will inevitably augment the reimbursement obliga-tions of those payers from whom costs had previously been shifted.

In short, a basic schizophrenia of purpose confuses the efforts of many programs and introduces fundamental problems in the evaluation of their results. However, before further analyzing these and other types of issues associated with hospital rate regulation, it will be helpful to review the major features of the various rate-setting programs functioning in the United States as of the end of 1975.

An Overview of Current Rate-Setting Programs

Blue Cross plans and state governments administer most rate-setting programs; in three localities hospital associations do so. The University of South Carolina is conducting a rate-setting experiment in sixteen hospitals.

Under special contract provision, twenty-two of the nation's seventy-four Blue Cross plans currently negotiate or establish Blue Cross rates or charges for their member hospitals. These plans, listed in Table 1, unless designated as pilot programs cover virtually all the hospitals in their region or state. Four Blue Cross plans—Indiana, Kentucky, Missouri and North Carolina—establish charge rates that hospitals voluntarily apply to their self-pay as well as to their Blue Cross patients. The Medicare program, under special waivers, accepts the prospective payment rates set by Blue Cross plans in Western Pennsylvania and Rhode Island as well as by the University of South Carolina program.

Nine states have rate-setting laws. The types of agency that perform the function and the types of payers whose rates they cover are shown in Table 2.[2] It will be seen that four states have independent commissions, with a structure roughly similar to that of Maryland's; five others administer rate setting through some existing state government agency. The unique private-public structure in New York and Rhode Island will be described later.

The unit of payment chosen for control is usually, but not always, that which had been customary for the payer affected. Although the largest number of programs use hospital charges as

[2] An attentive reader comparing Tables 1 and 2 will discover that Colorado and Connecticut have separate rate-setting programs, administered both by Blue Cross plans and by state government. The Colorado Blue Cross plan covers only a few hospitals; in Connecticut, the two programs are estimated to control about 65 percent of hospital revenues.

230

TABLE 1

Blue Cross Plans with Rate-Setting or Review Programs as of January 1976[a]

State or Area within State	Name of Blue Cross Plan	Number of Short-term General and Other Special Hospitals Covered	% Plan Area Population Enrolled in Blue Cross
Connecticut	Connecticut Blue Cross	40	51
Indiana	Indiana Blue Cross	115	38
Kentucky	Blue Cross Hospital Plan	107	43
Missouri:			
Kansas City area	Blue Cross of Kansas City	57	34
New York:	(under state regulations & approvals)		
New York City	Blue Cross-Blue Shield of N.Y.C.	185	73
Upstate	7 upstate plans; as consortium	140	59
North Carolina[b]	Blue Cross and Blue Shield of N.C.	133	34
Ohio:			
Cincinnati area	Blue Cross of Southwest Ohio	35	59
Oklahoma	Blue Cross and Blue Shield of Okla.	40	24
Rhode Island	(with State Office of Budget)		
	Blue Cross of Rhode Island	15	80
Wisconsin	Associated Hospital Service	149	34
Colorado	Colorado Hospital Service	8 (pilot)	36
Michigan	Michigan Hospital Service	12 (pilot)	58
Ohio:			
Cleveland area	Blue Cross of Northeast Ohio	2 (pilot)	56
Pennsylvania:			
Pittsburgh area	Blue Cross of Western Penn.	17 (pilot)	56
Wilkes-Barre area	Blue Cross of Northeastern Penn.	2 (pilot)	57

SOURCES: Communication with Blue Cross Association, January 30, 1976; Hospital Statistics, 1975 edition (1974 data from the American Hospital Association Annual Survey), American Hospital Association, Chicago, 1975; Blue Cross Association Enrollment and Utilization Report, third quarter, 1975.

[a]Blue Cross plans in Delaware and New Mexico also have rate-review and negotiating provisions in their contracts but are not included here because implementation, so far, has been minimal.

[b]Voluntary compliance.

the payment unit, the per diem unit is used in programs that control the largest number of hospitals. Payment by the case and capitation have been tried only in small experiments involving a few hospitals (Arthur D. Little, 1974c; Sigmund, 1968).

Enabling statutes specify the types of providers and payers whose rates are to be regulated. In most states, the rates of nursing homes as well as hospitals are covered. Table 2 shows that the share of total hospital revenues affected by state rate-setting bodies varies considerably; only in Arizona and Rhode Island is the proportion clearly commanding. The absence of control on a hospital's total revenue allows it to make up for an unusually tight rate from one payer by inflating charges to others. The University of South

TABLE 2
Hospital Rate Setting Activities of State Governments as of December 1975

State	Type of State Agency	Number of Hospitals Covered	Type of Payer Rates Currently Regulated	Estimated % of Hospital Revenues Affected
Arizona[a]	Dept. of Health Services	75	Charges to self-pay pts. Blue Cross	85
Colorado	Department of Social Services	89	Medicaid	8
Connecticut	Independent commission	40	Charges to self-pay pts.	30
Maryland	Independent commission	54	Blue Cross Charges to self-pay pts.	55
Massachusetts[b]	Independent commission (full-time commissioners)	133	Medicaid; Charges to self-pay pts. & others	45
New Jersey	Dept. of Health with concurrence of Dept. of Insurance	104	Blue Cross Medicaid	55
New York	Dept. of Health with concurrence of Dept. of Insurance; recommendation from Blue Cross plans	320	Medicaid Blue Cross	55
Rhode Island	State Budget Director with R.I. Blue Cross	15	Blue Cross Medicare Medicaid	90
Washington	Independent commission	119	Charges to self-pay pts. Workmen's Compensation	50–55

SOURCES: Telephone interviews with state agencies, December 1975; January 1976; Hospital Statistics, 1975 edition, American Hospital Association.

[a]Hospital rate review is mandatory under Arizona law, but compliance is voluntary. (To date there has been almost 100 percent compliance.)

[b]The Massachusetts Rate Setting Commission has approval power over the terms of Blue Cross contracts; since the current contract incorporates controls on charges consonant with the state's charge control law for self-pay patients, the 45 percent figure understates the commission's overall leverage.

Carolina's sixteen-hospital experiment is the only place where the rates set cover 100 percent of the payers.

In a later section we will review some of the principal cost containment targets and the mechanisms these programs have developed for reviewing hospital costs and budgets and for projecting rates. First, however, we will discuss certain questions of structure and organization that affect their administrative feasibility and limit or strengthen their power.

Who Sets the Rates?

Successful implementation of a hospital review and rate-setting system requires that there be a sound legal or contractual mandate, an effective organizational base, adequate resources of budget and staff, power to enforce decisions, and a feasible and appropriate rate-setting and appeals process. In most of these matters the issue of who sets the rates is crucial.

Issues Surrounding Rate Setting by State Governments

The clear legal authority given by state legislatures to regulate hospital rates, together with the statement of purpose that usually prefaces such laws, obviously provides a far stronger framework for regulation than do the voluntary contractual arrangements of the Blue Cross plans. The message is clear to all parties that action must and will be taken, and that it will continue over time.

The place within the structure of state government where the rate-setting responsibilities are placed is important, although it will not be discussed at length, since what may be most appropriate depends heavily on the particular history of organizational relationships within each state. Hospital associations prefer the independent commission model. They object on principle to having any one of the major third-party payers, such as a state department administering Medicaid, given the responsibility for setting rates, claiming that for a major purchaser of service to determine the price at which it buys that service constitutes a clear conflict of interest (AHA, 1972).

The case for rate-setting commissions is also made on grounds of independence from the direct political interference to which regular agencies of state government are usually exposed. Such independence, of course, also complicates the process of public accountability unless there is an accompanying public disclosure law.

In states with large numbers of hospitals, rate-setting responsibilities appear to demand full-time, well-paid commissioners; so far only the Massachusetts law provides them. The composition of commission membership is obviously important to both its acceptance and its effectiveness. Systematic analysis of what constitutes desirable numbers, types, and proportions of consumer and provider representation has yet to be made.

The commission structure predisposes toward certain problems in the rate-setting and appeal process. John Dunlop, the former Secretary of Labor, commenting on regulation in other types of industries, recently cited two of these (Dunlop, 1975). First, the traditional regulatory approach discourages the posture of negotiation; the rule-making and adjudicatory procedures prescribed in administrative practice laws mitigate against the development of mutual accommodation among conflicting interests. Second, the regulatory process

> ... involves legal game-playing between the regulatees and the regulators; the tax law is a classic example, but it is typical of regulatory programs in general. The regulatory agency promulgates a regulation; the regulatees challenge it in court; if they lose, their lawyers may seek another round for administrative or judicial challenge.

Meanwhile time passes—the regulatory lag. And legal services become one more factor in hospital costs. The stakes in legal battles are high, particularly during the first few years of a new regulatory commission's life, since the case precedents that are set will set the limits on its future activities. It is not improbable to suppose that more time and skills may be devoted to beating the system in the courts than are devoted to improving efficiency in the hospitals.

Placement of the rate-setting function within an established state agency may provide more flexibility. If that agency also has concurrent responsibilities for other regulatory functions affecting hospitals, such as licensing, inspections, planning, and certificate of need, such placement should minimize duplications of hospital reporting requirements and avoid regulations written at cross purposes. Most important, a centralizing of regulatory functions should force the agency to formulate some coherent overall health policy and regulatory strategy for the jurisdiction it covers. In such a context, rate setting could become an effective tool for coordinated policy implementation, particularly if such an agency also sought to forge links to PSROs for utilization and quality controls and to HSAs for planning (Dowling and Teague, 1975).

Opportunities for synergism through the concentration of regulatory powers may be more apparent than real, however, since problems of noncommunication and bureaucratic rivalry can impede coordination among the separate offices within a single large agency almost as effectively as they do among the offices of separate agencies. For example, the 1975 Moreland Commission exposed an almost total lack of interchange between the nursing home inspection and the rate-setting divisions of the New York State Department of Health (New York State Moreland Act Commission, 1975).

Wherever the rate-setting function may be located within state government, certain endemic problems are likely to handicap its effective implementation. One is the familiar bricks-without-straw phenomenon, where state legislatures pass laws that require state agencies to perform new functions, but fail to pass the budgets that are needed for proper implementation. This was dramatically illustrated in New Jersey in 1971 where an unusually well-drafted law centralized a host of health regulatory functions, including hospital rate setting, in the State Department of Health—with no new funding (Somers, 1973). In consequence, for two years the department was able to assign only one full-time staff member to carry the rate-review responsibilities for New Jersey's 104 hospitals.

Currently, programs that promise to contain hospital costs have sufficiently high political visibility to make extreme under-budgeting of this kind unusual, but even now most state rate-setting executives feel severely handicapped by budget constraints. The Maryland commission, after eighteen months of operation, has not yet been able to conduct rate reviews of all the Maryland hospitals. Looking ahead, with many state governments entering severe fiscal crises, one cannot be sanguine about funding continuity even at present levels.[3]

Another set of endemic problems arises from state civil service regulations governing job classifications, salary scales, recruitment, examinations, and promotions. In many instances these seem almost programmed to discourage the employment of rate-setting staff with capabilities to carry out the complex and important responsibilities with which they are charged. It is tribute to the devotion and imagination of rate-setting program administrators that

---

[3]Rate-setting commissions can, if their enabling law permits, raise the revenue for their operations from special assessments on hospitals which can then include them as costs allowable for reimbursement. This type of arrangement, endorsed by the AHA guidelines, is criticized by some legislators because it removes the public accountability of the rate-setting body. One way out is to have assessments support the program but flow through a special state fund ewhich can be used only with the approval of the legislature.

they manage as well as they do. However, most of the leaders in state rate-setting bodies today are unusual people, attracted by the challenge offered for developing programs in a new and important regulatory area. It is doubtful that many current incumbents will want to be at these same posts five years hence, and that replacements of the same caliber will be available. Again, looking to the future, one must speculate whether there is anything intrinsic to hospital rate regulation that is apt to make its long-run core staffing prospects much different from any other type of state regulatory body.

Even though state legislatures grant formal authority to rate-setting bodies, there are very real political constraints on the amount of power these bodies can actually exercise. If their actions prove to be sufficiently unpopular, laws can be changed, or already slim appropriations further cut. As the history of community battles over certificate of need has so well documented, constituents of legislators are markedly ambivalent about their community hospitals: they want costs to be controlled overall, but at the same time, they want their own hospital to be fully equipped and staffed to give them the care they need at the moment they need it. By the same token, they fight proposals for service closings.

The problem appears to be common to other types of regulatory bodies as well. Noll, in a Brookings Institute report on regulation (1971), observes:

> One measure of success of the [regulatory] agency is continued operation of the regulated sector. Widespread service failure is likely to be blamed on the agency, and is therefore to be avoided even if the cost exceeds the costs of the service failure.

Finally, there is the familiar problem of the capture of regulatory agencies by the industries they regulate. Noll offers the following explanations of this phenomenon:

> There is little political gain in effective regulation. Once a regulatory agency has been established to deal with an issue of public concern, public attention is apt to shift to new issues. While the stake of the public may still be high, it is diffused.

> [However] . . . most regulatory issues remain of continuing deep interest to the regulated industry. Its economic viability may rest on the agency decisions. The industry's motivation to fight unfavorable decisions is very high. . . .

> [A] . . . measure of success is the failure of the courts or the legis-
> lature to override agency decisions on either procedural or substantive
> grounds. An agency that tries to minimize the chance of being over-
> ruled must, when the interests of the regulated firm and the public are
> at odds, be overly responsive to the interests of the regulated. It wants
> to be sure it cannot legitimately be accused of being unfair to the
> groups that are most likely to challenge its decisions.

According to this observer, whether the agency is independent or
located in the executive branch of the government, or whether it is
headed by a single administrator or is collegial, does not seriously
affect its essentially pro-industry proclivities in the long run (Noll,
1971).

Hospital associations, however, sensitive to the political
climate, usually recognize the importance of efficiency objectives to
a greater extent than do their individual hospital members. Even if
regulatory policy is dominated by the industry, Ginsburg observes
(1976), this difference in perspective should result in a lower price
than if there were no regulation.

Blue Cross Programs

Programs administered by Blue Cross have two large advantages
over those administered by state government: they can usually command the budget, staff, and computer resources they feel to be
necessary to implement their rate-review processes in an equitable
manner, and they can be more flexible in the rate-setting processes
they design. Program costs are paid for out of subscriber premiums.
As long as the plan's board of trustees is satisfied that the program
is cost-effective, funding will continue. Furthermore, because Blue
Cross programs are not subject to the job classification restraints of
civil service, they can attract to their rate-review staffs people with
intimate knowledge and understanding of hospital operations, such
as ex-hospital controllers and accountants, who know what areas of
inefficiency to look for and who can successfully defend their decisions during appeals. Finally, Blue Cross programs have much more
flexibility than state programs. They are free to design rate-setting
processes that incorporate various mixes of educational,
negotiational, and formalistic approaches, and to modify these approaches over time in the light of subsequent evaluation.

On the other hand, the Blue Cross programs labor under their own special handicaps. In most states, participation is entirely voluntary; hospitals may decide not to participate at all. Or, once participating, if they feel the program is too strict, they may withdraw. (They have rarely done so, but this may only reflect their best guesses as to likely alternatives.) Second, lacking a legal mandate for their programs, Blue Cross plans may not be able to secure all the types of data they might wish from the hospitals on which to base their rate decisions. Finally, they are likely to receive scant recognition from their subscribers for their efforts. As with other types of cost-containment efforts by Blue Cross plans, the costs of running such programs inevitably appear in larger administrative budgets—making the plans open to charges of "inefficiency" by critics and competitors who assume no such responsibilities.

The Model of a Mixed Public-Private Structure

Since Blue Cross and state government rate-setting programs each have certain specific strengths and weaknesses, the possibility of their cooperation in carrying out rate-setting responsibilities offers an attractive alternative. In this model, the legal authority for hospital rate setting and for the securing of necessary data on which to base rate decisions comes from state laws, but the limited staff and budget usually available to state government agencies can be augmented by sharing implementation responsibilities with Blue Cross, which can bring a more appropriate level of resources to the task. This type of complementary activity is currently taking place in three of the nine states with rate-setting laws.

In Massachusetts, Blue Cross auditors are regularly detailed to work in the state rate commission office to supplement the core staff; they review hospital costs reports and conduct a large proportion of the commission's hospital audits. In New York state, the Department of Health establishes the regulations that determine the rate-setting process for Blue Cross as well as for Medicaid, promulgates standard hospital reporting forms, and makes final decisions on all rates and rate appeals. But the department permits the eight Blue Cross plans to conduct their own analyses of member hospitals' costs and submit recommendations on future Blue Cross rates for member hospitals.

In Rhode Island, under state law the state Director of the Budget has final authority to approve hospital budgets, but Rhode

Island Blue Cross staff conducts most of the analyses on which the budget negotiations are based. The Budget Office has access to all such analyses, as well as to the data on which they are based, and thus needs only a small staff with which to conduct monitoring activities and special studies. The Budget Director's staff representative participates in hospital budget negotiations side by side with Blue Cross officials.

These sorts of partnerships may serve to diffuse the heat of possible opposition to tough rate-setting decisions that might well weaken or destroy either of the partners were they to act singly. On the other hand, political risks always attend a state government agency's dependence on outside technical assistance.

Having noted these various types of structural constraints on currently operating rate-setting programs, let us examine their objectives and the mechanisms they employ to pursue them.

Rate-Setting Objectives and Processes

We saw earlier that third-party payers, legislators, and hospitals have looked to hospital rate setting as a means to accomplish different purposes. In the interest of space, we will not consider here the hospitals' goal of achieving fair share payments by third-party payers, but will confine our discussion to the goals of containing increases in hospital prices and of containing increases in overall expenditures for hospitalization without attendant sacrifice of access or quality.

The central issue is how to set rates in a manner that will neither underpay nor overpay, but will encourage each institution to increase the efficiency with which its services are provided. One overriding obstacle to accomplishing this is lack of any reliable way to define or measure the efficiency of most patient care services of hospitals. Another lies in the large number of hospitals to be regulated and their great diversity in patient mix; case severity mix; medical staff training levels; scope and quality of services; size, age, and characteristics of physical plant and equipment; financial reserves and endowments, and so on. So far, as we have already noted, many of these basic types of data are either not available or not used. Even when the required data become available, it will be some time before techniques to weigh and correlate the differences among hospitals are sufficiently refined to permit reliable judgments as to whether given levels of costs are justifiable or whether they reflect inefficiencies.

Thus, most rate-setting bodies must carry out their mandates to contain costs with few clearly defined notions of where specific spending excesses may lie. The tripartite mission of many hospitals—teaching and research as well as patient care—serves further to complicate their task. Finally, rates must be set in the realistic context of whether hospitals can, in fact, control many types of costs that rate setters may identify as unjustifiable. They soon come to recognize, for example, the very limited power of hospital administrators and trustees to change the cost-inducing behavior of their physicians.

Specific Cost-Containment Objectives

The objectives to be pursued by rate-setting programs are usually set forth in state enabling laws and as part of preambles to Blue Cross contracts or contract amendments. Characteristically they state that:

- rates (or budgets, or charges) should be related to the efficient production of hospital services of good quality;
- excess hospital costs that may be associated with duplications of services and facilities should be discouraged.

Several also provide that:

- increases in hospital rates should be linked to increases in the prices of goods and services in the general economy.

Only in the 1975 Rhode Island experimental program under a Social Security Administration contract are rates set within the limits of some overall ceiling on an increase of total expenditures for hospital care in a geographic region. The rate-setting program and the hospital association arrive at the percentage figure for this state-wide maxi-cap annually, through a strenuous process of negotiation some months before the hospitals submit their budgets for review. Subsequently, the reviewers negotiate each hospital's budget within the limit of the total increase—with the freedom to give higher increases to some and lower to others. Here, for the first time in the United States, rate-setting bodies are being forced to make choices in cost allocations among hospitals, rather than considering each case entirely on its own merits in an open-ended situation.

State rate-setting bodies usually have considerable latitude in translating the broadly stated objectives of enabling legislation into regulations and guidelines that either implicitly or explicitly specify particular targets for cost containment. Such regulations usually state certain intermediate rate-setting goals and set out mechanisms for achieving them that appear to be politically, administratively, and technically feasible in the context of their local environment. Blue Cross contract provisions, on the other hand, usually specify objectives explicitly and spell out the rate-setting process in full detail.

Almost all programs try to hold down capital costs through cooperation with certificate-of-need programs; their own major program efforts focus on the control of operating costs. Targets for cost containment usually include one or more of the following, in descending order of frequency:

- control of *increments to interest and depreciation* from unapproved facility construction or expansions;
- control of *increments to operating costs* from new medical programs, additions to personnel and supplies in existing programs and services, expanded fringe benefits, contracted services, and so on;
- encouragement of *improved management*, better internal budget and control systems;
- encouragement of the *phasing out of underutilized beds and services*;
- detection of *inefficiencies in base costs*, particularly in the hotel and support service departments;
- identification and *reduction of departmental cross-subsidies*.

Rate-setting programs may or may not explicitly spell out such target objectives. Often, their actual goals must be ascertained from interviews with program executives, from analysis of regulations or rate-review guidelines, and from observation of the rate-review process. Furthermore, there appear to be considerable differences in the intensity with which these various goals are actually pursued.

The types of containment *not* pursued through rate setting should also be noted. Only Rhode Island's program attempts to identify and reduce excessive lengths of patient stay. With this single exception, none of the programs uses its rate-setting power to reduce hospitalization costs that might be associated with inappropriate patient care management such as unnecessary surgery, unnecessary tests or drugs, or delays in treatment scheduling. Nor do the programs adjust rates to reward quality controls that minimize the extra hospital costs associated with complications resulting from hospital infections, from drug synergisms, or from other iatrogenic conditions. Again, although most program executives privately deplore the often six-digit remuneration of hospital-based physicians such as radiologists and pathologists, in this area too, controls are rarely attempted.

In short, as noted at the onset, rate setting rarely attempts to influence the huge segment of hospital costs generated by physician actions.

Scant effort is made through rate structure to promote hospital-based alternatives to inpatient care—such as day surgery units, home care programs, or preadmission testing. Widespread introduction of such services, designed to reduce overall expenditures for hospitalization and overall medical costs would, of course, force up the per diem or other unit costs for the more complex cases still requiring acute-care inpatient services. If the rate-setting body is evaluated according to its success in moderating increases in unit prices, over the course of time such actions would be counterproductive in terms of its own institutional viability.

Methods of Determining Rates

There is no established wisdom to guide hospital rate setting. Most programs are still struggling to develop a satisfactory process; they make changes in their methods almost yearly. Basically, however, in every program next year's hospital rates will in one way or another be based on this year's rates; modifications of natural trends will be relatively modest. No program starts the rate-setting process with the concept of zero budgeting.

Rate setters reach their decisions in one of a number of ways:

- special reviews of the costs, budgets, and volume of each individual hospital in the light of its own characteristics;
- interinstitutional comparisons;
- rate increases tied to movement of economic indicators;
- recommendations of planning agencies;
- some combination of these methods.

In all but a few programs rates are set annually, for all hospitals, either as of a given calendar date or at the beginning of the hospital's fiscal year.

Cost-Budget Reviews   The Blue Cross and hospital association programs tend to establish rates on the basis of cost and budget reviews that focus primarily on cost trends within the individual hospital. Reviews usually include line-item scrutiny of all budgeted additions to facilities, services, and personnel, and close analyses of cost trends in each hospital department. This rate-setting method reflects in part the preferences of hospitals, in part the belief that a strenuous but equitable review process itself serves to make hospital officials more cost conscious, to force the setting of internal priorities for expansion requests, and to motivate hospital managers to improve their own budgeting and to exercise better internal controls. Once the reviews have been conducted and budgets or rates approved, the hospital is usually free to make budget transfers within the bottom line amount. Most programs try to avoid infringing on management prerogatives.

Interhospital Comparisons   State programs tend to rely heavily on interinstitutional comparisons. Adopting one or another method of classifying hospitals into comparison groups, they perform analyses by service, department, and/or cost center. Employing screening methods, these analyses identify statistical outliers of preestablished parameters around the mean or median of each hospital group. Most programs then individually review the more costly outlier hospitals or hospital departments, giving opportunity for justification before establishing the final rates. Others, notably the New York state programs, automatically adjust the rates of outlier hospitals downward to the preestablished ceiling[4] (Bauer and Clark, 1974d).

The same types of information are used for individual reviews and interinstitutional comparisons, although each program has designed its own report requirements to suit its own objectives and methods. Hospitals submit annually some type of uniform cost and budget report to the reviewing agency. At a minimum, this includes

[4]New York does not ask for budget projections from the hospitals. It calculates future rates solely on the basis of cost trends from the prior to the current year, and projected inflation rates. Massachusetts employs this type of formula to set its Medicaid rates, but employs different methods to control charges for self-pay patients.

general statistical and financial descriptors of the hospital and counts and projections of its activity measures (patient days, clinic visits, and so on). At a maximum, the report may include detailed descriptors of medical staff, teaching programs, scope of services, contracts and leases, long-term capital budgets. The report packages run from twelve to forty-eight pages of schedules. As of December 1975, only one program (again, Rhode Island) sought any patient-related information on case mix or the age or sex of the patients for whom the hospital was caring. This program obtains standard reports derived from abstracts of the records of all patients discharged from Rhode Island hospitals each year, using the Professional Activities Study report system.

Limiting Rate Increases to the Rate of Inflation   The New York, Massachusetts, and Western Pennsylvania programs explicitly tie hospital rate increases in allowable costs to corresponding wage and price trends in the general economies of their regions. Elaborate indices have been designed for use in making projections. Automatic adjustments are usually made at quarterly or six-month intervals during the rate year, to adjust the rates to the actual movement of the designated economic indicators. During the early years of the two New York programs affecting New York City hospitals, adjustments for underprojections were not routinely made. This was one of the several contributing causes of their widespread fiscal distress, documented by Rossman (Hospital Association of New York State, 1975).

Most of the other programs, while not employing formal economic projection indices, informally adopt some rule of thumb percentage increase in rate that they will consider to be reasonable in their budget reviews for the coming year, a target that serves the same purpose but that is more flexible. Hospitals that are dissatisfied may request special cost and budget reviews based on interinstitutional comparisons.

Increments to Operating Costs   Budget increments for operating costs due to changes in facilities or services during the prospective rate year can be easily identified through the use of appropriately designed reporting forms. The problem lies in determining, on a line-item basis, whether or not the proposed new expenditures are necessary. Programs that conduct individual hospital reviews reach these decisions before setting the hospital's rates; in a formula system, they are reached after the rates have been set, through individual hospital appeals. In either case, decisions must ultimately be reached on the basis of subjective judgment of the reviewers. The process is almost always time-consuming and fraught with emotion and is the source of the greatest tension between the parties at interest.

Decisions on adding to the rate the cost of interest and depreciation for new facilities are usually left to planning agencies; if a certificate of need or formal approval is forthcoming, the rate-setting agency usually agrees to make the necessary rate adjustment. Since in many areas the effectiveness of planning agency reviews is questionable, such controls are often more apparent than real. Some rate-setting programs, however, notably those of Washington, New York, and Rhode Island, work in close collaboration with planning agencies in mutually reinforcing arrangements (Bauer and Altman, 1975).

A few programs, such as Maryland's, reserve the right to make independent determinations on capital expansions, arguing that even though a community need for an additional hospital facility or service may have been found to exist, the capability to pay for it through the reimbursement rate may not. In such cases, the community and the hospital must raise the operating funds for the added service in addition to the necessary capital.

The New York state program is particularly stringent in regard to new services and facilities. In general, its formula for rate projection adjusts *only* for wage and price increases, except when new costs are authorized after a process of formal appeals. This assumes that the identical hospital product is to be produced in 1977 as was produced in 1970, when the cost control program began.[5] Even when appeals for changes in facilities or services are granted, since rate projections in New York are based solely on historical costs rather than budgets, support for a new program will not be fully included in the rate until several years have elapsed. In Massachusetts no new operating costs are recognized for one full year. Such refusals to subsidize start-up costs also discourage expansions.

Identifying Out-of-Line Costs in the Base Year Most rate-setting programs are fully aware that simply projecting a hospital's base

[5]Blue Cross plans in upstate New York, however, include a factor to allow for changes associated with new technology.

costs forward to construct future rates provides license for the indefinite perpetuation of existing inefficiencies. A weakness of rate-setting methods that rely on statistical screens to identify hospitals for special review is that they have no means to detect inefficiencies in the hospitals that fall within their allowed cost parameters: that is, they assume that low costs are equated with efficiency rather than other factors such as case mix, quality differences, or exogenous factors. Individual budget reviews offer more possibilities, but most reviewers admit that with the kinds and quality of data and analytic tools presently available to them, their power to detect all but grossly out-of-line situations is severely limited. Only the university sponsored program in South Carolina employs industrial engineering consultants to work with hospitals to identify and correct specific areas of low productivity. (In both rate-setting and nonrate-setting states, however, individual hospitals are, on their own, increasingly using management science consultants to improve internal operating efficiency.)

Phase-Outs of Underutilized Beds and Services A number of programs try to attack the problem of continued low occupancy. Some, like those in Massachusetts and New York, impose rate penalties when average occupancy rates fall below preestablished minimum levels, for example, 80 percent for medical-surgical, 70 percent for pediatrics, and 60 percent for obstetric services. By establishing rates that fail to subsidize excess costs from underutilization, they hope to encourage appropriate bed reductions. Other programs try to achieve this purpose indirectly through their interhospital comparisons of unit costs, to identify services where utilization is low but staffing remains high. To detect these kinds of inefficiencies requires that the true unit costs of direct services be compared. This means that for purposes of the analysis, at least, the traditional cross-subsidization of services within hospitals, whereby revenues from departments like the laboratory make up losses from departments like the emergency room, must be eliminated. Also, direct costs are isolated for comparisons before indirect cost allocations are made.

Some Obstacles to Achieving Cost Containment with Equity

As we have seen in the foregoing section, the several different types of processes used in rate setting employ different types of methodologies and demand different types of information.

To reach decisions on new facilities and new medical programs requires guidelines and supporting data for determining community need, and reliable methods for projecting the capital and future operating costs attendant on hospital expansions.

To tie future hospital rates directly to the movements of wages and prices in the general economy of an area requires the development of an economic index constructed of items selected and weighed to reflect the particular types and mix of labor and supply items hospitals use to produce their services, and reliable data reported at frequent intervals for small areas. Although technical difficulties surround each of these tasks, the early 1970s have witnessed considerable progress (Gort et al., 1975; Berger and Sullivan, 1975). A major block to further refinement is the lack of Bureau of Labor Statistics wage and salary data for small geographic areas, since important variations in these factors may exist even within the boundaries of counties and of metropolitan areas. Inequities in projections that are inevitable during periods of rapid inflation can be compensated for by quarterly or semi-annual adjustments in rates during the prospective year. Unexpected factors over which hospitals have no control, such as the recent rise in malpractice insurance premiums and in fuel prices, can also be handled by periodic across-the-board rate adjustments.

The major problem with tying rate increases to inflation increases is that the mechanism does nothing to improve hospital operating efficiency. On the contrary, unless linked to a hospital review process as in the Western Pennsylvania Blue Cross plan, it protects and perpetuates any existing inefficiencies by projecting their costs into the future. At the same time, such formula projections make no allowance for innovations that may contain or reduce long-term episodes of illness and thus case costs, if such innovations demand short-term expenditures that drive up the unit costs of particular types of patient services. Again, however, a sensitive review and appeals process, though cumbersome, can mitigate this danger.

Occupancy minimums designed to encourage hospitals to phase out underutilized services or effect mergers with other hospital services are easy to promulgate. But any hospital service reduction generates strong resistance by physicians since their livelihood may depend on continued access to that hospital. Therefore, unless utilization minimums are accompanied by moves toward opening up staff privileges and by regular feedback from effective utilization reviews, physicians can respond by ordering unnecessary volumes of care in order to avoid ceiling penalties. Again, the program may be able to demonstrate success in moderating unit prices, but the defensive actions taken may serve to increase the community's total expenditures for hospital care.

Whether the kinds of *indirect penalties on underutilization*, such as Maryland's, will work better remains to be seen. Much still remains to be learned about the complex art of volume prediction and volume adjustment; it is an area where hospitals can play many types of defensive games. In general, hospitals whose unit costs rise because of uncontrollable shortfalls from the predicted volume eventually obtain rate adjustments; those whose unit costs decline because of volume increases up to the limits of allowable parameters (if any), benefit.

To assess hospital efficiency calls for enormous leaps forward from where we stand today in our methodological capabilities.

Individual budget reviews, while offering important possibilities for achieving desired kinds of change in hospitals, are usually criticized for lacking objectivity, since decisions are reached on an ad hoc "best judgment" basis. Hospitals that can muster the accountants and physicians to plan an effective case, it is argued, have unfair advantage. However, the same criticism holds for the special reviews given to "outlier" hospitals identified by statistical screens. It also applies to the large volume of hospital appeals under a formula rate projection such as New York's. This is because rate setters under any method of review lack reliable standard performance measures on which to base their decisions. In the end, the reviewers must reach their decisions according to the plausibility of each particular case on the basis of the best evidence they can muster.

The lack of performance standards by which to measure hospital efficiency is the most intractable problem in rate-setting methodology. Most programs during their first years hopefully set out to develop such standards to guide them in setting rates that are "reasonably related to the efficient provision of hospital services of good quality." However, if one accepts a definition of "efficiency" to mean using the most economical, timely, and efficacious mix of labor, materials, and skills to generate a particular product of a given quality, the inherent problems these rate setters face in trying to develop standards become clear.

First, in the patient care services of hospitals it is usually impossible to identify, much less quantify, the actual product that is being produced, that is, specific degrees of improvements in health status and/or alleviation of suffering of the patients who come to the hospital for care. Even were these products to be defined, it is far from clear in many instances just what types, mixes, and timing of labor, materials, and skill inputs are efficacious in producing them (Cochrane, 1972). Finally, as we noted earlier, whatever monitoring of quality does exist, such as through medical audits and PSRO studies, is not reported to rate-setting bodies. Thus rate setters find themselves reduced to using surrogate measures of product, of process, and of quality—such as "patient days," "number of tests," and "accreditation"—measures whose inadequacies have long since been demonstrated (Berki, 1972; Institute of Medicine, 1974; Rutstein, 1974). The pervasive temptation for rate setters simply to equate low cost per unit of service with "efficient production of hospital services of good quality" is only too understandable.

Lacking the ability to develop performance standards for patient care services, and reluctant to impinge on physician prerogatives, rate setters often content themselves with trying to control the more peripheral types of costs that are incurred in the hotel and maintenance departments of the hospital. Even here, however, few reliable performance standards exist. Again, the output measures are widely agreed to be unsatisfactory (Bauer, 1975). For example, when reviewers detect twofold differences between two hospitals' housekeeping costs per square foot, they may have spotted genuinely inefficient deployment of resources in the high-cost institution—but on the other hand, closer examination may reveal that the spread in costs reflects only differences in architectural layout, in building construction, and in traffic volumes. Management studies in individual hospital departments can indeed spot areas of inefficiency and develop standards that may point the way to savings (Hardwick and Wolfe, 1972). On the other hand, substantial cost containment from rates adjusted according to preestablished regionwide performance measures has yet to be demonstrated (Wolf, 1973; Elnicki, 1975).

Attempts to identify hospital inefficiencies by using inter-hospital comparisons have been fraught with several other types of difficulties. First, because of the wide diversity of hospitals, it is difficult to identify the key variables and to account properly for them in making comparisons. Second, both the scope and quality of the information reported from hospitals leaves much to be desired.

For rate-setting programs that rely on comparative analysis to screen for inefficiency, *equitable selection of the comparison hospitals is essential*. There are various classification schemes by which to group hospitals (Bauer, 1974b). Most use only very crude variables such as size, urban versus nonurban location, and teaching status. This leads to considerable debate and special pleading during individual hospital reviews, as each institution brings forth data to show the many important respects in which it differs from its comparison group hospitals. In formula-type processes it leads to large volumes of appeals and lawsuits. Considerable refinement of grouping systems has been made in recent years, however. Some systems classify hospitals on the basis of detailed data on a few key variables, such as complexity of hospital services (Berry, 1973) or service complexity plus numbers and types of teaching programs (Shuman et al., 1972). The Shuman and Wolfe system has been successfully employed by the Blue Cross of Western Pennsylvania for several years.

Another approach, developed by J. Phillips at the American Hospital Association, captures and weighs a large number of both exogenous and endogenous variables through cluster analysis. A version of this more sophisticated grouping method is currently being used to group the 119 hospitals in the Washington State Hospital Cost Commission's program (Baker, 1975).

No rate-setting program yet classifies hospitals directly according to the complexity of the medical problems with which they deal.

Lack of patient-related data is the most serious single deficiency in the information available to rate setters. Without access to diagnostic case mix and operative procedure profiles, they risk the continual danger of setting rates too high for hospitals whose work demands low levels of input and of setting rates too low for tertiary-care institutions. With the advent of patient discharge abstract data that must be generated for use by PSROs, this lack may soon be at least partially remediable. The New Jersey and the Maryland rate-setting programs plan to use such data to factor case mix into their rate decisions as soon as possible (Thompson et al., 1975).

Taking the methodology of case-mix analysis from the stage of research to application in rate setting will be difficult, however (Rafferty, 1971; Lave and Lave, 1971; Feldstein and Schuttinga, 1975). Diagnosis per se does not adequately reflect work-load demands in hospitals—the real problem lies in finding measures of case complexity. Few classification schemes to measure differences in patients' requirements for care that can be related to costs have yet been developed, although work is in progress (Diggs and Easter, 1974; Thompson et al., 1975; Cooney, 1974). In the absence of better measures, most programs take the teaching status of hospitals as a gross surrogate for both case mix and case complexity. Some, as already noted, also use complexity of services and composition of medical staff.[6]

Finally, *the quality of the cost and activities data* that rate-setting bodies receive in reports from hospitals is notoriously weak. Although the rate-setting bodies design standard schedules on which the data is to be reported, lack of uniform accounting and reporting practices in the hospitals usually make the resultant figures useless for comparative analysis. This problem not only results in honest confusion, but offers able hospital controllers wide scope to exercise skills in "reimbursement accounting."

In a noteworthy exception to this general rule, the California Health Facilities Commission has over a considerable number of years developed first a detailed uniform accounting system, then a uniform reporting system, and finally a uniform budgeting system, each with very detailed accompanying manuals. Hospitals began to use the system for the first time in 1975. The states of Washington and Arizona have adopted the same system with slight modifications. While it is too soon to know what effects these systems will have on the quality of the data reported by the hospitals, it illustrates that progress is being made in a difficult and important area. Finally, under Section 1533(d) of Public Law 93-641 (the National Health Planning and Resources Development Act), the Department of Health, Education, and Welfare is charged with developing uniform accounting and reporting systems for the nation's hospitals. Criteria to guide such development have been

---

[6]Lave and Lave (1971) found that institutional characteristics of size, teaching status, and a number of advanced services explained only about 25 percent to 45 percent of the variation in their case-mix measures and thus concluded that these could not be considered good surrogates.

formulated (Bauer, 1975) and a new accounting system has been developed.

In summary, the techniques for setting rates that will serve to contain hospital costs yet be equitable to both the public and the provider are still quite primitive. However, serious developmental efforts are being made to improve them.

Risks and Incentives

The degree of risk inherent in any program depends largely on the equity of its rate-setting process, the tightness of its rates, and the hospital's ability to secure additional revenue—whether from payers whose rates or charges are uncontrolled, from increased volume, or from favorable adjustments and appeals. As we have noted, all these factors vary considerably from one program to the next—depending on particular laws, regulations, or contract provisions.

A closer examination allows us to distinguish two quite separate types of risks, those to which the hospitals are deliberately exposed by the program to encourage them to contain costs, and those to which both hospitals and rate setters are unintentionally exposed from malfunctioning of the rate-setting process itself.

Deliberate Risks

The overall rationale for rate setting, as we have seen, is to put the hospital at risk for living within a rate calculated at a point that will discourage inefficient operation but that will meet the hospital's financial requirements for continuing to produce services at previous levels of quality and access.

If a given rate-setting methodology is sufficiently sophisticated to permit reviewers to identify the extent of excess costs stemming from inefficiencies in hospital operation, such as failure to adjust staffing to swings in occupancy, the presence of expensive "sweet-heart" contracts with relatives of investor-owned hospital proprietors (or nonprofit hospital trustees), or failure to phase out underutilized services, rate adjustments can impose financial hardships on that hospital if it fails to mend its ways. Unless it can make up the rate difference from other revenue sources, the hospital will have to cut out its inefficiencies; the cost-containment objectives of the program will be achieved.

In real life, however, sources of inefficiency are rarely so clear cut, and, as we have seen, the reviewers have only limited means to detect them. In particular, with the present state of the rate-setting art, reviewers will discover many "out-of-line" situations, but hospitals will be able to explain most of them away. They will usually be able to show that their outlying costs have resulted from incomplete or unreliable data used in the rate reviewers' comparative analyses, or be able to point to real differences in patient mix, resource complexity, service quality, or one of many more legitimate explanatory variables. In consequence, most rate-review bodies after a few years of bloodletting experience devote most of their attention to limiting increments to hospital costs rather than to the much more difficult task of detecting on-going inefficiencies in the base of these costs.

Risks from an Inadequate Rate-Setting Process

The limitations of rate-setting methodology put both hospitals and rate setters at risk. First, and most obvious, the rate may underpay some hospitals, failing to meet their financial requirements for rendering services without detriment to the quality of or the access to proper patient care. This danger may be more apparent than real, however, since safeguards are usually available. A program's adjustment and appeals process is, of course, the principal means of mitigating the effects of inequitable rates. Some third-party payers such as Connecticut Blue Cross offer risk-sharing arrangements. They agree to make up some fixed percentage of a hospital's loss if its actual costs turn out to exceed its revenues from the prospectively established rates; in turn, the hospital agrees to share any savings that it might accrue under the rate. Other programs, such as those of Maryland and Indiana, allow hospitals to request rate increases at any time, rather than, as in most programs, confining reopenings to fiscal year endings. Finally, rate setters often informally sweeten the rate for a hospital's next rate year to make up for any justifiable losses in the prior year. In short, most programs employ a variety of means to relieve the plight of the hospital that can demonstrate that it is genuinely underpaid because of some weakness in the rate-setting process.

The risk of *overpaying* hospitals is equally real, but seldom discussed. Setting rates that are too high in relation to the type, quality, and appropriateness of services rendered brings cost consequences to the rate-setting program and the public that are especially serious because they are likely to remain undetected. While the underpaid hospital can be counted on to make its case heard, offering a chance for rectification, the hospital that is overpaid through the processes of an inequitable system can be guaranteed to be silent. Common examples of overpayment are found in:

- hospitals with a less complex case mix than that of comparison group hospitals;
- hospitals whose case mix becomes progressively less complex over time;
- hospitals that were inefficiently operated when the rate-setting program began and thus started with an excessively high rate base;
- hospitals where the quality of care deteriorates;
- hospitals that deliberately inflate volumes of admissions, tests, procedures, patient days beyond what patients need in order to achieve low unit costs and thus avoid being caught as outliers in interhospital cost comparisons.

One can only speculate as to whether the cost savings effected from rate reductions for assumed or detected inefficiencies in some hospitals outweigh the overpayments to others.

A poor rate-setting process and methodology also expose a rate-setting body to political risks. First, its credibility is damaged since any adjustments it gives to unjustly underpaid hospitals tend to make its prospective reimbursement system look more and more like retrospective cost-based reimbursement. Thus, while in any given year the rate setters may be able proudly to show the public that they are keeping hospital cost increases down to a commendable X percentage increase, over a longer period of time subsequent rate adjustments will result in a quite different and less impressive overall record. In its own defense, any rate-setting body will want to keep its rates tight and its adjustments minimal, even at the expense of equity.

This in turn, however, exposes it to other kinds of risks—retaliations by hospitals, for whom revenues are lifeblood. Hospital retaliation can and does take the form of defensive accounting practices, lawsuits, cancellation or nonrenewal of Blue Cross contracts, and/or political action to change the enabling laws under which state rate-setting bodies function.

Incentives for and against Cost Containment

In examining the kinds of incentives that are set in motion by rate setting it is necessary to recognize two quite different classes. Some types of incentives, whether rewards or penalties, are expressly designed into a program to encourage greater hospital efficiency. Others, often perverse, emerge unexpectedly as unintended consequences of the program's own structure, or from its failure to recognize or deal with the special nature and goals of hospitals as organizations. It is useful to distinguish between structural and behavioral types of incentives.

As we have seen, early advocates of rate setting believed that hospitals would be motivated to increase efficiency by the possibility of retaining any savings they could effect by keeping spending under the allowed rates. In fact, hospitals do not respond to the possibility of making such windfall profits. Their financial officers quickly learn that their institution's future rates are calculated primarily on the base of its historical and current year spending; to reduce this spending base would, therefore, run completely counter to its long-run interests (Messier, 1975). Thus, in most programs, the true operative incentives are for each hospital to spend exactly to the limit of each year's allowed rates or budget—and as much more as it can reasonably expect to justify through the program's adjustment and appeals process.[7] Where group comparisons are made, it behooves them to calculate spending toward the top of the allowable spending parameter for their group. Over time, of course, this escalates the group average year by year.

Where penalties for underutilized services are imposed through downward rate adjustments, the obvious incentives are, as we have seen, for physicians to alter their admissions and ordering practices to keep beds filled. However, in services such as obstetrics where demand cannot be artificially stimulated, such controls may work well. In New York state, 483 obstetric beds were phased out in one period from January 1973 to March 1974 (Meitch, 1974).

---

[7] It is possible that such counterincentives to improve efficiency may be less strong in rate-setting programs that pursue the objective of meeting total hospital financial requirements in each year's rate, allowing a reasonable margin of working capital and a factor for growth. Examples are programs in the state of Washington, the Cincinnati region, and Indiana.

As Dowling has explicated (1974), what kinds of incentives will be set in motion also depend on the type of payment unit the rate-setting program employs—per diem, per service, per case, and so on. Many of these incentives, unfortunately, run counter to the objectives of containing overall hospital expenditures. For example, as we have already noted, a tight per diem rate designed to keep unit costs low encourages increased lengths of stay and volumes of procedures, whether or not these are medically justified. In New York state, for example, where the tightest limits on per diem increases have been imposed, the average length of stay exceeds that of any other state in the nation. Unfortunately, although the shortcomings of per diem and charge payments are by now well recognized, most of the feasible alternatives also offer their own potentialities for establishing perverse incentives.

Most observers believe that the mere existence of hospital rate setting, regardless of type, has a positive effect on administrators and trustees, stimulating them to pay closer attention to hospital costs and to upgrade the quality of financial management. On the other hand, the advent of a new program often signals hospitals to make a hefty increase in rates before the program comes into effect, in order to maximize the base from which their future rates will be projected.

One possible source of future difficulty, already experienced by rate-setting bodies in some Canadian provinces, is a changed framework of incentives within which hospital labor negotiations take place. To the extent that the managers of individual hospitals feel they have nothing but trouble to gain from hard bargaining, either the costs of higher wages and increased fringe benefits will be passed through the new rate as "uncontrollable" costs, or the rate-setting body will find itself in the position of bargainer, since it alone has the authority to decide what final terms it will allow (Messier, 1975).

In general, the overriding emphasis on high utilization of hospital inpatient services, and lack of support in the rates for start-up cost of alternative forms of care, such as hospital-based home health services, militate against efforts of progressive hospitals to experiment with or move toward a changing role in their community health system. Fortunately, however, a few programs, such as Rhode Island's, actively encourage such system-improvement innovations.

Besides these structural types of incentives, intentional or perverse, most budget review programs regard their rate-setting process itself as a positive instrument for effecting behavioral change. The program's requests for detailed cost and budget data, its individual review sessions, and its cost and volume monitoring reports during the rate year are usually designed in some fashion to strengthen internal management controls in hospitals and to promote cost consciousness.

Case studies in Indiana and Cincinnati and in the New Jersey program prior to 1975 indicate that the new visibility of their operations and the scrutiny by knowledgable external reviewers may well motivate better management (Bauer and Clark, 1974a, b; Arthur D. Little, 1974e). Operating on the assumption that most administrators have strong personal concerns with job security and opportunities for promotion, these programs (largely designed by hospital associations) structure their rate reviews so that hospital managers are questioned on their performance by informed fellow administrators and by trustees, and thereby demonstrate their degree of professional knowledge and competence. Most such reviews are confined to costs directly under administrator control, in particular those for the hotel services of hospitals.

Some state programs also view the rate-setting process as a vehicle for inspiring organizational change within the hospitals. For example, the Washington program requires each hospital and each department head to submit a narrative account of its cost-saving management objectives for the coming year, with quantitative progress toward these objectives to be reviewed when the next year's budget is submitted.

State disclosure laws that expose hospital costs to public scrutiny offer another type of positive incentive for cost containment. Success depends on whether the press and consumer groups know how to ask the right questions from the cost data, how to interpret the answers, and how long they maintain their interest.

We have already noted the unanimity with which both Blue Cross and state agency rate setters choose almost completely to ignore the influence of the hospital medical staff on hospital costs. To the author's knowledge, no program has made any attempt to gear incentives to raise the cost consciousness of physicians, to work with utilization review committees on problems of unnecessary utilization, or to bring the sacrosanct question of open staff privileges into rate-review discussions. Some rate-setting organizations appear to operate on the fiction that administrators and trustees could, if they only wanted to, take any necessary action to influence physician cost-affecting behavior. Other programs, however, consciously use the processes of rate-setting reviews to encourage mofification of the traditional balance of power within hospitals. Few administrators and trustees themselves want to add unnecessary, loss-producing services, but are often pressured to endorse the wish lists of all their service chiefs rather than risk offense to any one of them. The requirements of the external rate-review system can provide a foil to force their medical staffs to order their new spending priorities and to cost out the consequences (Bauer and Clark, 1974c; Bauer, 1974a). Rate setters become the necessary scapegoats.

Requirements for five-year capital budgets from each hospital also force the setting of internal hospital priorities, and give rate setters and planning agencies an opportunity both to anticipate and to evaluate expansion requests in terms of population needs and the services already being provided by potential referral hospitals. If sensitively and judiciously applied, rate setting combined with other forms of external regulation could increasingly provide conscientious hospital trustees and managers with the muscle they need to make unpopular cost-saving management decisions—a substitute for the lever that the profit factor provides to corporate managers.

Conclusions

State and regional experience during the 1970s indicates that in and of itself, hospital rate setting is by no means the way to salvation. Federal policy makers were wise not to have prematurely rushed into this plausible-sounding route to cost containment. Setting rates for thousands of hospitals of diverse character at the point that will induce greater "efficiency" and that will at the same time protect the legitimate concerns of third-party payers, providers, patients, and the bill-paying public is easier legislated than accomplished. The methodology for implementing a task of this delicacy is still at a primitive stage. Worse, well-intentioned mistakes in designing either the structure or the processes of rate setting may be counterproductive; quite possibly they may actually stimulate increases in overall hospital care expenditures. This should not be surprising; it is the perennial risk associated with any new type of intervention in complex social systems.

At the same time, most rate-setting programs appear to be learning from their initial experiences. They are continually improving their methodologies and enlarging and improving the information base on which they are reaching rate decisions. Nevertheless, in the absence of a broader policy of health regulation, expectations of cost containment through most of the types of rate-setting programs currently in operation should be kept modest, commensurate with the modesty of their programs' own operational objectives, namely, to thwart the spiral of hospital inflation by discouraging duplicative expansions and overbedding, and to encourage types of potential cost savings in areas of hospital functioning not affected by physician decisions.

Rate-setting programs are not charged with responsibility either to identify or to control the vast bulk of excess hospital costs that spring from basic discontinuities in the system through which patients now obtain their health services. Nor can they be responsible for excess costs stemming from the ways in which society has chosen to organize and finance these services. In fact, rate setting per se is just a highly complicated tinkering operation, plugging up leaks in one small section of a rudderless ship that is cracking at the seams.

In the future, perhaps, it may play a far more powerful role. Continuing untrammeled health care costs may eventually force the nation to adopt some coherent overall health care policy to improve the processes of resource allocation in line with principles of cost effectiveness. Implementing such a policy will require new coordinated approaches and cooperative activities between and among organizations now providing care and those influencing its provision via planning, utilization review, quality monitoring, and payment. In preparing for such a role hospitals and rate setters have joint interests in developing far more refined methods of defining and measuring what hospitals do for the money they spend, and far more refined methods of accounting for that money.

The working links that have been forged between planners and rate setters vary in strength from one program to the next. The Rhode Island experience demonstrates that such a partnership can be used to promote system-wide objectives. Within the overall limit of hospital spending increases imposed by the annual maxi-cap, the rate-setting body approves spending for new programs in hospitals in strict conformance with written listings of priorities of statewide community need established by the planning agency.

As yet there are no similar links between rate-setting programs and utilization review and quality monitoring organizations such as PSROs. A national health policy designed to improve the cost effectiveness of hospital care would seem to call for their development. This would raise the sights of rate setters from narrow considerations of the unit costs of producing given types of hospital services to decision making enriched by information on the appropriateness, quality, and, one hopes, eventually, the efficacy of those services.

Speculating on the possibilities of building these various types of cooperative relationships designed to improve the health status of the population while containing costs is a heady exercise. While acknowledging the possibility that in the real workaday world, the organizational and technical problems that inevitably accompany efforts to implement such new tasks may again turn to defeat the good intentions of those who pose the proposition, this approach still appears to be the best of any likely alternatives. Failure to move forward incrementally toward greater cost effectiveness of health care can only, by default, precipitate far cruder measures, such as across-the-board hospital rate freezes and cuts in health insurance benefits. Such solutions to the complicated problems of containing costs of the multibillion-dollar hospital industry would, of course, single out the ill and disabled citizens in our society to bear the consequences of reduced accessibility, comprehensiveness, and continuity of good quality medical care.

References

American Hospital Association. 1972. *Guidelines for Review and Approval of Rates for Health Care Institutions and Services by a State Commission.* Chicago.

Arthur D. Little. 1974a. The Prospective Reimbursement Program of Connecticut Blue Cross. Processed.

———. 1974b. The Prospective Reimbursement Programs in the State of Colorado. Processed.

———. 1974c. The Prospective Reimbursement Program of Blue Cross of Northeast Pennsylvania. Processed.

————. 1974d. The Prospective Hospital Rate Review Program for Blue Cross of Wisconsin Payments to Hospitals. Processed.

————. 1974e. The Prospective Reimbursement Program of Blue Cross of Southwest Ohio. Processed.

————. 1974f. The Prospective Reimbursement Program of Blue Cross of Northeast Ohio. Processed.

Baker, Francis. 1975. *The Washington Hospital Commission's Method of Grouping Hospitals for Reimbursement.* Washington State Hospital Commission, Olympia, Washington.

Bauer, Katharine G. 1974a. *The Combined Budget Review and Formula Approach to Prospective Reimbursement by the Blue Cross of Western Pennsylvania.* Harvard Center for Community Health and Medical Care (April).

————. 1974b. *Classifying Hospitals for Purposes of Prospective Reimbursement.* In fulfillment of contract SSA-PMS-74-336, United States Department of Health, Education, and Welfare, Social Security Administration (August).

————. 1975. Uniform Reporting for Hospital Rate Reviews: Criteria to Guide Development and Proceedings of a 1975 Conference. Processed.

Bauer, Katharine G., and Altman, Drew. 1975. *Linking Planning and Rate Setting Controls to Contain Hospital Costs.* Division of Resource Development of the Public Health Service, Department of Health, Education and Welfare, Region II, New York, New York (October).

Bauer, Katharine G., and Clark, Arva R. 1974a. *The New Jersey Budget Review Program.* Harvard Center for Community Health and Medical Care (March).

————. 1974b. *The Indiana Controlled Charges System.* Harvard Center for Community Health and Medical Care (March).

————. 1974c. *Budget Reviews and Prospective Rate Setting for Rhode Island Hospitals.* Harvard Center for Community Health and Medical Care (February).

————. 1974d. *New York: The Formula Approach to Prospective Reimbursement.* Harvard Center for Community Health and Medical Care (March).

Berger, Laurence B., and Sullivan, Paul R. 1975. *Measuring Hospital Inflation: A Composite Index for the Measurement and Determination of Hospitals in the Commonwealth of Massachusetts.* Lexington, Mass.: Lexington Books, D.C. Heath & Co.

Berki, Sylvester E. 1972. *Hospital Economics.* Lexington, Mass.: Lexington Books, D.C. Heath & Co. pp. 31–77.

Berry, Ralph E. 1973. "On grouping hospitals for economic analysis." *Inquiry* 10 (December): 5—12.

Cooney, James. 1974. *Type of Medical Care Classification System.* Chicago: Hospital Research and Educational Trust.

Cochrane, A.L. 1972. *Effectiveness and Efficiency: Random Reflections on Health Services.* London: The Nuffield Provincial Hospitals Trust.

Diggs, Walter W., and Easter, James A. 1974. "Incremental hospital and nursing home pricing." *Inquiry* 11 (December): 300—303.

Dowling, William L. 1974. "Prospective reimbursement of hospitals." *Inquiry* 11 (September): 163—180.

Dowling, William L., and Teague, Nancy. 1975. *Proposed Relationships among Regulatory Programs to Improve the Health Care System.* School of Public Health, University of Washington.

Dunlop, John. 1975. *New York Times* (Sunday, November 9), p. 70.

Elnicki, Richard A. 1975 "SSA—Connecticut hospital reimbursement experimental cost evaluation." *Inquiry* 12 (March): 47—58.

Evans, Robert G., and Walker, Hugh D. 1972. "Information theory and the analysis of hospital cost structure." *Canadian Journal of Economics* 5 (August): 405.

Feldstein, Martin, and Schuttinga, James. 1975. *Hospital Costs in Massachusetts: A Methodological Study.* Discussion Paper No. 449, Harvard Institute of Economic Research, Cambridge, Mass.

Feldstein, Paul. 1968. "An analysis of reimbursement plans." In Department of Health, Education, and Welfare, *Reimbursement Incentives for Hospital and Medical Care: Objectives and Alternatives.* Washington, D.C.: Government Printing Office.

Ginsburg, Paul B. 1976. *Regulating the Non-Profit Firm: Hospital Price and Reimbursement Controls.* Department of Economics, Michigan State University.

Gort, Michael, et al. 1975. Report on the Hospital Price Index for Greater New York. Prepared for the Associated Hospital Service of New York.

Hardwick, C. Patrick, and Wolfe, Harvey. 1972. "Evaluation of an incentive reimbursement experiment." *Medical Care* 10 (March-April).

Hospital Association of New York State. 1975. Fourth Annual Voluntary Hospital Fiscal Pressures Survey. Hospital Association of New York State, Albany, New York (October).

Institute of Medicine. 1974. *Advancing the Quality of Health Care: Key Issues and Fundamental Principles.* A Policy statement. Washington, D.C.: National Academy of Sciences.

Kovner, Anthony R., and Lusk, Edward J. 1975. "State regulation of health care costs." *Medical Care* 13 (August): 619–629.

Lave, Judith R., and Lave, Lester B. 1971. "The extent of role differentiation among hospitals." *Health Services Research* 6 (Spring): 15–38.

Meitch, George. 1974. Communication with Katharine Bauer (March 7).

Messier, Edward A. 1975. "Prospective reimbursement is no panacea." *Hospital Financial Management* 5 (September): 24.

National Advisory Commission on Health Manpower. 1968. Report. Washington, D.C.: Government Printing Office.

New York State Moreland Act Commission on Nursing Homes and Residential Facilities. 1975. *Regulating Nursing Home Care: The Paper Tigers*. Report No. 1 (October).

Noll, Roger G. 1971. *Reforming Regulation: Studies in the Regulation of Economic Activity*. Washington, D.C.: The Brookings Institue. pp. 20–21.

Rafferty, John A. 1971. "Patterns of hospital use: An analysis of short run variations." *Journal of Political Economy* 79 (January-February): 154–165.

Rutstein, David D. 1974. *Blueprint for Medical Care*. Cambridge, Mass.: M.I.T. Press.

Shuman, Larry; Wolfe, Harvey; and Hardwick, C. Patrick. 1972. "Predictive hospital reimbursement and evaluation model." *Inquiry* 9 (February): 17–33.

Sigmond, Robert M. 1968. "Capitation as a method of reimbursement." In Department of Health, Education and Welfare, *Reimbursement Incentives for Hospital and Medical Care: Objectives and Alternatives*. Washington, D.C.: Government Printing Office.

Somers, Anne R. 1973. *State Regulation of Hospitals and Health Care: The New Jersey Story*. Blue Cross Reports, Research Series 11:9.

Thompson, J.D.; Mross, C.D.; Fetter, R.B. 1975. "Case mix and resource use." *Inquiry* 12 (December): 300–312.

U.S. Department of Health, Education, and Welfare. 1975. An analysis of state and regional health regulations. Health Resources Studies. HRA No. 75-611:2-4. Washington, D.C.

Waldman, Saul. 1968. "Average increase in costs—and incentive reimbursement formula for hospitals." In Department of Health, Education, and Welfare, *Reimbursement Incentives for Hospitals and Medical Care: Objectives and Alternatives*. Washington, D.C.: Government Printing Office.

263

Wolf, Gerrit. 1973. A Behavioral Analysis of the Connecticut Incentive Reimbursement Experiment. Mimeographed. Yale University Administrative Sciences (January).

This paper will appear in the forthcoming book, *Hospital Cost Containment*, edited by Michael Zubkoff and Ira E. Raskin. New York: PRODIST for the Milbank Memorial Fund.

Address reprint requests to: Katharine G. Bauer, Harvard Center for Community Health and Medical Care, 643 Huntington Avenue, Boston, Mass. 02115

Inflation and
Hospital Capital Investment

PAUL B. GINSBURG

Hospital capital investment is affected by general inflation and policies designed to combat it in the short run, yet contributes to inflation, through its effect on hospital prices, in the long run. The latter relationship has received substantial attention in government, since it is an important part of the rationale for hospital planning and regulatory activities. The former relationship has not received attention before because of past price stability in the United States. It is the subject of the first and larger part of this contribution.

Impacts on Hospital Investment

In discussing the impact of inflation on hospital capital investment, it is essential to consider whether a reduction in investment is a good or bad thing. The hospital capital market does not resemble the concept of an efficient allocator of resources, and thus it is possible that too much or too little capital is being supplied to the industry. A number of factors tend to induce overinvestment. One is the subsidy effect of health insurance. Since health insurance pays a large part or all of the hospital bills of most individuals, the price they face is a small fraction of the cost of producing hospital care. Empirical studies have supported the notion that this induces the use of too many bed days and too expensive a variety of medical care (Feldstein, 1973). Hospitals are induced to build more beds and be

In *Health: A Victim or Cause of Inflation?*, edited by Michael Zubkoff. New York: PRODIST, 1976.
Note: References for this article are on p. 435.

less conscious of cost than if the full price was borne by patients. A second factor increasing investment is that hospitals have access to free but limited capital in the form of grants, both from the private sector and from government. Finally, a large proportion of hospital revenue is obtained from reimbursement of costs. Since reimbursors tend to pay interest and depreciation charges attributed to their patients in full, an incentive to use capital is alleged to exist.

On the other side of the issue, while nonprofit hospitals have access to grant capital, they do not have access to profit-seeking equity capital. Netting out, their access to capital may be lower. Also, while reimbursement pays capital costs in full, it may make it difficult to earn a surplus to accumulate equity for investment. Thus a "shortage" of capital funds can be apparent to administrators while at the same time economists maintain that "too much" capital investment is taking place. The subsidy effect of health insurance can expand demand for health care facilities, while the nature of the hospital capital market prevents institutions from raising the funds necessary to satisfy these demands. Consequently, should the following analysis show that inflation reduces investment, there is no consensus as to whether this is a cause for concern or rejoicing.

Another issue that must be noted prior to assessing the effects of inflation is the importance of the distribution of capital funds across regions, among hospitals within a region, and among services within a hospital. The hospital capital market does not appear to allocate funds in accordance with the demand for services, or the marginal efficiency of investment. Lenders tend to require hospitals to obtain a substantial portion of the funding for an investment project from equity sources. Since grants and retained funds, the sources of equity, are not interest elastic, the hospital faces a constrained access to capital funds which may or may not be binding. Consequently, access to private donations can be of crucial importance in determining total access to capital funds (Ginsburg, 1972).

As an example of this pattern, hospital donors tend to be from the upper middle and upper income brackets, to choose hospitals that they use, and to favor pediatric and cancer facilities. Consequently, those hospitals located in or near upper income communities specializing in these or services favored by other donor groups have the most extensive access to capital funds and probably command a greater share of resources allocated to the industry than they would if allocation strictly followed the demand for services.[1] Inflation will affect these distribution patterns, at least in the short run, and this relationship will be examined along with the impact on total investment.

Inflation

In a "textbook" world of perfect markets and perfect knowledge of the future, inflation would have *no* effect on the *real* level of hospital investment. The prices of capital and labor would increase at the same rate, as would the price of hospital services. The fact that the hospital does not maximize profits but has objectives such as the quantity and quality of care, prestige, and other factors does not change this conclusion.

Of course, we do not live in a textbook world. Markets (particularly hospital capital markets) are not perfect, and people do not know with certainty what future prices will be. As a result, general inflation appears to *reduce* real hospital investment and increases the role of access to equity capital in the distribution of investment across regions, institutions, and services.

Much of the impact of inflation on real hospital investment occurs as a result of changes in the supply of capital funds to hospitals. As mentioned above, hospitals obtain capital funds from private grants, government grants, retained funds (depreciation and earnings), and borrowing. The last source has increased in importance over time, as is shown by summary data from American Hospital Association surveys on financing of *construction* projects (Marine and Henderson, 1974; refer to Table 1).

[1] The Hill-Burton program, which has made capital grants, loans, and loan guarantees to hospitals and other health care facilities since 1947, was designed to redress some of the imbalances between access to equity capital and "need" for hospital facilities. A formula directed most Hill-Burton funds to low-income states. Rural areas within these states were favored until the mid-1960s, when urban hospitals in need of modernization began to be assisted. See Lave and Lave (1974) for a recent evaluation of this program.

Paul B. Ginsburg

TABLE 1   Sources of Capital for Construction Projects:
Nonfederal Short-Term Hospitals
(in percentages)

	1969	1973
Private grants	15.1	10.4
Government grants	26.1	15.7
Retained funds	23.8	16.4
Borrowing	35.0	57.5

Source: Marine and Henderson (1974).

In most capital markets, lenders cope with risk by requiring collateral and/or requiring equity participation in financing. In hospital capital markets, since collateral is not of great value (the market for used hospitals is not well developed) the equity participation is substantial and innovative underwriters have dropped the use of the mortgage and instead take a lien on hospital revenues as collateral. Of course such a lien is worthless if there is no net cash flow, so the equity requirement takes the form of requiring expected cash flow available for repayment of the loan to exceed the required repayments by some multiple. Since access to debt appears to be interest inelastic and directly related to equity raised by the hospital we analyze the effects of inflation on the supply of funds through inflation's effect on access to debt, given an amount of equity, and on its effect on hospital equity.

Inflation affects access to borrowed funds through its effect on nominal interest rates. When borrowers and lenders expect future price increases, interest rates rise. These high nominal rates of interest reduce access to debt capital in a number of ways. Life insurance companies are important lenders in the hospital bond market. However, during periods of high interest rates, policy holders exercise options for loans from their policies at fixed rates of interest. As a consequence, reduced funds are available to lend to hospitals. In a classical competitive market, a small increase in interest rates on hospital bonds should attract other lenders into this market. However, hospital bond underwriters maintain that the capital market is sufficiently specialized so that this does not occur in the short run, and in addition to an interest rate increase, lenders demand a greater equity participation on the part of the hospital. As

268

a result, at least in the short run, the cost of debt capital is increased and access is reduced.

Access to debt is reduced by high nominal interest rates in states where usury laws limit what hospitals can pay for loans. High interest rates caused by inflation push hospital bond rates above these ceilings. While this will not influence the total supply of debt capital to hospitals since funds will go to other states, the distribution of hospital investment across states may be affected.

Access to borrowed funds is also reduced through a reduction in the *valuation* of the hospital's equity which is necessary to support debt. Consider the requirement of a multiple of cash flow available for repayment for each dollar of repayment scheduled. As nominal interest rates increase, scheduled repayments increase. However, only if the full amount of the expected inflation reflected in these interest rates is projected for hospital revenues by the consultants hired by underwriters, will projected funds available for repayment keep pace with repayment requirements. If hospital consultants are conservative in projecting inflation in hospital revenues, then hospital equity will not support as much debt.

Aside from increasing the proportion of a project that the hospital must finance through equity, inflation works to decrease the real value of an institution's equity funds.

Retained funds are affected most importantly. The stock of retained funds may lose value because of falling prices of investments in stocks and bonds (due to increasing interest rates) and because of erosion of purchasing power of fixed income securities. This phenomenon will affect hospital endowment funds as well as funded depreciation and retained surpluses. One of the most important mechanisms by which inflation reduces real equity funds available for investment is through a *reduction* in real cash flow. This occurs through the cost reimbursement mechanism which is responsible for a major share of hospital revenue. Hospitals are reimbursed for the cost of capital goods by payment of interest and depreciation by the third-party payer. However, only depreciation based on historical cost is paid. Once a piece of capital is in place, depreciation charges calculated in this way do not vary with changes in replacement costs. As a result, inflation reduces the real value of depreciation reimbursement by third-party payers and thus real cash flow.

Philanthropy is affected by inflation via the impact of inflation on the stock market—a relationship not altogether clear. If stock prices decline, as in the present inflationary period, paper wealth of potential donors declines and opportunities to escape taxation of capital gains through donation of appreciated stock are reduced. Thus, as in the current experience, philanthropy could decline in the short run via effects of inflation on stock prices.

With the phasing out of the Hill-Burton program, most public capital grants currently obtained are from local governments. While most of these grants go to institutions controlled by these municipal or county governments, recently voluntary hospitals have also been recipients. To discuss the effect of inflation on these grants, one must consider its effects on the budgets of these governments, an issue outside the scope of this paper.

Thus far we have noted a number of mechanisms by which inflation affects access to capital funds by hospitals. Many are relevant only in the short run. Use of historical cost in reimbursement of depreciation is a notable exception. The longer inflation continues, the more adjustments are likely to occur, and the smaller is the effect on investment. In the long run, the result for perfect markets—that inflation does not affect real investment—is expected. The empirical importance of these market imperfections which lead to this qualitative result is not known. In the absence of appropriate time series data on sources and uses of hospital capital funds, we can only rely on informed opinions of underwriters, fund-raising counselors, and hospital consultants that these phenomena do have quantitative importance.

If inflation reduces overall capital investment in the short run, what can be said about the distribution of this reduction? According to the analysis here, those hospitals with most access to equity funds will be least affected by the reduction in access to debt. Some hospitals have sufficient equity funds so as not to be constrained at all in their investment plans by access to capital, and these will be affected least. Those services within the hospital most attractive to philanthropists or local governments might be cut least. Also, those services producing the greatest cash flow per dollar of capital should be favored.

If we turn from the supply of funds to the demand for capital investment, we find fewer important effects of inflation. Above, the problem of reimbursement of depreciation based on historical cost was noted in conjunction with the effect of inflation on real cash flow. Since an erosion in the future value of equity capital invested in plant and equipment can be expected, hospitals may be loath to use their equity capital to finance investments. Instead, current cash flow can be used to subsidize current services not requiring capital. For example, the hospital may want to expand emergency services or subsidize additional teaching or research programs. Since inflation is expected to erode equity invested in plant and equipment, it is rational to redeploy these funds toward uses not taxed by inflation. Note that this trade-off is not strictly a current versus a future one. Retained funds can be invested in financial assets so that they can subsidize certain services over a lengthy period of time.

People knowledgeable in hospital financing have also mentioned that high interest rates deter hospitals from investing. If we assume that only money interest rates are high, and real interest rates are unchanged by inflation, it is not obvious why this should occur. One explanation offered is that high interest rates cause expectations that rates will be lower in the future—a type of thinking basic to Keynes's analysis of the demand for money. A second explanation is that people have not yet adjusted to living with inflation, and are uneasy about depending upon future cash flows increasing with inflation.

A third explanation is that while debt repayments are increased in money terms by inflation, they are constant in money terms over the length of the loan and thus decline in real terms. This situation presents a problem in hospital pricing. In order to keep the real price of hospital care constant over time, losses must be incurred in the early years of the loan while surpluses are earned in the later years. The hospital may not have the ability to finance these early losses for repayment. Thus, the standard repayment schedule of loans and bonds may force a substantial increase in the price of hospital care initially in order to cope with the high initial repayments. This could put the institution at a competitive disadvantage.

Clearly a potential innovation to deal with chronic inflation would be loan repayment schedules which are constant in real dollars.

To sum up, while in a world of perfect markets and certainty, inflation should affect neither total hospital investment nor its distribution among hospitals and among services, imperfections in hospital capital markets alter this conclusion. A substantial number of mechanisms were outlined by which inflation can affect real hospital capital investment. All of these mechanisms work in the direction of causing inflation to reduce investment. Further, inflation reallocates hospital investment toward those institutions possessing the most equity capital and toward those projects which generate the most equity capital.

Anti-Inflationary Policies

Many of the mechanisms by which inflation affects hospital investment occurred because interest rates are higher during inflation. Tight money, by pushing interest rates still higher, will further reduce capital investment via all of these mechanisms. More usury constraints will be encountered, more policy holders will borrow from their life insurance, the increase in required repayments of loans will demand greater equity capital, the stock of which will be reduced by tight money, and so on.

Tight money has additional impacts, however. This policy raises the real rate of interest as well as the nominal rate. An increase in the real rate of interest reduces investment even in a textbook economy. Hospitals are induced to substitute labor and supplies for capital. Thus plans for an automated meal delivery system may be shelved as orderlies continue to deliver meals, or nursing staff may be substituted for electronic patient monitoring systems. Not only will capital be reduced relative to other hospital inputs, but the cost of hospital care will be increased. If the demand for services of an individual hospital is not completely inelastic, the increased cost of investment would cause a reduction in output. This would induce a further reduction in hospital capital investment. Thus tight money reduces investment not only by aggravating the effects of high nominal interest rates, but also by increasing the real costs of capital investment.

A final effect of tight money works through the decline in economic activity. While I am not aware of any research that has measured the impact of cyclical income and unemployment changes on the demand for hospital care, one presumes that a decline in economic activity reduces the demand for hospital care. If this is the case, then we have an additional reduction in demand for investment caused by tight money.

Increases in taxes or reductions in government spending will impact on hospital investment in a manner quite different than tight money. First let us note that since most hospitals do not pay taxes, there is no direct effect of tax increases. Also, since most hospitals are nonfederal, spending cuts should not have a direct impact either. An exception would be if Medicare or Medicaid financing were affected by spending reductions—this would reduce the demand for hospital services and reduce investment as a result.

Contractionary fiscal policy should reduce both the real and nominal rates of interest in the economy. This will tend to stimulate investment through all of the mechanisms outlined above in connection with inflation effects and tight money effects. In this respect, contractionary fiscal policy will have generally the opposite effects of tight money. On the other hand, the decline in economic activity will tend to reduce investment via the demand for hospital care. While one cannot determine the net impact a priori, my judgment tells me that the effects of reducing interest rates are far more important than the effects of a decline in economic activity. Thus it appears that contractionary fiscal policy will increase hospital capital investment.

Wage and price controls are the most difficult anti-inflationary policy to deal with. There is little agreement about their effects on the economy, and the effect of direct controls on hospitals is highly dependent upon the details and interpretation of the regulations (see my earlier contribution to this volume). Assume that controls are successful in holding down general prices and wages. This should reduce the demand for money and as a result reduce interest rates. A reduction in interest rates should stimulate hospital investment for all of the reasons discussed above. However, part of this effect may

273

be reversed by the fact that controls tend to hold wages down more effectively than they do prices, particularly when prices of hospital construction and equipment are considered. Prices of goods that are not standardized are the most difficult to regulate. The relative decline in labor prices may offset part of the effect of lower interest rates.

General controls on wages and prices would undoubtedly be accompanied by special regulations for hospitals. These would affect hospital investment, but the direction is dependent on the details of the regulation. For example, regulations could induce either an increase or a decrease in length of stay, with important effects on the demand for beds. The fact that exceptions could not be granted for prospective price increases needed to cover expenses of new facilities cut off all lending to hospitals for a period during Phase II. Nevertheless, to generalize, controls should reduce capital investment for a number of reasons. On the supply of funds side, controls over hospital prices increase the risk involved in lending to hospitals. This will increase the premium hospitals must pay in interest and cause lenders to demand greater equity participation from hospitals. On the demand side, limits on prices will probably cause hospitals to drop plans to build facilities and buy equipment for expensive new services. Hospitals will have an incentive to avoid duplication of equipment. Procedures used for exceptions requests will tend to increase the power of state planning agencies and further reduce investment. These reasons for a decline in hospital investment with controls should be more important than the effects of lower interest rates induced by general controls.

To summarize the discussion of the effects of anti-inflationary policy on capital investment, fiscal and monetary policies result in opposite changes in the interest rate, and similar changes in economic activity. Thus, fiscal policy favors an increase in capital investment while monetary policy favors a decline in it. General wage and price controls if successful will reduce interest rates and avoid a decline in economic activity. However, the effects of hospital controls are believed to be more important, causing investment to decline.

Impact on Inflation

Capital investment in hospitals contributes to general inflation via its effects on hospital costs. However, the effect is not direct. Hospital cost data make it clear that interest and depreciation are a small part of hospital costs and cannot be considered an important cause of cost increases directly. However, the indirect effects may be substantial. A new wing in a hospital must be heated, maintained, and insured. Nurses, orderlies, and technicians must be employed. Similarly a new piece of equipment requires use of space, wages for technicians, and expenditures for supplies. Thus, capital investment may add little directly to operating costs, but can require vast amounts of operating expenses indirectly. Consequently when the question of inflationary impact is raised, costs associated with the services produced from plant and equipment purchases must be evaluated.

Discussion of inflation in hospital costs requires a unit of output by which to divide costs. Knowledge that expenditures for hospital care increased by 10 percent in one year tells us little about inflation unless we know how output changed. The ultimate output of the hospital is the marginal change in the health status of patients attributed to services performed by the hospital. It is necessary to know how the change in the patient's health status that occurred during and after the hospital stay compares with what would have happened in an alternative setting, such as a home stay. Needless to say, measurement problems, both in assessing health impacts and in aggregating diverse impacts, make such a concept impractical as an operational tool. However, conceptually, the notion is crucial to the discussion of the inflationary impact of investment in facilities and equipment. There will be cases when new capital increases cost per *day* of hospital care but is not considered inflationary and others where cost per day is not affected but the impact is inflationary. This notion of the ultimate output of the hospital will assist in judging these situations as inflationary or not.

Assume that a hospital expands its number of beds, but the community already has sufficient stock of beds to meet the demand

275

for patient days. Presumably this adds to the cost of hospital care without an increase in output of services and thus is inflationary. However, assume that the beds left empty by this expansion were truly obsolete and not equipped to deliver effective care. Then the output of the hospital system would have increased and the expansion may not be inflationary. On the other hand, if the older beds are not obsolete, and physicians decide to admit more people to the hospital and expand lengths of stay, the inflationary impact will be even greater than the additional fixed costs of maintaining superfluous beds. However, in this last case, which is most difficult to recognize, cost per day need not increase, so that the inflationary impact goes unnoticed.

Let us now consider an example with equipment. Imagine that a hospital purchases a second x-ray machine that is identical to its initial facility. If the new equipment (or functional old equipment) is underused, then its purchase will have an inflationary impact. If an increase in x-rays is associated with the additional equipment, the difficult question must be asked as to whether the additional tests improve patient care or not. Are x-rays ordered unnecessarily such as for defensive medicine or to increase hospital revenue, or do they improve the quality of care? Consequently, additional services can either be inflationary or not, depending upon the effectiveness of these marginal services.

Now consider a facility which permits a new service to be performed. If the service is already available in the community at an underused facility, this move appears inflationary. It is in this area that health planning has probably had its greatest success. However, what if this facility is the only one in the community offering the service? It may still be underutilized. This is a very difficult case, since the medical benefits of the service must be weighed against the cost. If the benefits are large, then the increase in cost per day may reflect not inflation but a large increase in output not adequately reflected by the patient day measure.

As a final example, consider purchase of a new dishwasher that substitutes for dishwashing labor. The impact of such an investment on costs is the easiest to assess since there is little change in the nature of the product. Aside from the computer, equipment additions in nonmedical departments have seldom been considered to inflate hospital costs.

Those examples have shown a principle that whether or not capital investment contributes to inflation depends upon comparison of net improvements in health from the services produced with costs. Facilities that are underused *tend* to be inflationary, while facilities producing additional services that are used, whether they be bed days, x-rays, or exotic treatments, are either inflationary or not depending upon their net medical benefits. Often assessing the medical benefits of commonly used medical procedures is highly difficult as ethics prohibits designation of a control group. Clearly some investment projects are inflationary and others are not. Estimates of the proportion of investments adding to costs would be a heroic effort which probably would not be accepted. Instead policy should design mechanisms which weed out inflationary projects.

Policy Alternatives

In the United States, governments are already quite active in influencing capital investment. Through the Hill-Burton program, the federal government has influenced the number and quality of hospital beds and their distribution. Through comprehensive health planning agencies, capital projects have been reviewed publicly. When disapproved, they have been denied Medicare reimbursement for depreciation and interest, and in states with certificate of need laws, have been vetoed entirely. In order to reduce capital projects that contribute to inflation, a number of alternatives are available.

One is to continue health planning and certificate of need. The presumption behind this type of program is that a committee of providers and consumers in a local area or a state can determine which projects have merit and which do not. While this is not the place to evaluate the effectiveness of such a program (Havighurst, 1974), two serious problems in this area have impressed me in my participation as a member of such an agency. One is that there is an absence of practical criteria to guide citizens in judging the merits of projects. The other is that consumer representatives have seen their role as one of maintaining or expanding access to health facilities rather than reducing the cost of health care.

A second alternative is reform of hospital reimbursement. Currently many states or regions within states are experimenting with reimbursing hospitals prospectively rather than on the basis of costs (Dowling, 1974). When working properly, such a system gives hospitals incentives to avoid capital projects that inflate costs. These systems are imperfect, and the focus on cost per day or per admission has shortcomings. While prospective reimbursement in theory strengthens hospital incentives to boost productive efficiency and avoid waste, it may not be a complete substitute for planning as a control mechanism. The prospective rate is often only one instrument, and its goals are multiple. Thus while an incentive for elimination of unnecessary services is given, the same formula may give incentives to expand days of care and build additional beds.

A third alternative is to alter the incentives for individuals' consumption of hospital care. Feldstein's (1971) proposal for very large deductibles in public health insurance and Newhouse and Taylor's (1970) variable subsidy insurance plan give the patient an incentive to avoid hospitals whose high costs are not reflected in superior service or essential amenities. To the extent that patients are sensitive to price in selecting hospitals, the institutions will have an incentive to avoid inflationary capital investments. While this approach is particularly attractive, eliminating subsidies for the purchase of health insurance is necessary for it to work, and this does not appear on the political horizon. Incentive reimbursement is probably the second-best solution.

Research

Given the lack of consensus with regard to the adequacy of overall funding for capital investment, empirical studies of the impact of inflation on investment have limited usefulness. This lack of usefulness is compounded by the fact that inflation affects real hospital investment only in the short run.

With regard to the effects of investment on inflation in hospital costs, more fruitful research opportunities exist. One avenue is the assessment of the medical benefits of time spent in the hospital and of specific medical services performed. Economists tend to think that technicians (physicians in this case) know the production function (the relationship between medical services and health), but according to Cochrane (1972), this is not the case.

Instead of deciding if capital financing is adequate and starting a new grant program if it is not, researchers should be working closely with government to evaluate and improve programs in planning, reimbursement, and insurance in order to improve the allocative abilities of the hospital capital market. Researchers are all too often absent in the design of programs of planning and reimbursement control, at least in early stages. By urging the elimination of ineffective programs and suggesting designs for more effective programs, the allocation of resources in the health care industry can be improved and cost inflation reduced.

The Role of PSROs
in Hospital Cost Containment

JAMES F. BLUMSTEIN

The Social Security Amendments of 1972 institutionalized peer review, through Professional Standards Review Organizations (PSROs),[1] as a means of promoting cost consciousness and assuring quality maintenance in federal medical programs. Composed exclusively of licensed physicians in an area, a PSRO is to review medical care provided to federal beneficiaries under the Medicare, Medicaid, and Maternal and Child Health programs. No funds appropriated for these federal financing programs can be disbursed for the provision of health services if those services are subject to review by a PSRO and that PSRO, applying professionally developed norms of care (§1320c-5), disapproves of the services (§1320c-7(a) (2)). This chapter will consider the contribution, if any, PSROs can make to hospital cost containment.

PSRO Responsibilities and Structure

Although the jurisdiction of PSROs is limited to reviewing the disbursement of federal health dollars under the Medicare, Medicaid, and Maternal and Child Health programs, they are seen as

[1] The PSRO law is codified at 42 United States Code §1320c et seq. For convenience, references will hereinafter omit mention of the United States Code, designating only particular sections of the statute.

In *Hospital Cost Containment: Selected Notes for Future Policy*, edited by Michael Zubkoff, Ira E. Raskin, and Ruth S. Hanft. New York: PRODIST, 1978.

prototypes for extension to private sector activities (Decker and Bonner, 1974). Where a PSRO disapproves of services, it must notify the practitioner or provider and also the individual who would have received or did actually receive the services. There is an elaborate hearing procedure (§1320c-8) by which any provider or recipient entitled to benefits can seek reconsideration by the PSRO, appeal to the State Council where one exists, appeal to the secretary of DHEW, and obtain judicial review where more than $1,000 is involved.[2]

PSROs are charged with the responsibility for review of the professional activities within their geographical area of "physicians and other health care practitioners and institutional and noninstitutional providers of health care services. . ." (§1320c-4(a)(1)). They must determine whether health care services and items for which payment may be made under Medicaid and Medicare (a) are or were medically necessary, (b) meet professionally recognized standards of quality, (c) or could be effectively provided on an outpatient basis or more economically in an inpatient facility of a different type (§1320c-4(a)(1)). A PSRO need only review health care services "provided by or in institutions," unless the PSRO itself, with the approval of the secretary of DHEW, seeks to expand its review capability to other health services (§1320c-4(g)). PSROs also must "utilize the services of, and accept the findings of, the review committees" of institutions in the area, provided that such institutions have demonstrated to the PSROs' satisfaction "their capacity effectively and in timely fashion" to carry out the required reviewing procedures (§1320c-4(e) (1)).

At the outset, PSRO designations are made on a conditional basis (§1320c-3(a)) for a trial period not to exceed two years (§1320c-3(b)). During this initial phase, DHEW need only require a PSRO to perform limited review functions within its capability; but by the end of the trial period, a PSRO can be considered qualified for permanent designation only if it is "substantially carrying out, in a satisfactory manner, the activities and functions" required of PSROs (§1320c-3(b)).

[2]A separate and distinct hearing procedure is involved where a sanction is sought to be imposed on a provider (§1320c-9).

The PSRO legislation alters the nature of the utilization review process. The very clear mandate is that a PSRO be composed of licensed physicians practicing in the area (§1320c-1(b)(1)(A)(ii)). Also, the law specifically addresses what former Senator Wallace Bennett, its sponsor, felt was a major irritant in the utilization review procedure under Medicare—namely, the resentment by the medical profession of having nonmedical personnel make utilization review decisions (U.S. Congress, 1972:256). The Medicare legislation required hospitals to have utilization review procedures but specified that hospital staff committees need contain only two physicians. Moreover, claims review by financial intermediaries often involved insurance company personnel in reviewing and questioning medical procedures prescribed and performed by physicians. Senator Bennett believed that "clerical personnel could not and should not make decisions as to the quality and necessity of medical services" (Congressional Record, 1972a:S16111). Accordingly, under the law no PSRO can allow anyone but a duly licensed physician to make final determinations with respect to the "professional conduct" of any licensed physician or with respect to "any act performed by any duly licensed doctor of medicine . . . in the exercise of his profession" (§1320c-4(c)).

Quite clearly, review by PSROs is intended to shift utilization control authority expressly and uniquely to physicians themselves so that "physicians can assume full responsibility for reviewing the utilization of services" (U.S. Congress, 1972:257), and is "based upon the premise that only physicians are, in general, qualified to judge whether services ordered by other physicians are necessary" (U.S. Congress, 1972:256).

Although the legislation provides for the establishment of local PSROs, the act also creates certain oversight mechanisms to advise PSROs and review their activities. In states having three or more PSROs, DHEW must establish a Statewide Professional Standards Review Council. The Statewide Council is to be composed of one representative from and designated by each PSRO in the state, two physicians chosen by the state medical society, two physicians chosen by the state hospital association, and four persons "knowledgeable in health care" who presumably are to represent consumer interests. Two of these consumer representatives must be recommended by the governor of the state before the secretary of DHEW can select them for the Statewide Council; the secretary can appoint the other two representatives from the state on his own (§1320c-11(b)).

If the appointment procedure is well defined, the duties of the Statewide Council are somewhat uncertain. The function of the Statewide Council is to "coordinate the activities of, and disseminate information and data among" the PSROs within the state, but the only specific coordinating function mentioned in the statute is the development of "uniform data gathering and operating procedures" so as "to assure efficient operation and objective evaluation of comparative performance of the several areas" (§1320c-11(c)(1)). This coordinative role is linked with a responsibility to assist DHEW in "evaluating the performance" of each PSRO in the state and to help DHEW find or organize a qualified replacement PSRO where necessary. The Statewide Council's reporting reponsibility is to the secretary of DHEW; it has "no direct authority over PSROs," but PSROs are expected to cooperate with Statewide Councils to "facilitate communication and cooperative arrangements among the PSROs in the State" (U.S. DHEW, 1974b:§530).

States that have Statewide Councils will also have advisory groups furnishing input to the council (§1320c-11(3)(1)). In states without Statewide Councils, these advisory groups will operate directly under the jurisdiction of the PSRO; the selection process is to be determined by DHEW regulation (§1320c-11(3)(2)). Since the council's provider members are all physicians, the advisory group represents an official mechanism which allows nonphysician provider viewpoints to be expressed at the statewide level. Where Statewide Councils exist, PSROs themselves have the option of establishing a formal relationship with an advisory body, subject to DHEW approval (U.S. DHEW, 1974b:§540); but in such states, PSROs are under no obligation to maintain any such formal tie.

In addition to the Statewide Councils and state or local advisory bodies, the PSRO legislation provides for the establishment of a National Professional Standards Review Council (NPSRC). This national body poses a major potential threat to the autonomy of

local physicians. The regional structure of the peer review procedure was a gesture toward retention of regional control and maintenance of regional differences in medical practice. Nevertheless, as
former Office of Professional Standards Review director Dr. Henry
Simmons early realized, where certain procedures are by general
consensus recognized to be of no use or are actually counterproductive, there is little reason to allow regional determinations of
necessity or appropriateness. This tension between local or regional
autonomy on the one hand and imposition of technological efficiency in disbursement of federal funds on the other is one that
is left unresolved by the language of the act and predictably
has generated pointed and probing questions by the medical
association.

The NPSRC is charged with the responsibility of providing for
the development and distribution of information and data to PSROs
and Statewide Councils. These materials "will assist such review
councils and organizations in carrying out their duties and functions"
(§1320c-12(e)(2)). The National Council also will review the operations of PSROs and Statewide Councils to determine their effectiveness and comparative performance (§1320c-12(e)(3)), and make
studies and recommendations to DHEW and to Congress about how
to accomplish the objectives of the act more effectively (§1320c-
12(e)(4)). Membership in the NPSRC is limited to eleven physicians, a majority of whom must be selected by DHEW only if
recommended by "national organizations recognized by the Secretary as representing practicing physicians" (§1320c-12(b)). The
department is also required to include as members physicians who
have been recommended by consumer groups and other health care
interests.

The provisions regarding composition of the NPSRC are clearly
aimed at assuaging the sensitivities of physicians since all members
must be doctors, and organized medical groups representing practicing physicians must recommend a majority of the members.
Nevertheless, the ambiguity of the NPSRC's charge raised medical
association eyebrows because of the possible usurpation (in the eyes
of the AMA) of local autonomy by the national body.

The act provides for three different kinds of reviewing procedures which can be construed as sanctions. First, a PSRO can disapprove of health services and thereby deny federal payment of claims based upon provision of those services (§1320c-7). This disapproval must be based on criteria set out in the act under norms adopted by the PSRO (§1320c-4(a)(1) & (2)). Any beneficiary, recipient, provider, or practitioner dissatisfied with a claim determination (a) can seek reconsideration by the PSRO; (b) where a Statewide Council exists and $100 or more is at stake can appeal to the Statewide Council; and (c) where $100 or more is at stake can appeal to the secretary, who is obligated to provide a hearing. If $1,000 or more is at stake, an appeal to the courts is allowed (§1320c-8).

Secondly, a PSRO can report to the secretary (through the Statewide Council, where one exists) that a provider or physician has violated a duty imposed by the PSRO legislation (§1320c-6). If the secretary finds that the practitioner or provider has demonstrated an unwillingness or a lack of ability substantially to comply with his statutory obligations, then he can impose one of two penalties. He can either (a) exclude or suspend the provider from eligibility to provide health services on a federally reimbursable basis, or (b) require that the provider pay back to the government the excess charges (not to exceed $5,000). Either of these alternative penalties can be imposed only upon a finding (1) that the provider has failed in a substantial number of cases substantially to comply with the obligations imposed on him under the act, or (2) that he grossly and flagrantly violated any obligation in one or more instances (§1320c-9(b)(1)). Before imposition of any penalty, the provider is entitled to a hearing before the secretary and to judicial review of the secretary's final decision (§1320c-9(b) (4)).

Finally, the secretary can terminate a contract with a PSRO upon a finding that it is not "substantially complying with or effectively carrying out" its agreement with DHEW. In making this determination, the secretary must give notice in accordance with regulations he establishes and provide a formal hearing to the PSRO (§1320c-1(d)(2)). Statewide Councils, where they exist, will assist the secretary in evaluating the performance of the PSRO and help him locate or organize a substitute where an agreement is terminated (§1320c-11(c)(2) & (3)).

James F. Blumstein

The PSRO's Reviewing Procedures

The PSRO law mandates that each PSRO "apply professionally developed norms of care, diagnosis and treatment . . . as principal points of evaluation and review" (§1320c-5). These norms are to be based on "typical patterns of practice in its regions" and are to include "typical lengths-of-stay for institutional care by age and diagnosis" (§1320c-5). The statutory provision makes it clear that PSRO educational efforts and reviewing activities are to be more than a series of ad hoc decisions, and the development and application of norms have been described as the "keystone to the PSRO program" (Gosfield, 1975:29).

The PSRO Program Manual, the primary source of authority for understanding DHEW's implementation of the law, establishes three categories for guiding PSRO operations. "Norms" are defined as reflecting typical practice; "criteria" are expertly developed guidelines against which actual practice can be measured; "standards" are professionally developed statements of an acceptable range of deviation from a norm or criterion (see also U.S. DHEW, 1973:§709). Although there is no mention of the concepts of "criteria" or "standards" in the statute itself, these constructs reflect DHEW's response to the statute's mandate that professionally developed norms accommodate actual patterns of practice.

Under the statutory provisions, the "professionally developed norms" must include "the types and extent of the health care services which . . . are considered within the range of appropriate diagnosis and treatment" for particular illnesses or health conditions (§1320c-5(b)(1)). In the formulation of these norms, "differing, but acceptable, modes of treatment and methods of organizing and delivering care" must be taken into account; and the norms adopted must be "consistent with professionally recognized and accepted patterns of care."

This language does appear to support the view that the PSRO program was aimed in part to improve techniques of practice in areas where "actual norms" diverge from "professionally developed" norms. From the legislative history, which reflects the concern for excessive utilization of unnecessary services (Havighurst and Blumstein, 1975; Blumstein, 1976), it is reasonable to conclude that the act's sponsors thought such imposition of expertise would likely cut down on unnecessary care. To the extent that physicians are prescribing care which has no benefit to patients, or which may even be counterproductive, then the "waste" control objective may be achieved through articulation and communication of professionally developed norms. Presumably, the "professionally recognized and accepted patterns of care" would effectively curtail wasteful procedures that are ordered by providers who have not been able to keep up with the latest developments.

Unfortunately, from a cost-containment perspective, this expectation would appear ill-founded. First, as a practical political matter, traditional physician concerns for professional autonomy have predictably led to erosion of national control over the development of norms. The statute nowhere grants a PSRO the authority to "develop" norms; rather the PSRO must "apply" (§1320c-5(a)) and "utilize" (§1320c-5(c)(2)) norms prepared under the supervision of the National Council (§1320c-5(c)(1)). It is the duty of the National Council to "provide for the preparation and distribution" to each PSRO of "appropriate materials indicating the regional norms to be utilized. . . ." The act contemplates NPSRC approval of regional norms "based on its analysis of appropriate and adequate data" (§1320-5(c)(1)).

Where the "actual norms of care" in a PSRO area are "significantly different from professionally developed regional norms of care," the act requires the NPSRC to inform a PSRO of the divergence. The statute then calls for a period of discussion and consultation between the National Council and the PSRO. This provision seems to be a clear expression of legislative intent to impose a professional standard of practice on regions where "typical patterns of practice" do not conform to professionally developed norms prepared at the national level. If the PSRO can show a "reasonable basis" for usage of other norms, then it can apply those norms, provided the National Council approves (§1320c-5(a)). This procedure would conform to the view that an accommodation with regional practice should be made; but the regional PSRO would have to justify its deviant practice standards, presumably as meeting special regional needs, or at least as not imposing unnecessary ("wasteful") services at increased cost. Thus, the PSRO legislation would seem to require that PSROs apply and utilize the nationally approved and professionally developed norms unless they secure approval from the NPSRC to deviate from that standard (Havighurst and Blumstein, 1975:47–51).

It appears that DHEW initially took this position. In a question-and-answer pamphlet published in December 1973—prior to release of the PSRO Program Manual—DHEW's Office of Professional Standards Review (OPSR) stated that "[e]ach PSRO will establish standards and criteria of care that reflect acceptable patterns of practice in the PSRO's area." The office went on, however, to indicate that the NPSRC "must approve norms used by a PSRO that are significantly different from professionally developed regional norms" (U.S. DHEW, 1973).

Perceiving and reacting to this apparent threat to local decision-making, the AMA raised the question, "Who would have the right to set norms and how would they be determined?" (U.S. DHEW, 1974a:2). This was obviously seen by OPSR as a very delicate issue. In response, OPSR sought to persuade the medical association that the "clear intent is to use norms, criteria, and standards developed by physicians in the PSRO area" (U.S. DHEW, 1974a) and that the PSROs would retain the "overall responsibility for the development, modification and content of norms, criteria and standards . . ." (U.S. DHEW, 1974b:§702.2). Clearly, OPSR felt under heavy pressure to come out on the side of greater local autonomy in the setting of practice norms.

The PSRO Manual reflects this decision not only in the section quoted in the OPSR Memo but also in section 709.1, which discusses development of norms. Whereas the act specifies that the National Council shall distribute materials "indicating the regional norms to be utilized" by PSROs, the manual states that the NPSRC will provide, when available, "sample sets of norms and criteria to each PSRO" (U.S. DHEW, 1974b:§709.11). The manual calls upon each conditional PSRO to review as early as "feasible" the model sets of norms "in order to adopt or adapt them for their use" (U.S. DHEW, 1974b:§709.12). Then the manual underlines the word "alternatively" and notes that the PSRO can choose "to develop its own criteria and standards and/or select its own norms." Nowhere in the section on PSRO responsibilities is there any mention of approval by the National Council, as contemplated by the act.

This position was hardly an oversight. Former DHEW Secretary Caspar Weinberger explicitly stated at PSRO Oversight Hearings in May 1974 that he believed PSROs had the authority to set norms and that if DHEW or the NPSRC in fact had that power, he would support a statutory change to remove that authority (Gosfield, 1975:55). Thus, it seems that DHEW concluded that it must rewrite the statute in order to live with the AMA. Simultaneously, the department's stance significantly waters down even the waste control authority of the NPSRC to require use of professionally developed norms by PSROs.

A second problem with the cost-containment assumptions of PSRO sponsors is that "waste control" objectives are not necessarily consistent with cost-containment goals. A program that successfully curtails unproductive or counterproductive care may not deal with broader—more fundamental—questions. Some care may be effective (that is, marginally improves the likelihood of cure or diagnosis) but uneconomic (that is, benefits do not outweigh costs). Since these procedures make a positive contribution to improved health, a purely professional standard could reasonably permit high-cost measures to be taken even if the incremental benefits are relatively small. If "waste control" is seen purely as a concept that eliminates unproductive or counterproductive care, then it is very possible that PSROs could increase rather than decrease aggregate costs.

This is a point that OPSR stressed in its early sales pitch to physicians: total cost may rise under PSRO, but this will not mean failure. The office was forced to recognize the potential conflicts between cost-containment objectives and a program limited to "waste control." But for whatever reasons, DHEW seems to have opted for "waste control," while still talking about potential cost savings (Havighurst and Blumstein, 1975:41–45).[3]

Utilization review generally incorporates an economic dimension (Stuart and Stockton, 1973), where the label "unnecessary" can

[3] For a discussion of a similar conflict in program objectives between family planning proponents and population control advocates, see Blumstein (1974).

also mean "of insufficiently high priority to warrant an expenditure." A judgment must be made in these situations whether to permit (with federal reimbursement) or require (through malpractice standards) a certain procedure in a given situation. Consider the case where a person in his twenties complains of growing near-sightedness. The symptom continues for a number of years and he ultimately goes blind. Should a physician routinely test for glaucoma in this situation when the likelihood of its occurring in persons under the age of forty is, say, 1 in 25,000? A standard based purely on technical factors might say one thing, while a consideration of cost might lead to a different conclusion (*Helling* v. *Carey*, 1974). This type of concern, however, balancing costs and benefits, cuts against the grain of the medical profession, accustomed as it has become to unchallenged underwriting by the deep pockets of third-party payers.

The PSRO statute itself calls for imposition of economic factors in the formulation of norms. Delivery of medical services can be conceived as a production process that combines a variety of inputs in order to achieve a certain outcome (Blumstein and Zubkoff, 1973). Under traditional economic theory, a production process that does not utilize inputs in a combination that brings about a given result in the least costly way is inefficient. In medical care, as in other processes, there is often a variety of treatments or combination of treatments that will bring about a desired outcome. Utilizing resources in such a way as to minimize the cost for a specified result is one way to define efficiency. One of the explicit charges to a PSRO is to determine whether health services can be provided on an outpatient rather than on an inpatient basis, or whether the services can be provided on an inpatient basis in a less costly facility (§1320c-4(a)(1)(C)). This is implicitly a responsibility to determine whether the "production process" proposed by the attending physician is an efficient one or whether, "consistent with appropriate medical care," an alternative process would utilize fewer scarce medical resources.

Improvement in the technology of producing medical outcomes is a broadly accepted goal. The controversy is who will decide what methods are effective and efficient (Blumstein, 1976). Opposition to this function of the PSRO is partly explained as professional resentment to outside supervision or control of a process that has typically been insulated from external review (Rivkin and Bush, 1974:315–324). Currently, only egregious cases, which wind up in court as malpractice cases or before disciplinary boards of medical societies, subject a physician to significant external review. A more principled objection to the exercise of this production function review by PSROs is that techniques of measurement are insufficiently refined so that a single efficient production technology is an unrealistic goal at this stage. Establishment of detailed and possibly rigid protocols for treating specific illnesses and a heavy-handed reviewing organization could lock in a specific production technology, thereby hampering experimentation or innovation.

The effectiveness and efficiency objectives, however, are not the same as faced in the glaucoma testing case posed earlier. Where unproductive, counterproductive, or inefficient care is being provided, costs can be cut without consumer sacrifice (though professional autonomy is being threatened). The glaucoma testing situation is different in that failure to test will actually result in increased health risk for some people. It is this type of problem that a cost-containment program must face if it is to keep aggregate expenditures under control. Yet a program like PSRO that emphasizes improved production function technology really does not address squarely this very basic question—whether certain expenditures are worth their cost (Fein, 1973; Fuchs, 1973, 1974; Havighurst and Blumstein, 1975; Lave and Lave, 1970).

A third problem with PSRO cost-containment assumptions is the use of and reliance on professionally developed norms of care. It is clear that formulation of norms will be a critical determinant of a PSRO's ability to pursue cost-containment goals (Gosfield, 1975:29). But the emphasis on a professionally developed standard seems likely to result in norms that impose the best available practice as the expected level of quality—with its attendant high cost. Former Assistant Secretary for Health Dr. Charles C. Edwards indicated the force of the "professional quality imperative" when he said that PSROs can be a "vehicle for change whereby the best and most effective care becomes the standard of care" (Edwards, 1973). Such an outcome could result in a mandated format of medical practice

that inadequately considers forgone alternative expenditure opportunities. "Indeed, instead of serving as watch dogs on behalf of the
public at large, PSROs might well become potent, and virtually
unopposed, political instruments for increasing rather than containing costs" (Havighurst and Blumstein, 1975:66). This is evidently
what has happened in West Germany with its counterpart to the
PSRO program (Stone, 1974).

In addition to the impetus of the "professional quality imperative" in the formulation of norms, the formula for establishing norms
provides an opportunity for expanding quality objectives, at the
expense of cost-containment goals. Ironically, the statute implicitly
contemplates development of PSRO norms which might fall below
standards of customary medical practice in a PSRO area. Since this
would entail a risk of malpractice susceptibility for practitioners
following those more cost-conscious PSRO norms (King, 1975;
Holder, 1975), the statute immunizes providers who apply PSRO
norms from any form of civil liability (§1320c-16(c)). As long as
providers comply with PSRO norms and standards in effect in the
region where care is rendered, and apply those norms and standards
with due care, they cannot be held liable for malpractice under state
law (George Washington Law Review, 1974).

The malpractice immunity makes sense if PSRO norms were
likely to establish more cost-conscious standards of practice for
providers than currently exist under state malpractice law. But the
PSRO statute, especially as implemented by DHEW, seems to set
current practice patterns as the minimum upon which to build.
"Criteria" are to be developed by national specialist groups under
contract with DHEW, and they are likely to require more sophisticated patterns of treatment (even while weeding out some "wasteful" procedures). Thus, the manual and the statute call for establishment of a range of acceptable care, but the bottom of the range is
likely to be current practice, while the "professional quality imperative" will tend to push the upper end of the range to more elaborate
coverage. At the very least, the PSRO statutory references to
"professionally developed norms of care" seem to dictate a higher
standard than currently exists under traditional malpractice law,
which relies on "customary" practice (King, 1975). The implementa-

tion formulation developed by the PSRO Program Manual would seem virtually certain to assure this result, encouraging providers who practice at the lower end of the established range to "improve" their standards by modifying their patterns of practice. If this prediction is accurate, then the malpractice immunity provision may be less significant than PSRO strategists initially thought.

While professionalism and quality goals provide an impetus for "upgrading" patterns of care at public expense, professional self-interest also cuts in the same direction. Composed of physicians who practice predominantly in a fee-for-service environment, PSROs are unlikely to look kindly on cost-containment objectives when they threaten physician incomes. This is especially true when a patient is a public beneficiary whose welfare is increased by improved quality of medical treatment and who loses a benefit if he or she does not undertake a treatment whose net health effect is positive, even if very costly. This allows the physician to have a congruence of interests with the patient, providing the "best" care unconcerned with and unconstrained by cost factors. The coincidence of the physician's pecuniary interest with the patient's welfare maximization interest is a comfortable one for the provider, alleviating the need for soul-searching about improper motivation for self-interest. Yet, this factor of self-interest has been recognized as a lurking influence in standard-setting: "Obviously there is minimal possibility of such low cost-oriented norms because the physicians establishing norms have a financial incentive to extend Medicare and Medicaid coverage to as many services as possible" (Gosfield, 1975:54, n. 37).

Impact of PSRO Authority and Structure

The problems that PSROs will have in achieving cost-containment objectives arise not only from the format and control of the standard-setting and reviewing process but also from their range of authority and their structure.

Delegation

The PSRO law stemmed in part from the Senate Finance Committee's conclusion that hospital utilization review procedures had not succeeded in curtailing excessive use of hospital services. A primary legislative concern was the apparent conflict of interest represented by internal institutional reviewing committees. Testimony showed that physicians who had a financial interest in a hospital often sat on the utilization review committee; also, because of the attendant fiscal hardship, hospitals had an institutional stake in avoiding low occupancy rates. Some evidence even supported the view that the rigor of the reviewing process decreased as the hospital's occupancy rate fell.

The Finance Committee's concern with conflicts of interest found its way into the statute. Physicians with staff privileges in a hospital may participate in reviewing services provided by that institution, but they "ordinarily should not be responsible" for that review (§1320c-4(a)(5)). Similarly, a physician is not permitted to review services provided to a patient "if he was directly or indirectly involved in providing such services" (§1320c-4(a)(6)(A)); nor can a physician review services provided by or in an institution "if he or any member of his family has, directly or indirectly, any financial interest in such institution, organization, or agency" (§1320c-4(a)(6)(B)). Nevertheless, in the final version of the act, each PSRO was required to "utilize the services of, and accept the findings of, the review committees" of provider institutions if they satisfied a PSRO that they were doing an effective job (§1320c-4(e)(1)).

While hospital review committees must apply norms established by PSROs, the manual allows PSROs to grant permission to hospitals to use their own guidelines (U.S. DHEW, 1974b:§709.42). This provision undermines much of the desired independence sought for the reviewing process. By September 1976 fewer than 30 percent of all hospitals under PSRO review held "nondelegated status"—that is, were permitting PSRO personnel directly to perform the reviewing function (U.S. DHEW, 1977:30). However, it is possible that some good can still come from the new procedure.

Presumably, if PSRO norms are applied, even by a hospital committee under delegated status, the review will be less idiosyncratic, reflecting a broader practice pattern (Havighurst and Blumstein, 1975:51). Also, PSROs have a duty to keep track of each institution's performance under delegated review status (U.S. DHEW, 1974b:§720.01); and as part of its overall responsibility for collecting and comparing data and profiles of care, a PSRO will be able to exercise some oversight.

Another plus might be the effect of delegated status on the practice in health maintenance organizations (HMOs). PSROs have jurisdiction over HMOs, and an argument can be made that the process norms being developed by PSROs are suited primarily for a fee-for-service milieu and are incompatible with the prepaid group practice mode of delivery (Havighurst and Bovbjerg, 1975; but see Gosfield, 1975:89–94). Through the delegation amendment to the act and the even more permissive provision in the manual, it is possible that some of the more onerous effects of PSRO review on HMO care might be curtailed.

Of course, it is questionable whether PSROs will have any reason to act so munificently toward HMO providers (Havighurst and Bovbjerg, 1975). And the delegation amendment certainly raises questions about the effectiveness that PSROs will have, for it seems that internal committees still continue to play the critical reviewing role as before.

Structural Aspects

The mission of PSROs, as reviewing institutions, is to determine whether a provider has furnished adequate quality care to a specific Medicare or Medicaid beneficiary and whether the government should pay for that care. It has no jurisdiction to consider trade-offs among competing allocative priorities within the health sector (for example, curative vs. preventive care) or between health and other items. PSROs' cost-containment goal has apparently become that of eliminating unproductive or counterproductive care—that is, barring payments where there is no net benefit to the patient. While PSROs have authority to enforce improvements in production technology, including requiring outpatient in lieu of inpatient treatment or inpatient care in less costly facilities (§1320c-4(a)(1)(c)), they do not have authority to reinvest these savings to spend in other ways to promote other health objectives. This is a particularly difficult structural disincentive to cost containment where PSROs are asked to curtail admittedly efficient and useful procedures on the grounds that they are of insufficiently high economic priority when balanced against competing claims on scarce resources.

It is helpful to introduce the concepts of "micro-" and macro-" quality at this point. Macro concerns emphasize the "effectiveness of the health-care sector as a whole in maintaining or improving the health status of the . . . population as a whole" (Reinhardt, 1973:177). Micro-quality, on the other hand, would place primary emphasis on the technical quality of the medical services actually provided to individual patients (Reinhardt, 1973:177). Assuming that the health industry knew how to produce either macro- or micro-quality efficiently, there would be a trade-off between achieving either goal. Given a level of resources, a health policy planner would have to face the question of determining which measure of quality is more important and which therefore should receive more weight and command additional resources.

In this context, the limited jurisdiction of PSROs poses an extremely difficult institutional problem. From a societal viewpoint, there is a very real trade-off between goals of micro- and macro-quality. There can be no objective statements about the "overall quality" of alternative allocation decisions because, for any given resource constraint, "any overall index of quality must be a weighted sum of micro- and macro-quality, and these weights can be established only through political consensus" (Reinhardt, 1973:180). Thus, one's evaluation of a health system often depends on the relative weights assigned to differing concepts of quality.

Since a PSRO does not have an option to reallocate resources, and its choice is limited to approval or disapproval of federal reimbursement for specific medical services, it is warranted in concluding that its micro-quality goal is being promoted once it determines that a medical procedure arguably will make a positive contribution to a patient's health. What such a decision ignores, unfortunately, is that society does have an option to reallocate funds to macro goals if it chooses. But reorientation to macro objectives or reallocation to important nonmedical priorities is not within the institutional competence of a PSRO, and the legislation establishes no incentive for a PSRO to be sensitive to these other societal needs.

Indeed, the PSRO legislation promotes just the opposite. Since

PSROs are organized regionally, a hard-nosed PSRO may be imposing lower standards of micro-quality on patients in its region without their receiving any tangible benefits in return. Both Medicare and Medicaid are entitlement programs whereby patients are reimbursed if they incur eligible expenses. As an organizational matter, there is no mechanism established to assure that patients in a PSRO's area will reap any reward from forgoing very expensive medical services. Savings imposed by one PSRO remain in the common pool for expenditure elsewhere or are returned to the federal treasury. These funds, therefore, are disbursed broadly, not to those who cut expenditures to reduce costs. This is an especially strong consideration and disincentive to economize where patients (and providers) in one region can accurately point to nearby PSROs which are applying more lenient standards.

In addition, the constituency to which regional PSROs are accountable includes physicians and other providers in their area. DHEW has very little maneuverability in applying sanctions to an ornery PSRO because of legislative limitations on the conditions for termination and designation as a qualified organization. On the other hand, the PSRO law gives physicians, institutional, and other providers standing to challenge PSRO judgments. Therefore, it is fair to assume that pressure on PSROs will come almost entirely from those who have a stake in maximizing micro-quality. Formal challenge procedures have been created to guarantee patients review of PSRO denial of payments, and patient interests are likely to be aroused when they are hit with medical bills that are deemed ineligible under a federal program. Providers will also press claims to reimbursement for services since many patients under Medicare or Medicaid are unable to make good on payments for already rendered care (*Mount Sinai Hospital of Greater Miami* v. *Weinberger*, 1974).

Not only is there no incentive for PSRO patients to restrain pursuit of micro-quality irrespective of cost because they will not benefit tangibly from such restraint, but also each PSRO itself has no institutional reason to face up to the difficult general allocative problems that society must confront with regard to public expenditures in the aggregate. Thus, while often promoted as a cost-containment tool that examines economic as well as medical perspectives, utilization review as carried out by PSROs may exacerbate already existent pressures for focusing on micro-quality. PSROs may therefore serve as extremely forceful political institutions influencing federal health and spending priorities generally and helping to shape definitions of quality of care. Rather than serving to contain aggregate costs, they may very well become extremely potent political lobbies that perpetuate current perspectives on medical spending and promote adoption of high standards of quality at the expense of other important social goals (Stone, 1974; Stuart and Stockton, 1973:342-343).

Regulatory Authority

The Senate supporters of PSROs identified two factors that had contributed to cost increases in the Medicare and Medicaid programs: rises in the unit prices of services, and increases in the number of services provided to beneficiaries (U.S. Congress, 1972:254). PSROs have no jurisdiction to consider pricing decisions, and therefore their effectiveness as cost-containment institutions is inherently limited. Moreover, to the extent that determinations of medical necessity include a socioeconomic judgment (Stuart and Stockton, 1973), limitations on PSRO power to concern itself with price inevitably inhibit its ability to perform a resource allocation function.

The narrow scope of PSRO authority also leaves it no role in the planning process. PSROs will generate data on utilization rates and profiles of practice and patient care; and some cooperative arrangement with the areawide Health Systems Agencies—HSAs—being set up under the National Health Planning and Resources Development Act of 1974 will be necessary (U.S. Congress, 1975). But the HSA regions have not been established to conform to PSRO regions (even though the Health Planning Act called for coordination of PSRO areas and health services areas to the "maximum extent feasible.") And there seems to be a conflict brewing between HSAs and PSROs with regard to their respective data-gathering roles (Butler et al., 1977).

In addition, the Health Planning Act requires states to establish a certificate-of-need program which applies to "new institutional health services," defined as services provided through health care facilities and health maintenance organizations. The certificate-of-need requirement vests planning and regulatory activities in another limited function organization, which will authorize expenditures on capital items. Under traditional forms of pricing arrangements, institutions will be permitted to earn a rate of return on approved capital outlays. With this approval, providers will have a much stronger claim in negotiating with PSROs that usage of the facilities should be permitted.

The Health Planning Act reflects a federal move toward more regulation in the health area, but functions typically performed by a regulatory body are now dispersed among multiple agencies. Utilization decisions for federal beneficiaries are made by PSROs; capital outlay decisions will be made by a statewide certificate-of-need body in consultation with areawide planning agencies (HSAs); and pricing decisions will be made by a third set of decision makers, typically government health officials or fiscal intermediaries.

Neither PSROs nor certificate-of-need agencies, furthermore, have any institutional incentive to curtail overinvestment or overutilization (Havighurst, 1973). This is an especially noteworthy problem for PSROs since their funding comes directly from DHEW and is unrelated to their performance in curtailing excessive utilization. Also, PSROs do not have a fixed budget to administer—either as an absolute amount or a target—so that their utilization review decisions will be made in part in a vacuum, which inevitably means the "yes-no" perception is exacerbated at the expense of the "either-or" viewpoint (Havighurst and Blumstein, 1975). Without some prior specification of a budget for a region, it becomes difficult to assess how individual decisions should be made, giving due consideration to cost factors.

Thus, the regulatory apparatus being set up in the health field will suffer even greater disadvantages than the regulatory bodies in other industries (Posner, 1971). Given the fragmentation, financing, and functional specialization, there is likely to be even less incentive and less opportunity to affect costs and to weigh different health objectives. Expansion of PSRO authority, on the other hand, has its risks, and further governmental involvement in supervising doctor-patient encounters runs the risk of invading privacy (Springer, 1975; Boyer, 1975), though not impermissibly so in the PSRO case, *Association of American Physicians and Surgeons v. Weinberger* (1975). This overall pattern must be part of an evaluation of the likely effectiveness of PSROs as a cost-containment instrument for hospital services and should encourage policymakers to search for additional mechanisms for pursuing cost-containment objectives.

References and Acknowledgments

Initial work on PSRO research was supported by the Common-wealth Foundation and by grant number HS 01539 from the Bureau of Health Services Research, Health Resources Administration, U.S. Department of Health, Education, and Welfare. The preparation of this study was supported by the Vanderbilt Institute for Public Policy Studies and also by the Department of Community Medicine, Dartmouth Medical School.

American Medical Association
   1972   Peer Review Manual. Chicago: American Medical Association.
Andreano, R., and B. Weisbrod
   1974   American Health Policy. Chicago: Rand McNally College Publishing Company.
Association of American Physicians and Surgeons v. Weinberger
   1975   395 F. Supp. 125 (N.D. Ill.), *affirmed* 423 U.S. 975.
Berki, S.E.
   1972   Hospital Economics. Lexington, Mass.: Lexington Books, D.C. Heath & Co.
Blumstein, J.F.
   1974   "Foundations of federal fertility policy." Milbank Memorial Fund Quarterly/Health and Society 52 (Spring): 131–168.
   1976   "Inflation and quality: The case of PSROs." Pp. 245–295, 375–380 in Michael Zubkoff, ed., Health: A Victim or Cause of Inflation? New York: Prodist for Milbank Memorial Fund.
Blumstein, J.F., and M. Zubkoff
   1973   "Perspectives on government policy in the health sector." Mil-

bank Memorial Fund Quarterly/Health and Society 51 (Summer): 395-431.

Boyer, B.B.
1975   "Computerized medical records and the right to privacy: The emerging federal response." Buffalo Law Review 25: 37-118.

Butler, L.H., et al.
1977   Cooperation between Health Systems Agencies and Professional Standards Review Organizations. San Francisco: Health Policy Program, University of California School of Medicine.

Cochrane, A.L.
1972   Effectiveness and Efficiency: Random Reflections on Health Services. London: The Nuffield Provincial Hospitals Trust.

Congressional Record
1972a   Remarks of Senator Bennett. 118, No. 152 (September 27): S16111-16112.
1972b   Remarks of Senator Long. 118, No. 168 (October 17): S18479.

Decker, B., and P. Bonner
1973   PSRO: Organization for Regional Peer Review. Cambridge: Ballinger Publishing Company.

Edwards, C.C.
1973   "Improving the nation's health care system." Address before the National Association of Blue Shield Plans. Chicago: October 25, 1973.

Fein, R.
1973   "On achieving access and equity in health care." Pp. 23-56 in John B. McKinlay, ed., Economic Aspects of Health Care. New York: Prodist for Milbank Memorial Fund.

Fuchs, V.R.
1973   "Health care and the United States economic system—an essay in abnormal physiology." Pp. 95-121 in John B. McKinlay ed., Economic Aspects of Health Care. New York: Prodist for Milbank Memorial Fund.
1974   Who Shall Live? Health, Economics and Social Choice. New York: Basic Books, Inc.

George Washington Law Review
1974   Note, "Federally-imposed self-regulation of medical practice: A critique of the Professional Standards Review Organization." George Washington Law Review 42: 822-849.

Gosfield, A.
1975   PSROs: The Law and the Health Consumer. Cambridge: Ballinger Publishing Company.

James F. Blumstein

Havighurst, C.C.
1973   "Regulation of health facilities and services by 'certificate of need.'" Virginia Law Review 59 (October): 1143–1232.
Havighurst, C.C., and J.F. Blumstein
1975   "Coping with quality/cost trade-offs in medical care: The role of PSROs." Northwestern Law Review 70 (March–April): 6–68.
Havighurst, C.C., and R. Bovbjerg
1975   "Professional Standards Review Organizations and Health Maintenance Organizations: Are they compatible?" Utah Law Review (Summer): 381–421.
Helling v. Carey
1974   519 P.2d 981.
Holder, A.R.
1975   Medical Malpractice Law. New York: John Wiley & Sons, Inc.
InterStudy
1973   Assuring the Quality of Health Care. Minneapolis: InterStudy.
Jeffers, J.R., et al.
1971   "On the demand versus need for medical services and the concept on shortage." American Journal of Public Health 61 (January): 46–63.
King, J.H.
1975   "In search of a standard of care for the medical profession: The 'accepted practice' formula." Vanderbilt Law Review 28: 1213–1276.
Koos, E.L.
1954   The Health of Regionville. New York: Columbia University Press.
Lander, L.
1974   "PSROs: A little toe in the door." Health/PAC Bulletin 59 (July/August).
Lave, J.R., and L.B. Lave
1970   "Medical care and its delivery: An economic appraisal." Law and Contemporary Problems 35 (Spring): 252–266.
Mount Sinai Hospital of Greater Miami v. Weinberger
1974   376 F. Supp. 1099 (S.D. Fla.).
Posner, R.A.
1971   "Regulatory aspects of national health insurance plans." University of Chicago Law Review 39 (Fall): 1–29.
Reinhardt, U.
1973   "Proposed changes in the organization of health-care delivery:

An overview and critique." Milbank Memorial Fund Quarterly/ Health and Society 51 (Spring): 169–223.

Rivkin, M.O., and P.J. Bush
1974   "The satisfaction continuum in health care: Consumer and provider preferences." Pp. 304–332 in Selma J. Mushkin, ed., Consumer Incentives for Health Care. New York: Prodist for Milbank Memorial Fund.

Simmons, H.E.
1973   "PSRO's—An opportunity for medicine." Address before the American Public Health Association, San Francisco, November 7, 1973.

1974a   "PSRO and the quality of medical care." Address before the Indiana Medical Association, May 16, 1974.

1974b   "Federal policy on health manpower." Pp. 81–87 in Institute of Medicine, Manpower for Health Care. Washington, D.C.

Springer, E.W.
1975   "Professional standards review organization: Some problems of confidentiality." Utah Law Review (Summer): 361–380.

Stevens, R.
1971   American Medicine and the Public Interest. New Haven: Yale University Press.

Stone, D.
1974   "Professionalism and accountability: Controlling health services in the United States and West Germany." Working Paper #8742, Center for the Study of Health Policy, Institute of Policy Sciences and Public Affairs. Durham: Duke University.

Stuart, B., and R. Stockton
1973   "Control over the utilization of medical services." Milbank Memorial Fund Quarterly/Health and Society 51 (Spring): 169–223.

Tancredi, L., and J. Woods
1973   "The social control of medical practice—Licensure versus output monitoring." Pp. 327–353 in John B. McKinlay, ed., Economic Aspects of Health Care. New York: Prodist for Milbank Memorial Fund.

Theodore, C.
1974   "Towards a strategy for evaluating PSROs." Westchester Medical Bulletin (November).

U.S. Congress
1972   U.S. Senate Committee on Finance, Report 92-1230, 92d Congress. Washington, D.C.: U.S. Government Printing Office.

James F. Blumstein

1975   National Health Planning and Resources Development Act of 1974. Public Law 93-641 (January 4, 1975). Statutes at Large 88: 2225.

U.S. Department of Health, Education, and Welfare
1973   Publication No. (OS) 74-5001 (December). Reprinted in 2 CCH Medicare and Medicaid Guide: ¶12,885.
1974a   OPSR Memo No. 4 (April).
1974b   P.S.R.O. Program Manual. Washington, D.C.: OPSR.
1977   PSRO Fact Book. Washington, D.C.: Office of Health Standards · and Quality, Health Care Financing Administration.

Welch, C.
1973   "Professional review organizations—problems and prospects." The New England Journal of Medicine 289 (August): 291-295.

The Impact of
Certificate-of Need Controls
on Hospital Investment

DAVID S. SALKEVER

THOMAS W. BICE

Certificate-of-Need (CON) controls over hospital investment have been enacted by a number of states in recent years and the National Health Planning and Resources Development Act of 1974 provides strong incentives for adoption of CON in additional states. In this study, we review the questions that have been raised about the effectiveness of CON controls and then we develop quantitative estimates of the impact of CON on investment. These estimates show that CON did not reduce the total dollar volume of investment but altered its composition, retarding expansion in bed supplies but increasing investment in new services and equipment. We suggest that this finding may be due to (1) the emphasis in CON laws and programs on controlling bed supplies and (2) a substitution of new services and equipment for additional beds in response to financial factors and organizational pressures for expansion. Finally, we caution against the conclusion that CON controls should be broadened and tightened, though our results might be so interpreted, because of the practical difficulties involved in reviewing and certifying large numbers of small investment projects.

Introduction

In the wake of rapid post-Medicare cost inflation, investment controls have emerged as important regulatory mechanisms for moderating the rise in health services expenditures. These controls take two forms: (1) legal prohibitions of unnecessary capital investment, and (2) financial controls, whereby a health care institution's eligibility to receive capital or operating funds relating to an investment project is dependent upon the approval of designated planning agencies. Presently, both types are widespread. Legal prohibitions are in effect through certificate-of-need (CON) laws in twenty-four states, and similar legislation has been proposed in seven other states (Lewin and Associates, Inc., 1974). Moreover, with the passage of P.L. 93-641, the National Health Planning and Resources Development Act of 1974, CON was slated for adoption by all participating states.

Several types of financial controls have been applied. Under

Section 1122 of the Social Security Act, reimbursements under Titles V, XVIII, and XIX for depreciation, interest, and other costs associated with an investment project in excess of $100,000 may be denied if the project is not approved by designated planning agencies. Under contracts from the U.S. Department of Health, Education, and Welfare, thirty-seven states now conduct Section 1122 reviews. Similar provisions ("conformance clauses") link Blue Cross reimbursement to project review by planning agencies or Blue Cross plans themselves in nineteen states. In all states, eligibility for capital investment subsidies through the Hill-Burton program requires planning agency approval, as does participation in construction finance programs in forty-two states.[1]

This spate of controls emerged only very recently and without the benefit of systematic research as to its likely consequences. The major federal initiatives, Section 1122 and P.L. 93-641, were promulgated within the past four years, and all but five of the existing CON laws were enacted since 1970 (Curran, 1974). The reasons behind this wave of enthusiasm for investment controls have yet to be studied in detail. It is distressing to observe, however, that decisions to adopt controls were taken despite the total absence of evidence as to their efficacy or secondary effects. Thus, a thorough review of relevant literature by O'Donoghue and Policy Center, Inc. (1974:67) led to the conclusion that

> ...there is no evidence supporting the effectiveness or efficiency of capital expenditures regulation. On the other hand, it is equally true that there is no evidence indicating that such regulation is ineffective or inefficient.

Of course, the fact that investment controls are already in place does not obviate the need for such evidence. Indeed, since changes in the extent or structure of these controls are possible, and perhaps even likely, systematic assessment of their effects may contribute crucial information for policy formulation.

The major objective of this paper is to provide such information on the quantitative impacts of investment controls. Specifically, we assess effects of CON controls on investment in hospital facilities. The limited nature of this objective should be noted, in that our focus is on only a subset (i.e., hospital in-

[1]Our description of investment controls is from Lewin and Associates, Inc. (1974: Chapter 3), which is current as of April 1, 1974.

vestment) of all potential impact measures[2] and on one particular form of control (i.e., CON). There are, however, several considerations which justify concentration on CON. First, it is the strictest form of control in that failure to win approval for projects usually means that institutions are prohibited from carrying out proposed investments. In consequence, CON is likely to yield measurable impacts. Financial controls, by contrast, impose only monetary sanctions which may be either insufficiently severe to alter hospitals' investment behavior or compensated for by other sources of revenue. Second, the CON approach will probably soon emerge as the predominant form of investment control. As Section 1523 of P.L. 93-641 provides an incentive for non-CON states to adopt CON legislation, other forms of investment control will become redundant and probably fall into desuetude. On this point, Lewin and Associates, Inc. (1974:158) observed that nine of the 14 states which did not participate in the Section 1122 program already had CON laws and that

> ...their lack of interest in the program was based on a belief that Section 1122 review would not add to their existing authority or that 1122 procedural requirements would conflict with state administrative practices.

Our concentration on hospital investment also seems warranted on several grounds. In addition to entailing substantial resource costs, hospital investment triggers increases in utilization and operating costs.[3] In consequence, limitations on investment effect savings in operating as well as capital costs. Furthermore, since control of hospital investment is the principal concern of CON programs, we assume that their effects will be most profound in the hospital sector. By the same token, failure to detect such impacts would be compelling evidence of their ineffectiveness.

We begin with a survey of arguments regarding presumed effects of CON regulation. With these as a background for interpreting our findings, we describe our methods and results.

[2] For discussions of a fuller range of impact measures that would be relevant for a more complete policy evaluation, see May(1974: 58–59) and Brown (1969).

[3] The literature documenting the positive effect of bed supply on hospital use, the so-called "Roemer Law," is extensive. A recent contribution is in Feldstein (1971a). For evidence of the positive impact of equipment and facilities on use and costs, see Davis (1969; 1974) and Berry (1974).

Following these are discussions of the results and conclusions pertaining to policy implications, and suggestions for future research.

Effects of CON:
Critical Views from the Literature

The putative purpose of CON legislation is to restrain costs of health care by limiting unnecessary expansion of health facilities and of services rendered in them. Much of the recent literature expresses skepticism about CON's ability to accomplish this; three principal arguments are advanced. First, some doubt the willingness of agencies administering CON programs to effectively control investment. Second, some question these agencies' ability to accomplish this aim. Finally, concern is expressed about the possible unanticipated effects of CON laws on providers' investment plans.

The thesis that CON agencies will be unwilling to vigorously control hospital investment extends the "capture hypothesis" from experience in other regulated industries. Noting that a regulatory body becomes a focal point for industry lobbying and a prize worthy of capture, critics chronicle the process whereby it comes to serve the welfare of the regulated industry instead of the public interest (Havighurst, 1973: 1178–1179; Hilton, 1972). The political economy of health planning, some note, is particularly conducive to such capture, for the planning agencies that conduct CON reviews in most states include among their board members representatives of hospitals. They are thereby accorded easy access to agency personnel and to influence over agency policy (Lave and Lave, 1974: 169). Furthermore, hospitals are often an important source of financial contributions required for agency survival and growth. Pluralism falters, as the countervailing power of consumers in the review process is diluted by their reliance upon providers and agency staff for technical expertise (Havighurst, 1973: 1183–1184). Consequently, critics allege that CON regulation is employed primarily to block entry by new providers (e.g., hospitals and other potential competitors such as HMOs and surgicenters) rather than to restrain expansion of existing hospitals.

This line of argument suggests that CON programs will effectively control only one type of hospital investment, namely, the building of new hospitals.[4] Conceivably, it might even encourage expansion among existing hospitals by protecting them from competition for donor capital and patients. Were this so, the net effect on hospital investment would be only slightly restrictive at best.

Contrary to these expectations are two principal arguments that lead to the opposite conclusion. First, the existence of standards for review and requirements for public disclosure of rulings may militate against agencies' favoring existing providers at the expense of new entrants. Although such requirements permit considerable discretion in some states, and opportunities for obfuscation persist even when they are enforced, blatant discrimination against new entrants is presumably precluded. Second, existing providers may actually welcome CON control over their own investment opportunities. It may limit competition among hospitals (Posner, 1974) and enhance management's bargaining position vis-a-vis the medical staff.[5] By holding that they have little power to prevent CON agency disapproval of investment plans to which they themselves accord low priorities, administrators gain the power necessary to forestall such plans. (Schelling, 1963). In sum, the presumption that CON agencies serve the interests of existing providers, even when true, does not necessarily imply ineffective control of hospital investment.

The principal doubts about CON agencies' ability to control investment stem from the limited nature of CON coverage and the scarcity of agency resources. Although most CON laws require certification for new construction and for significant increases in bed capacity, other potentially important types of investment are not controlled. Several states exempt all projects below a minimum capital expenditure, which ranges from $10,000 in New York to $350,000 in Kansas. In some states, expenditures for equipment or expansion of existing services that do not involve enlargement of physical plant are excluded from review. Thus, while there is considerable variability in the provisions of laws, a substantial portion of investment activity is beyond the reach of CON, and this is particularly true of investment not requiring new construction or bed

[4]It is also frequently argued that, in addition to blocking new entrants, CON agencies will impose stricter controls upon disfavored existing providers, particularly proprietary hospitals.

[5]Curran's (1974) observation that medical societies, unlike hospital associations, have not been strong advocates of CON is of interest in this context.

increases (Havighurst, 1973: 1165-1166).[6]

CON agencies' ability to review thoroughly all projects requiring certification is limited by financial and personnel constraints (Stuehler, 1973). Again, the analogy to regulation in other industries points to provider domination (Havighurst, 1973: 1178). Sparing little expense in defending its requests for approval, a large and politically strong institution may easily convince an understaffed and underfinanced CON agency not to incur costs required to develop a compelling refutation. Accordingly, the agency will adopt the path of least resistance, that is, approval. However, this course of events is only one possibility. Pauly (1974a:158-159) argues, for instance, that the path of least resistance for the agency is to disapprove plans for new hospitals and bed expansions. The consequences of erroneous approvals—empty beds—are highly visible, while those of erroneous disapprovals (e.g., longer waits for elective admissions) are less so.

These observations raise a general point, namely, that in the presence of severe resource constraints, CON agencies will be forced to make decisions about priorities and to adopt either implicit or explicit rules of thumb. Pauly's view implies a "when in doubt, disapprove" rule for investments in new beds, which is consistent with moratoria on such expansion declared recently by several areawide planning bodies. However, a more permissive rule of thumb seems more likely for new services and equipment, particularly those which constitute innovations in medical practice. Moratoria on such investments or disapprovals after cursory reviews open the CON agency to the charge of capriciously depriving the citizenry of the fruits of medical progress. As for priorities, our previous discussion of the provider domination thesis contains some suggestions as to how these may be set. Furthermore, it may be reasonable to hypothesize that more agency resources will be devoted to the review of proposals for new beds than to reviews of new service and equipment requests. Empirical support for this expectation is provided by Bicknell and Walsh's (1975:1057) observations on the Massachusetts experience with CON, which revealed that facility improvement proposals not involving new beds usually did not "attract the closer, technically more sophisticated scrutiny...normally reserved for bed-related applications."

[6]Summaries of CON coverage are in Curran (1974: 93-97), Havighurst (1973: 1145-1146), and Lewin and Associates, Inc. (1974: 173-185).

Several authors note that the mere existence of a CON law may influence hospital investment plans, although it is not clear whether the effect is to deter or encourage growth. Bicknell and Walsh (1975: 1059) hold that it reduces investment, arguing that

> ...a certificate-of-need program, merely by its existence, may discourage construction and capital expenditures by causing an anticipatory reaction on the part of providers.

Others, noting that CON is similar to franchising, hypothesize the opposite effect. According to Havighurst (1973:1171, n.104), for instance,

> [t]here would seem to be a danger that the certificate-of-need process may actually stimulate hospital construction by causing applicants to accelerate their plans in order to pre-empt others.

This reasoning is also applied to decisions about costly innovations in services and facilities (Roth, 1974). Being the first hospital in an area to install a $400,000 EMI brain scanner becomes expecially important if the chances of approval of second and third requests are nil.

From this brief review of literature, we have reason to doubt the presumption that CON controls will negatively impact upon hospital investment. Indeed, several arguments lead to the opposite expectation. Moreover, they suggest that the effect of CON will vary among different types of investment. Specifically, limitations on coverage and considerations of agency priorities and rules of thumb imply that the effect on investment in bed expansion and new construction is likely to be more negative than the effect on investment in new equipment and services. Of course, the extent to which these various hypotheses are consistent with actual experience is an empirical question, and it is to this question that we turn in the remainder of this paper.

Methods

Two principal strategies are available for quantifying effects of CON: (1) a descriptive approach and (2) an analytic approach. Using the former, the investigator would review CON applications over some period and enumerate amounts of capital expenditure avoided by disapproval or agency-mandated modifications. (Obviously, adjustments would be required when dealing with competing applications.) Although the descriptive approach has the virtue of simplicity, Bicknell and Walsh (1975), who applied it in their Massachusetts study, note that it fails to capture projects which might have been undertaken in the absence of CON but for which applications were never filed because a rejection was anticipated. Another defect is that this approach overlooks investment not covered by CON law, although it is possible that it is indirectly affected by CON control. Finally, the most serious deficiency of the descriptive approach is that it inevitably must lead to the conclusion that CON reduces investment.

In this study, we employ the second strategy, that is, the analytic approach. In this approach, the effects of CON are estimated by statistically controlling for factors other than CON which influence investment. The obvious weakness of this method is that it may lead to spurious causal interpretations about CON's effects when relevant non-CON factors are omitted from the analysis. (To minimize this possibility, we specify models to include most factors other research has shown to affect investment.) At least, however, the analytic approach does not prejudge the direction of CON effects.

Estimates of the investment impact of CON are derived from cross-section, multiple-regression analyses of investment by non-federal, short-term general and other special hospitals. The data employed in the analysis pertain to the 48 contiguous states and the District of Columbia (49 observations in all). Estimates of CON impacts were obtained for three different measures of investment: change in plant assets, change in bed supply, and change in assets per bed. The first of these represents the total dollar value of investment while the third may be viewed as a measure of increases in sophistication or capital-intensiveness of facilities. All three measures were defined over the 1968–1972 period. This period was chosen on the grounds (1) that it included some exposure to CON in a number of states and (2) that the confounding influences of Section 1122, federal price controls, and Blue Cross conformance clauses were less important than in later years.

Following the approach taken in other studies of investment (Ginsburg, 1970; Muller et al., 1975; Pauly, 1974b), we employ a regression model of the general form:

$$I = b_0 + b_1 D + b_2 A + b_3 X, \qquad [1]$$

where

I = hospital investment

D = factors influencing demand for hospital services

A = availability of investment funds

X = other factors influencing investment,

and the b_i's are regression coefficients. Estimates of CON impacts are obtained by two procedures. First, we estimate an expanded version of equation [1]:

$$I = b_0 + b_1D + b_2A + b_3X + b_4C, \qquad [2]$$

where C is defined as the percentage of the four-year period from January 1, 1969, to December 31, 1972, during which CON controls were in effect.[7] In this equation, b_4 estimates the impact of CON. Our second approach estimates coefficients of equation [1] using data from non-CON states.[8] These estimates are then applied to data from CON states to obtain predicted values for the dependent variable, I. Differences between actual and predicted values of 1 for the 1968–1972 period for these states are interpreted as estimates of CON effects.

There is, of course, no perfect method for estimating CON impacts, and each of the two employed here has shortcomings. The former method assumes that the effect of CON is additive and proportional to the percentage of the four-year period in which controls were in force. We have no independent verification of these assumptions and it is at least possible that they may lead to erroneous conclusions. The latter method, while not requiring these particular assumptions, may still lead us astray if differences between actual and predicted investment in CON states are at-

[7]Dates of implementation used in determining the values of C were obtained from the descriptive study by Macro Systems, Inc. (1974), and were verified by telephone contacts with CON agency or planning-agency personnel in the individual states. Twenty states have non-zero values for C; only five (California, Connecticut, Maryland, New York, and Rhode Island) have values greater than 50.

[8]To obtain an adequate data base, some CON states with low values on C were included. For further detail, see the discussion of Table 4 in the next section.

tributable primarily to factors other than CON. This problem, however, is less important in the former method, which allows for differences between actual and predicted investment that are unrelated to CON. Since both methods are imperfect but complementary—in the sense that the major shortcoming of one is not shared by the other—we employ the prudent approach of applying both. The fact that both yielded similar results considerably strengthens our conclusions.[9]

Two specific forms of equations [1] and [2] are used in the regression analyses: (1) linear in percentage changes and (2) linear in logarithmic changes.[10] (Definitions of variables included in the regression equations are shown in Table 1; data sources are described in the Appendix.) The major advantage of these functional forms is that, while they are linear and additive, they incorporate the obvious restriction that the absolute impacts on investment of the CON variable (*C*) and of other "scale-free" independent variables, such as per capita income, should vary positively with the size of the state.

As the independent variables employed here are similar to those used in other studies, they require little comment. Demand variables, such as population size, income, and insurance, are included to capture the effects on investment of changes in demand for hospital services. The hypothesis that an increase in demand for services leads to an increase in desired capital stock, sometimes called the "accelerator hypothesis," predicts positive associations with investment. The occupancy rate may be viewed as a measure of demand pressure on available bed supply and, such, should be positively related to investment, particularly investment in new beds.[11] Net revenues, or the availability of internal investment funds, and Hill-Burton allocations, a measure of the availability of external investment funds, also impact positively upon investment

[9]Of course, several other methods of specifying CON impacts are possible. For example, quadratic (*C*²) or higher-order terms could be added to equation [2]. As time and resource constraints prevented our experimentation with other methods, we rely upon the consistency of findings reported below as evidence that other approaches would not have materially altered our qualitative conclusions.

[10]A third form with the logarithm of *I* as a linear function of absolute changes in the explanatory variables was also tested. Results are briefly discussed below in note 17.

[11]Ginsburg (1970: 104) suggests that the occupancy rate should be adjusted for size to account for larger hospitals' ability to function more comfortably at higher rates. Following his suggestion, we computed a size-adjusted occupancy rate from a size-

TABLE 1

Variables Included in the Analysis

	Percentage Change Equations		Logarithmic Change Equations	
	Form of Variable	*Name*	*Form of Variable*	*Name*
Dependent Variables				
Change in plant assets, 1968–1972	a	D2PA	c	D2LPA
Change in beds, 1968–1972	a	D2BD	c	D2LBD
Demand Variables				
Change in population				
1968–1972	a	D2POP	c	D2LPOP
1964–1968	a	D1POP	c	D1LPOP
Change in mean per capital income				
1968–1972	a	D2INC	c	D2LINC
1964–1968	a	D1INC	c	D1LINC
Occupancy rate in 1968	b	OCC	d	LOCC
Change in occupancy rate, 1964–1968	a	D1OCC	c	D1LOCC
Change in proportion of population with Blue Cross of Medicare hospital coverage				
1968–1972	a	D2BCM	c	D2LBCM
1964–1968	a	D1BCM	c	D1LCBM
Change in proportion of population with hospital insurance				
1968–1972	a	D2PH	c	D2LPH
1964–1968	a	D1PH	c	D1LPH
Change in number of physicians				
1968–1972	a	D2MD	c	D2LMD
1964–1968	a	D1MD	c	D1LMD
Change in number of specialists				
1968–1972	a	D2SP	c	D2LSP
1964–1968	a	D1SP	c	D1LSP
Availability of Funds Variables				
Ratio of total Hill-Burton allocations to 1968 plant assets				
1969–1972	b	R2HB	d	LR2HB
1965–1968	b	R1HB	d	LR1HB
1965–1972	b	RTHB	d	LRTHB
Ratio of total hospital net revenues to 1968 plant assets				
1968–1972	b	R2NR	d	LR2NR
1964–1968	b	R1NR	d	LR1NR
1964–1972	b	RTNR	d	LRTNR
Other Independent Variables				
Annual construction wages in 1970 (in thousands of dollars)	b	CW	d	LCW
Residents and interns per hospital bed, 1968	b	RI	d	LRI
Percentage of the 1968–1972 period with CON program in effect	b	C	d	C

a Percentage of change
b Level
c Change in logarithms
d Logarithm

by reducing the need for borrowing and other fund-raising efforts.[12] The number of residents and interns per bed is a compact, albeit crude, descriptor of average hospital type, included on the assumption that investment preferences vary among hospitals. Teaching hospitals, for example, may prefer expansion of scopes of services in response to increased demand over expansion of bed supply. Construction wages measure the cost of new capital, particularly new construction. Finally, independent variables relating to the 1964-1968 period are included to allow for lagged effects on investment.[13]

Results

The results of estimating investment regressions corresponding to equation [2] are shown in Tables 2 and 3. We begin our discussion of these results by considering the coefficients of *C,* which are of primary interest, since they represent the estimated effects of CON.

If CON programs have been effective in limiting total investment, this should be revealed by significantly negative coef-

---

occupancy regression and included this adjusted rate as an independent variable in several investment regressions. The results obtained were essentially similar in all respects to those obtained using the unadjusted occupancy rate.

[12]The view that availability of external grant funds should affect investment has recently been challenged by Pauly (1974b: 9). He argues that the *marginal* cost of investment funds, which is the critical financial variable in the determination of investment, is not affected by grant funds as long as any part of total investment is financed from borrowing. This argument depends, however; on the assumption that the per dollar cost of borrowing is constant, regardless of how much is borrowed. If this cost increases with the amounts borrowed, external grants would reduce the marginal cost for any given amount of investment, thereby increasing the amount invested.

[13]This simple method of accounting for lagged effects was employed by Pauly (1974b). We use it here because it avoids some practical and theoretical problems of other approaches. For example, proportional adjustment models (Feldstein, 1971a:866–868) imply that the initial impact of an explanatory variable is greater than its effect in subsequent years. In view of the long lags associated with certain types of hospital investment, this assumption is clearly inappropriate. Moreover, the usual method of estimating this sort of model by including lagged values of the dependent variable poses statistical problems which are not easily remedied when, as here, the number of observations is small. This difficulty also arises with more complicated lag models, such as polynomial distributed lags.

fieients for *C* in the total investment regressions (equations 2.1–2.3 and 3.1–3.3). In fact, these coefficients are all positive and all but one are insignificant. According to these estimates, CON programs clearly have not reduced total hospital investment.

However, the results for equations 2.4–2.9 and 3.4–3.9 indicate that CON programs have had a significant impact on the composition of investment. Specifically, the estimated coefficients of *C* in the bed-supply equations (2.4–2.6 and 3.4–3.6) are all negative and significant, indicating that CON restricted investment in new beds. By contrast, the corresponding coefficients in the assets per bed regressions (2.7–2.9 and 3.7–3.9) are all positive and significant. This suggests that CON programs have stimulated investment in modernization and in special equipment and facilities, thereby increasing assets per bed.[14] Moreover, the magnitudes of these estimated effects are relatively large. The coefficients in Table 2 imply that the effect of a CON program over the entire four-year period is to reduce the growth in beds by 5.4 to 9.0 percent and to increase assets per bed by 15.2 to 19.7 percent. Correspondingly, the coefficients in Table 3 imply a reduction in beds of about 3.5 percent and an increase in assets per bed of about 10 percent. A comparison with the mean increases in beds (9.3 percent) and assets per bed (37.7 percent) reveals that these estimated effects are indeed substantial.

Turning to the results for the demand variables, we observe that the coefficients for changes in population and insurance coverage are generally in the expected positive direction. The impact of insurance on assets per bed seems slightly stronger than its effect on bed supply. This agrees with Feldstein's (1971b: Chapter 4) thesis that growth of insurance increases hospital per diem costs by causing hospitals to upgrade "styles of care." However, changes in income had no appreciable effect on investment, and,

---

[14]Our coefficient estimates probably understate the positive effect of CON on these categories of investment because of the ways in which plant-asset data are recorded. Plant assets are generally defined at book value (i.e., the value at the time of construction or purchase) or a book value minus accumulated depreciation. Thus, increases in the costs of construction and facilities should lead to increased assets per bed with the addition of new bed capacity. However, if CON has reduced the growth of bed capacity, as our data suggest, this should also reduce the growth in assets per bed. Obviously, the positive effect of CON on other types of investment was strong enough to offset this reduction and to yield positive and significant coefficients for *C* in equations 2.7–2.9 and 3.7–3.9.

TABLE 2
Regression Coefficients for Percentage Change Equations
(*t*-statistics in parentheses)

Equation No.	2.1	2.2*	2.3	2.4	2.5*	2.6	2.7	2.8*	2.9
Dep. Var.	D2PA	D2PA	D2PA	D2BD	D2BD	D2BD	D2PAB	D2PAB	D2PAB
Constant	−0.197	−0.496	−0.392	0.076	0.294	−0.137	−0.263	−0.806	−0.150
C†	0.089 (0.75)	0.054 (0.48)	0.096 (1.04)	−0.090^c (3.12)	−0.083^b (2.44)	−0.054^b (2.19)	0.197^b (1.82)	0.152^b (1.52)	0.157^b (1.91)
D2POP	1.960^a (1.45)	1.404 (0.92)	1.362 (1.12)	0.367 (1.11)	−0.187 (0.40)	0.112 (0.34)	1.396 (1.11)	1.527 (1.12)	1.153 (1.07)
D1POP	2.633^b (1.77)	1.665 (1.13)	2.107^b (1.80)	0.579^a (1.60)	1.269^c (2.84)	0.202 (0.57)	1.720 (1.26)	−0.039 (0.03)	1.717^a (1.47)
D2INC	0.374 (0.80)	−0.044 (0.09)	0.239 (0.58)	−0.043 (0.42)	0.073 (0.47)	−0.084 (0.76)	0.415 (1.07)	−0.121 (0.27)	0.341 (0.94)
D1INC	−0.161 (0.36)	0.321 (0.67)	0.125 (0.32)	−0.267^b (2.42)	−0.116 (0.80)	−0.085 (0.83)	0.213 (0.51)	0.420 (0.98)	0.225 (0.66)
OCC††	−0.040 (0.57)		−0.014 (0.23)	0.038^b (2.24)		0.059^c (3.60)	−0.084^a (1.32)		−0.090^a (1.66)
D1OCC		−0.258 (0.43)			0.078 (0.43)			−0.350 (0.65)	
D2PH	0.718^b (1.93)		0.869^b (2.40)	0.061 (0.67)		0.136^a (1.40)	0.595^b (1.74)		0.628^b (1.95)
D1PH	0.350 (1.01)		0.441^a (1.35)	0.666 (0.78)		0.085 (0.98)	0.236 (0.73)		0.284 (0.98)
D2BCM		−0.297 (0.90)			−0.196^b (1.96)			−0.015 (0.05)	
D1BCM		0.207^a (1.63)			0.058^a (1.51)			0.115 (1.01)	
D2MD	−0.751 (0.75)			−0.478^b (1.96)			−0.091 (0.10)		

D1MD	-1.768[b] (1.88)	-1.854[b] (2.18)	0.462[b] (2.02)		0.262 (1.15)			-2.077[c] (2.75)
D2SP	-0.147 (0.20)					-2.255[b] (2.61)	0.431 (0.66)	
D1SP	-0.721 (0.91)			-0.441[b] (2.00) 0.359[a] (1.50)			-1.126[a] (1.59)	
R2HB	-0.935 (0.44)		-1.531[c] (2.92)	(0.95)				
R1HB	3.470[b] (1.75)		1.026[b] (2.12)	0.089 (0.44)		1.325 (0.67)		
RTHB	2.279[c] (3.37)	1.413[b] (2.36)			-0.218[a] (1.36)	1.736	2.023[c] (3.35)	1.608[c] (3.03)
R2NR	0.192 (0.78)		-0.033 (0.55)	-0.046 (0.72)		0.218 (0.96)		
R1NR	0.002 (0.01)	0.182 (0.61)	0.005 (0.06)		0.077 (0.96)	-0.024 (0.08)		0.042 (0.16)
RTNR	0.065 (0.31)						0.108 (0.57)	
CW	0.064[b] (2.10)	0.058[b] (1.97)	-0.021[c] (2.81)	-0.026[b] (2.53)	-0.023[c] (2.86)	0.086[c] (3.04)	0.086[c] (2.98)	0.083[c] (3.18)
R1	0.965[a] (1.46)			0.046 (0.23)			0.789[a] (1.34)	
R2	0.563	0.508	0.702	0.518	0.595	0.571	0.559	0.553

* Nevada excluded because of undefined values for independent variables.
† Coefficients shown are actual coefficients multiplied by 100.
†† Coefficients shown are actual coefficients multiplied by 10.
a Significant at the 0.1 level (one-tailed test)
b Significant at the 0.05 level (one-tailed test)
c Significant at the 0.005 level (one-tailed test)

TABLE 3

Regression Coefficients for Logarithmic Change Equations

(t-statistics in parentheses)

Equation No.	3.1**	3.2*	3.3	3.4**	3.5*	3.6	3.7**	3.8*	3.9
Dep. Var.	D2LPA	D2LPA	D2LPA	D2LBD	D2LBD	D2LBD	D2LPAB	D2LPAB	D2LPAB
Constant	-0.737	-0.736	-0.768	-0.121	0.743	-0.099	-0.858	-1.479	-0.669
C[†]	0.034 (0.82)	0.024 (0.56)	0.045[a] (1.48)	-0.034[b] (2.50)	-0.041[b] (2.69)	-0.018[b] (1.76)	0.068[b] (1.69)	0.065[a] (1.56)	0.063[b] (2.15)
D2LPOP	1.373[a] (1.43)	0.405 (0.42)	0.746 (0.84)	0.356 (1.12)	-0.216 (0.62)	0.237 (0.79)	1.017 (1.09)	0.621 (0.65)	0.509 (0.59)
D1LPOP	1.637[a] (1.59)	1.167 (1.07)	1.475[a] (1.62)	0.512[a] (1.50)	0.986[b] (2.52)	0.193 (0.63)	1.125 (1.22)	0.181 (0.17)	1.282[a] (1.46)
D2LINC	0.504[a] (1.37)	0.034 (0.08)	0.239 (0.67)	-0.066 (0.54)	-0.006 (0.04)	-0.124 (1.03)	0.570[a] (1.59)	0.040 (0.10)	0.362 (1.06)
D1LINC	-0.107 (0.27)	0.114 (0.26)	0.085 (0.27)	-0.294[b] (2.23)	-0.241[a] (1.51)	-0.088 (0.82)	0.187 (0.48)	0.355 (0.81)	0.173 (0.56)
LOCC	-0.122 (0.37)		-0.064 (0.20)	0.300[b] (2.70)		0.404[c] (3.81)	-0.422 (1.29)		-0.467[a] (1.54)
D1LOCC		0.038 (0.08)			0.057 (0.34)			-0.019 (0.04)	
D2LPH	0.494[b] (1.85)		0.616[b] (2.37)	0.069 (0.78)		0.137[a] (1.56)	0.425[a] (1.63)		0.480[b] (1.92)
D1LPH	0.374[a] (1.50)		0.389[a] (1.59)	0.065 (0.78)		0.056 (0.68)	0.310 (1.27)		0.333[a] (1.41)
D2LBCM		-0.186 (0.68)			-0.179[b] (1.82)			-0.007 (0.03)	
D1LBCM		0.316[b] (2.31)			0.084[b] (1.71)			0.232[b] (1.73)	

	(1)	(2)	(3)	(4)	(5)	(6)	(7)	(8)	(9)
D2LMD	-0.752 (1.04)			-0.447[a] (1.86)			-0.305 (0.43)		-1.484[b] (2.56)
D1LMD	-0.928[a] (1.32)		-1.317[b] (2.19)	0.407[a] (1.74)		0.167 (0.83)	-1.335[b] (1.95)		
D2LSP		0.006 (0.01)			-0.313[a] (1.46)			0.319 (0.54)	
D1LSP		-0.644 (1.01)			0.410[b] (1.80)			-1.053[a] (1.69)	
LR2HB	-0.063 (0.47)			-0.105[b] (2.35)			0.042 (0.32)		
LR1HB	0.211[a] (1.60)			0.073[a] (1.67)			0.138 (1.07)		
LRTHB		0.249[a] (3.37)	0.149[b] (2.31)		0.009 (0.33)	-0.032 (1.49)		0.240[c] (3.31)	0.181[c] (2.92)
LR2NR[††]	0.281 (1.08)			-0.030 (0.35)			0.311 (1.22)		
LR1NR[††]	-0.176 (0.70)		0.132 (0.63)	0.047 (0.56)		0.143[b] (2.02)	-0.222 (0.91)		-0.011 (0.06)
LRTNR[††]		-0.032 (0.08)			-0.071 (0.51)			0.039 (0.10)	
LCW	0.311[b] (1.91)	0.293[a] (1.62)	0.285[b] (1.78)	-0.168[c] (3.12)	-0.173[b] (2.67)	-0.161[c] (2.98)	0.479[c] (3.02)	0.467[b] (2.63)	0.446[c] (2.89)
LRI		0.480[b] (1.96)			0.084 (0.96)			0.396[a] (1.65)	
R^2	0.577	0.511	0.483	0.711	0.561	0.642	0.596	0.510	0.526

* Nevada, New York and Wyoming excluded because of undefined values for independent variables.
** Massachusetts and New York excluded because of undefined values for independent variables.
† Coefficients shown are actual coefficients multiplied by 100.
†† Coefficients shown are actual coefficients multiplied by 10.
a Significant at the 0.1 level (one-tailed test)
b Significant at the 0.05 level (one-tailed test)
c Significant at the 0.005 level (one-tailed test)

contrary to our expectations, changes in physician supply affected investment negatively. Finally, while the occupancy rate has no measurable impact on total investment, it apparently alters the composition of investment by increasing bed expansion and reducing other types of investment. Ginsburg (1970: Chapter 6) reports an identical finding from his study of individual hospitals over the 1961–1965 period.

Among the other variables, construction wages was the most significant. Its negative impact on investment in beds implies that plans for new hospital construction are sensitive to cost factors. However, while an increase in construction wages reduces the physical quantity of new construction, it increases the unit cost. Our estimates show that the net effect of these influences on the total dollar value of investment (equations 2.1–2.3 and 3.1–3.3) is significantly positive. Also, the positive coefficients in the plant assets per bed equation reflect both the positive effect of construction wages on the unit cost of construction and perhaps a reallocation of investment funds from construction to equipment.

The coefficients for residents and interns per bed conform to expectations in that they are more strongly positive for plant assets per bed than for beds. The coefficients for the Hill-Burton variables display a similar pattern, which may reflect the program's recent emphasis upon modernization rather than expansion of bed capacity. Finally, we were unable to detect any appreciable effect of net revenues on investment.

Overall, our coefficient estimates conform to prior expectations, and the regressions explain substantial portions of the variances in the dependent variables. In addition, the coefficients of C are stable across regressions that vary in terms of functional form and the set of included explanatory variables. This attests to the validity of the estimates of CON's impacts in that they are not likely to be artifacts of having omitted other relevant independent variables.

To arrive at the second set of CON impact measures, we reestimated 12 of the regressions described above, deleting the independent variable C and exluding the five states where CON had been in effect throughout 1971 and 1972 (i.e., California, Connecticut, Maryland, New York, Rhode Island). The reestimated equations include: 2.2, 2.3, 2.5, 2.6, 2.8, 2.9, 3.2, 3.3, 3.5, 3.6, 3.8, and 3.9. We also reestimated equations 2.3, 2.6, and 2.9, deleting C and excluding the 11 states where CON had been in effect for five or more quarters during the 1969–1972 period. (These include the five states mentioned above, plus Minnesota, New Jersey, North Carolina, North Dakota, South Carolina, and Washington.) Coefficients from these 15 reestimated regressions were then used to predict changes in plant assets, beds, and plant assets per bed for the excluded states. Differences between predicted and actual values for these variables are shown in Table 4 for California, Connecticut, Maryland, New York, and Rhode Island.

The pattern of these deviations conforms precisely to the pattern of coefficients for C reported above. In almost all cases, actual increases in beds in these five CON states are less than predicted increases. Furthermore, increases in plant assets and in plant assets per bed are generally greater than predicted, but deviations for plant assets per bed are more consistently positive and larger relative to the standard errors of the predictions.[15]

A brief comparison of deviations among the five states may also be of interest, for CON programs in these states differ structurally. In California, for example, final authority for CON determinations rest de facto with area-wide CHP agencies. Maryland's state CHP agency renders final decisions, although area-wide agencies are important parts of the process. In Connecticut, New York, and Rhode Island, CHP agencies have only minor roles, and in New York the agency that issues certificates (the state health department) is also responsible for regulating hospital costs.

One might expect such differences to be related to the effectiveness of controls. Close interaction between CHP area-wide agencies and hospitals, we have noted, may facilitate provider domination and, in turn, less effective control where these agencies figure importantly in the review process. Conversely, where the major responsibility rests with a state agency concerned also with operating-cost implications of unnecessary investment (as in New

[15]Deviations between predicted and actual investment for the other six CON states in the regressions where they were excluded did not consistently follow this pattern. Only three of the six states had less growth in beds than predicted, but these three negative deviations were on average about twice as large as the three positive deviations. Four of the six deviations were also negative for growth in plant assets and in plant assets per bed. Here, however, average sizes of positive and negative deviations were essentially equal.

York), one might expect more stringent controls (Havighurst, 1973: 1180–1181).

Surprisingly, there is little correlation between the results shown in Table 4 and these structural characteristics. One of the two states where CHP(b) agencies are presumably most influential, California, was the least successful in controlling bed expansion while the other, Maryland, was most successful.[16] No state achieved visible success in controlling increases in plant assets and plant assets per bed.

We should be careful, however, not to overinterpret these findings, for comparisons among states based on a single set of deviations between actual and predicted values obviously lack reliability. They do suggest, however, that simple hypotheses about the relative effectiveness of CON programs based on comparisons of real or presumed structural characteristics may be misleading. The effectiveness of controls within a single state may depend greatly upon political forces, personalities involved, and special circumstances not readily visible from afar.

Discussion

In sum, our two methods of measuring CON's effects on hospital investment yield similar results. These results indicate that CON controls did not reduce the total dollar amount of investment during the 1966–1972 period, but significantly altered its composition by reducing growth in beds and increasing other types of investment. Employing several different regression models composed of different combinations of independent variables, we obtained stable results, which attest strongly to their probable validity.[17]

[16]Several difference between California and Maryland may account for this. In Maryland, a considerable portion of all hospitals are within the purview of the Baltimore metropolitan area CHP(b) agency, a relatively well-staffed and active body in which non-providers have played an important role. California's fragmentation of the state into twelve different CHP(b) regions may have encouraged leniency by allowing citizens in one area to pass on a share of the costs of additional investment to others throughout the state in the form of higher insurance premiums and taxes for Medicaid payments. These speculations are, of course, just that and, as such, invite more careful investigation.

[17]As mentioned above in note 10, a third regression model was also tested in which the dependent variables were expressed as logarithms of absolute changes (e.g., log [plant assets in 1972 minus plant assets in 1968]). Most independent variables were

TABLE 4

Deviations of Actual from Predicted Values
for Dependent Variables from Five CON States
(Standard errors for predictions in parentheses)

Dep. Var.	Equation No. **	California	Connecticut	Maryland	New York*	Rhode Island
D2PA	2.2	−0.013 (0.189)	0.183 (0.173)	0.040 (0.210)	0.180 (0.224)	0.026 (0.183)
D2PA	2.3	0.068 (0.175)	0.296 (0.167)	0.066 (0.183)	0.065 (0.168)	−0.005 (0.172)
D2PA	2.3†	0.031 (0.199)	0.293 (0.179)	0.042 (0.202)	0.080 (0.182)	−0.005 (0.186)
D2LPA	3.2	0.025 (0.054)	0.094 (0.050)	0.039 (0.058)		−0.049 (0.081)
D2LPA	3.3	0.040 (0.051)	0.112 (0.050)	0.020 (0.054)	0.037 (0.049)	−0.008 (0.067)
D2BD	2.5	−0.027 (0.058)	−0.053 (0.053)	−0.115 (0.064)	0.048 (0.068)	−0.053 (0.056)
D2BD	2.6	0.040 (0.045)	−0.033 (0.043)	−0.099 (0.047)	−0.034 (0.043)	−0.077 (0.045)
D2BD	2.6†	0.055 (0.047)	−0.027 (0.042)	−0.104 (0.047)	−0.018 (0.042)	−0.078 (0.043)
D2LBD	3.5	−0.012 (0.021)	−0.021 (0.020)	−0.042 (0.023)		−0.004 (0.032)
D2LBD	3.6	0.011 (0.018)	−0.016 (0.017)	−0.033 (0.018)	−0.016 (0.017)	−0.010 (0.023)
D2PAB	2.8	0.020 (0.169)	0.237 (0.155)	0.182 (0.188)	0.099 (0.201)	0.093 (0.164)
D2PAB	2.9	0.014 (0.155)	0.318 (0.147)	0.187 (0.161)	0.103 (0.148)	0.092 (0.152)
D2PAB	2.9†	−0.039 (0.173)	0.306 (0.156)	0.171 (0.176)	0.095 (0.153)	0.093 (0.152)
D2LPAB	3.8	0.037 (0.052)	0.114 (0.048)	0.081 (0.057)		−0.045 (0.078)
D2LPAB	3.9	0.029 (0.049)	0.128 (0.047)	0.052 (0.051)	0.053 (0.047)	0.002 (0.064)

* Omitted values resulted from undefined values for independent variables.
**Equation number refers to the equation in Table 2 or 3 whose specification corresponds to that used in deriving predictions.
† Eleven CON states were excluded from the regression used to derive these predictions. In all other cases only the five states whose deviations are shown here were excluded.

Furthermore, our empirical findings are consistent with expectations derived from critical analyses of CON. That investment in beds was more effectively controlled than other investment in services and facilities accords with expected implications of provider domination, limitations in coverage of CON laws, and the likely response of CON agencies (in terms of setting priorities and rules of thumb) to the scarcity of resources. On the other hand, findings that total investment was not reduced and that the growth in assets per bed was actually stimulated by CON are somewhat surprising. These may be due to the franchising aspects of CON regulation, which, as we have noted, may encourage pre-emptive investment, or to the added protection from competitive pressures that these laws afford to existing providers. But there are at least two other explanations which should be considered.

First, one can reasonably postulate that strong pressures for capital expansion are operative within the management structure of many hospitals. The managerial preference for expansion of facilities and services appears to be characteristic of virtually all organizations (Perrow, 1970: 152–153; Starbuck, 1965), but it is probably strongest in non-profit institutions (such as most hospitals) where the significance of profit as a criterion of success is diminished. Furthermore, in the case of hospitals, these preferences are reinforced by the desires of staff physicians for the most up-to-date services, equipment, and patient accommodations. Since external market pressures for cost control are weak and expected profitability is of minor relevance in setting investment priorities, administrators and trustees are likely to be respossive to these desires. Indeed, failure to do so may impair the hospital's ability to compete for patients. These considerations imply that if one means of indulging the expansionist preferences of management and the medical staff is blocked by regulatory controls, alternative means that are not subject to regulation will be found. If CON prevents a hospital from adding the additional beds desired by the specialists

expressed as absolute changes instead of percentage changes or logarithmic changes. In this model, availability of funds variables were more significant predictors of investment, while population change was less so. However, findings with respect to C were identical to those reported in Tables 2 and 3. As a further check on the stability of the coefficients of C, we executed several regressions omitting one or more independent variables. Again, these coefficient remained quite stable. Finally, it is reassuring to observe that Hellinger (in press), using a somewhat different model in his multiple regression analysis of interstate variations in plant assets, has also found that CON has no significant effect on total investment.

on its staff, it can "compensate" these physicians (and thereby retain their custom) by installing facilities for cardiac catheterization, renal dialysis, and the like. Our findings suggest that this may in fact have occurred.

Second, there is the possibility that, for an individual hospital, investment in beds and other types of investment may be interrelated financially. The marginal cost of raising investment funds probably increases with total investment. In the credit market, as a hospital's indebtedness rises, its ability to obtain additional funds on favorable terms decreases. In the "philanthropy market," the yield of fund-raising efforts must certainly decline as more donors are solicited or the same ones are repeatedly solicited. Therefore, if a CON program successfully reduces amounts of funds spent on one type of investment (e.g., expansion of bed capacity), the cost of funds for other types (e.g., modernization and sophisticated equipment) is reduced, causing increases in these other types.

This argument is shown in Fig. 1, where *AB* and *AC* are the

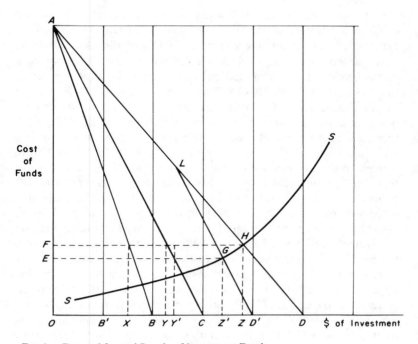

FIG. 1.   Demand for and Supply of Investment Funds.

hospital's demand curves for bed-investment and nonbed-investment funds, respectively, and SS is the funds supply curve. *AD*, the total demand for investment funds schedule, is the horizontal sum of *AB* and *AC*. In the absence of CON, equilibrium occurs at point *H*; the marginal interest cost is *OF* percent; total investment is *OZ*, of which *OX* is devoted to expanding bed supply; and *XZ* (= *OY*) is devoted to other investment. Suppose now that a CON program limits bed investment to *OB'*. The constrained total demand schedule is then *ALD'*, and equilibrium is at point *G*, with a marginal interest cost of *OE*. While investment in beds is reduced to *OB'* other investment increases to *B'Z'* (= *OY'*). The net effect on total investment remains negative, but it may be quite small. (This would occur if, for example, the segment of *SS* between *G*- and *H* is steeply sloped. When this segment is vertical, there is no decline in total investment.) Furthermore, the resultant decline in total investment may be further reduced or even eliminated by positive effects of pre-emptive investment and reduced competitive pressures.

As we have noted, our findings about the investment impacts of CON are both statistically robust and consistent with plausible expectations about the likely effects of CON regulation. However, in the absence of other studies offering corroboration and in view of the obvious policy implications of our findings, it is imperative that we attend to their possible limitations. One stems from our use of aggregated state data, which are not perfectly suited to our purposes. Planning and regulation ultimately occur in designated regions within states that are agglomerations of individual hospitals and localities which are probably quite heterogeneous. State aggregates, therefore, are averages across potentially quite diverse regions. Having relied upon published data, we have no independent means of assessing their reliability and validity, which is especially problematic regarding information on hospital plant assets and insurance coverage. Furthermore, we must note that our investment variables (changes in beds and changes in plant assets per bed) correspond imperfectly to the distinction between bed investment versus non-bed investment. A stronger test of our interpretations requires more precise measurement of non-bed investment in particular. Finally, non-random adoption of CON controls by states poses threats to the internal validity of our causal interpretations of CON's effects. States that adopted such legislation may differ systematically from others in terms of relevant dimensions not included in our analyses. If so, our causal reasoning would be spurious in some unknowable degree.

Because of these limitations, caution must be exercised in extrapolating our results to subsequent extensions of CON coverage. The self-selection of states into CON probably implies that our estimates will lead to upwardly biased effects when used to predict impacts in other states. Among those that subsequently adopt CON laws in response to P.L. 93-641, the restrictive impact on investment in beds will probably be less than reported here. Furthermore, as our results reflect only the effects of existing CON programs at a particular time, it would be incorrect to view them as necessary consequences of CON regardless of the nature of the review process and the circumstances in which it occurs. Indeed, the limited evidence presented here suggests that there is considerable variation in impact among existing programs. Finally, returning to our earlier caveat about the limited purpose of this analysis, we must note that CON is but one of several types of regulation currently in force or contemplated. Our findings cannot be used to predict the consequences of combining CON with other forms of investment, rate, and quality controls.

Policy Implications and Suggestions for Future Research

We have found that, while CON has controlled expansion in bed supply, it has stimulated other types of investment and, therefore, had little effect on total investment expenditures. One might be tempted to conclude that CON programs can be made more effective by tightening existing controls and extending them to cover all types of investment projects. The wisdom of this course of action is, however, by no means self-evident. Careful review of all certification requests, including the additional requests generated by extending the scope of CON, would require large additions to agency resources. Conceivably, the resources required for review might often exceed the costs of investment projects being reviewed. Such circumstances do not seem to constitute an optimal allocation of societal resources.

Other straightforward options are also undesirable in that they are either politically infeasible or at variance with CON's putative purpose, that is, to control cost inflation by deterring *unnecessary-investment*. For instance, CON agencies could adopt the general policy of denying certification for equipment and facilities except in cases where extreme and urgent need is demonstrable. Alternatively, substantial submission fees or even taxes on investment could be employed to discourage hospitals and other institutions from seeking certification. Although such measure have the superficial appeals of simplicity and economy, they are not particularly discriminating between needed and unneeded investments. Furthermore, they would most likely favor the large, wealthy institutions' interests even more than does the process currently in use.

The desirability of tightening or extending CON controls must also be considered within the total context of health-sector regulation. Realization of the impossibility of relying solely on CON to control health care costs (Bicknell and Walsh, 1975: 1060) leads to skepticism of arguments favoring such modifications of CON. Utilization controls and rate-setting policies which limit reimbursement for depreciation and operating costs relating to unneeded capital facilities may complement CON programs which focus almost exclusively on controlling bed supply.[18]

In concluding, we wish to stress our belief that the present study does not in itself provide an adequate basis for deriving specific programmatic policy options regarding CON. We have described several important limitations of our study which, we hope, can be eliminated in future research. In addition, there are other directions of complementary research that ought to be pursued if we are to attain a more complete understanding of direct and indirect effects of existing and proposed CON programs.

This paper is a part of a larger effort to assess CON's impacts on hospital operating costs and utilization and on investment in nursing homes, as well as on the types of investment reported here. Furthermore, using data from CHP(b) planning regions, we are examining effects of CON on bed supplies and the addition of specific facilities and services. Several other important questions invite investigation. For instance, study of CON's effects on the structure of the health care industry is warranted by the criticism that CON may block entry of new competitors, retard growth of

[18]In this regard, it is pertinent to recall that our results apply to a period (1968–1972) during which these other forms of control were relatively unimportant.

HMOs, and discourage investment in less costly alternatives to hospital care (e.g., surgicenters) (Havighurst, 1973). Longitudinal analyses of changes in CON's effects may also be revealing, for experience in other industries shows change in the behavior of regulators over time, in particular, a loss of reformist zeal and an increase in provider domination. With the recent adoption of other regulatory devices such as rate setting and PSRO, a detailed analysis of CON's interactions with them is especially relevant to current policy debate. Finally, as a means of verifying the reasoning behind our interpretations of findings reported here and for generating further insight, more descriptive studies like those reported by Bicknell and Walsh (1975) and Macro-Systems, Inc. (1974) are indicated. Having embraced CON as a cornerstone of nascent federal health policy, it is incumbent upon policy makers to evaluate carefully and extensively its effects. To do otherwise is inevitably to consign debate about CON to the realm of speculation, where undoubtedly the urge to regulate will prevail.

David S. Salkever, PH.D.
School of Hygiene and Public Health
The Johns Hopkins University
615 North Wolfe Street
Baltimore, Maryland 21205

Thomas W. Bice, PH.D.
Department of Sociology
Washington University
St. Louis, Missouri 63130

Support for this project is from the National Center for Health Services Research, U.S. Department of Health, Education, and Welfare, Contract Number HRA-106-74-57. The very competent research and computational assistance of William Harris, Margaret Solnick, and Barbara Vaeth is gratefully acknowledged.

Appendix

Data on beds, plant assets, net revenues, and occupancy rates in non-federal short-term hospitals were obtained from the *Guide Issues* of *Hospital, J.A.H.A.* Hospital insurance data were taken from the *Sourcebook of Health Insurance Data* (Health Insurance Association of America). Blue Cross hospital coverage figures were obtained from *Research and Statistics Notes* (Office of Research and Statistics, U.S. Social Security Administration) and from unpublished data provided by the Blue Cross Association. Medicare enrollment figures are published annually in *Medicare:*

Selected State Data (U.S. Social Security Administration). Construction wages were obtained from *County Business Patterns* (U.S. Dept. of Commerce) while per capita income and population figures were taken from *Sales Management: Annual Survey of Buying Power* (Sales Management, Inc.). Unpublished data on Hill-Burton allocations were provided by the U.S. Department of Health, Education, and Welfare. Finally, numbers of physicians, specialists, and residents and interns appear in *Distribution of Physicians* (American Medical Association). In certain instances, adjustments were made for missing data. These are described in a more extensive version of this appendix which is available upon request.

References

Berry, R.
  1974   "Cost and efficiency in the production of hospital services." Milbank Memorial Fund Quarterly/Health and Society 52,3 (Summer): 291–313.

Bicknell, W.J., and D.C. Walsh
  1975   "Certification-of-need: the Massachusetts experience." New England Journal of Medicine 292 (May 15): 1054–1061.

Brown, D.
  1969   Evaluation of Health Planning. Health Administration Perspectives No. A8. Chicago: Center for Health Administration Studies, University of Chicago.

Curran, W.J.
  1974   "A national survey and analysis of state certificate-of-need laws for health facilities." In Havighurst, C.C. (ed.), Regulating Health Facilities Construction. Washington: American Enterprise Institute for Policy Research.

Davis, K.
  1969   A Theory of Economic Behavior in Non-Profit, Private Hospitals. Ph.D. thesis, Rice University.

  1974   "The role of technology, demand and labor markets in the determination of hsopital cost." In Perlman, M. (ed.), The Economics of Health and Medical Care. New York: John Wiley and Sons.

Feldstein, M.S.
  1971a   "Hospital cost inflation: a study in nonprofit price dynamics." American Economic Review 61,5(December): 853–872.

  1971b   The Rising Cost of Hospital Care. Washington: Information Resources Press.

Ginsburg, P.B.
1970   Capital in Non-Profit Hospitals. Ph.D. thesis, Harvard University.

Havighurst, C.C.
1973   "Regulation of health facilities and services by certificate-of-need."
          Virginia Law Review 599(October):1143-1232.

Hellinger, F.
in   The Effect of Certificate of Need Legislation on Hospital Investment.
press   U.S. Social Security Administration.

Hilton, G.
1972   "The basic behavior of regulatory commissions." American Economic
          Review 62,2 (May): 47-54.

Lave, J.R., and L.B. Lave
1974   "The supply and allocation of medical resources: alternative control
          mechanisms." In Havighurst, C.C. (ed.), Regulating Health Facilities
          Construction. Washington: American Enterprise Institute for Policy
          Research.

Lewin and Associates, Inc.
1974   Nationwide Survey of State Health Regulations. Springfield, Virginia:
          National Technical Information Service (PB 236-660).

Macro Systems, Inc.
1974   The Certificate of Need Experience: An Early Assessment. Silver
          Spring, Maryland: Macro Systems, Inc.

May, J.
1974   "The planning and licensing agencies." In Havighurst, C.C. (ed.),
          Regulating Health Facilities Construction. Washington: American En-
          terprise Institute for Policy Research.

Muller, C., P. Worthington, and G. Allen
1975   "Capital expenditures and the availability of funds." International
          Journal of Health Services 5, 1(Winter): 143-157.

O'Donoghue, P., and Policy Center, Inc.
1974   Evidence About the Effects of Health Care Regulation. Denver: Spec-
          trum Research, Inc.

Pauly, M.V.
1974a   "The behavior of nonprofit hospital monopolies: alternative models of
          the hospital." In Havighurst, C.C. (ed.), Regulating Health Facilities
          Construction. Washington: American Enterprise Institute for Policy
          Research.

1974b   "Hospital capital investment: the roles of demand, profits, and physicians." Journal of Human Resources 9 (Winter): 7–20.

Perrow, C.
1970   Organizational Analysis: A Sociological View. Belmont, California: Wadsworth.

Posner, R.A.
1974   "Certificates of need for health care facilities: a dissenting view." In Havighurst, C.C. (ed.), Regulating Health Facilities Construction. Washington: American Enterprise Institute for Policy Research.

Roth, E.
1974   "Certificate of need as a part of comprehensive health planning." Unpublished paper. The Johns Hopkins Medical Institutions.

Schelling, T.
1963   The Strategy of Conflict. New York: Oxford University Press.

Starbuck, W.
1965   "Organizational growth and development." In March, J.G. (ed.), Handbook of Organizations. Chicago: Rand McNally.

Stuehler, G.
1973   "Certification of need—a systems analysis of Maryland's experience and plans." American Journal of Public Health 63 (November): 966–972.

Regulating the Bed Supply in Nursing Homes

JUDITH FEDER and
WILLIAM SCANLON

The Urban Institute,
Washington, D.C.

W HEN CONGRESS ENACTED MEDICARE AND MEDI-caid legislation in 1965, nursing home coverage was perceived as a minor adjunct to government insurance for medical care in acute illness. Today, nursing homes have become perhaps the major issue in public financing of health care for the elderly. In 1975, expenditures on such nursing home care were five times their 1966 level, an increase exceeding that for any other medical service in that period. As a result, nursing homes have come to absorb more than 25 percent of total health expenditures on the elderly, as compared with roughly 15 percent in 1966. Except for a brief period at its beginning, the Medicare program has contributed very little to nursing home financing. By default, as much as design, the federal-state Medicaid program has assumed responsibility for nursing home coverage (Chulis, 1977), and today pays for about half of all nursing home care; most of the other half is paid directly by the elderly themselves.

Expenditures for nursing home care loom large in the Medicaid budget—39 percent in 1977. Faced with fiscal pressures in the 1970s, many states have found themselves unwilling or unable to support these obligations and have taken measures to limit their liabilities. This paper analyzes the states' use of one such measure: restriction of the bed supply in nursing homes through "certificate-of-need" regula-

Milbank Memorial Fund Quarterly/*Health and Society*, Vol. 58, No. 1, 1980
© 1980 Milbank Memorial Fund and Massachusetts Institute of Technology
0160/1997/80/5801/0054-35 $01.00/0

tion. From an analysis of several states' experience, we will argue that direct regulation of this bed supply exacerbates rather than eliminates inefficiencies in the market for long-term care. We conclude that, if expenditure control is to be compatible with efficient and equitable allocation of resources, the states must use their payment policies to ensure that care is available to the persons who need it most.

Certificate-of-Need Laws and Nursing Homes

Before 1970, several states had enacted certificate-of-need (CON) laws, laws requiring state approval of the establishment or expansion of health facilities. By 1979, almost all the states had enacted such laws, which typically covered nursing homes (see Table 1). State

TABLE 1
States with CON Legislation

Year Enacted	States
Never	Idaho, Indiana, Louisiana
1970 and before	California, Connecticut, Maryland, New York, Rhode Island
1971	Arizona, Massachusetts, Minnesota, Nevada, New Jersey, North Dakota, Oklahoma, Oregon, South Carolina, Washington
1972	Florida, Kansas, Kentucky, Michigan, South Dakota
1973	Colorado, Tennessee, Virginia
1974	Georgia, Hawaii, Illinois
1975	Arkansas, Montana, Ohio, Texas
1976	Alaska*
1977	Alabama, District of Columbia, Iowa,* West Virginia, Wisconsin, Wyoming
1978	Delaware,* Maine, New Mexico, North Carolina
1979	Mississippi, Nebraska, New Hampshire, Pennsylvania, Utah, Vermont, Missouri

Source: DHEW, Health Resources Administration, Bureau of Health Planning, Division of Regulatory Activity, Certification Programs Branch, July 12, 1979.
*CON legislation went into effect the year after enactment.

action was undoubtedly influenced by passage of the National Health Planning and Resources Development Act in 1974, by which grants from the Public Health Service are contingent upon a state's enactment of CON legislation. For nursing homes, as for other health facilities, the regulation of capital expenditures has been justified as a means both to ensure a rational allocation of health care resources and to control total expenditures on medical care. But assumptions that typically justify the use of CON legislation may not apply in the nursing home market. Control of capital expenditures is intended to compensate for perceived inadequacies in the health care market—notably, the providers' ability to influence and stimulate demand. Providers' influence stems from widespread third-party insurance, which reduces or eliminates the consumers' concern with the cost of the service, and from consumers' inability to evaluate their need for medical services and the kind of services they require. In these circumstances, providers, who benefit financially from delivering more services, can increase the quantity and sophistication of the services they offer. Even if providers deliver only the services they believe to be of positive value, this value is likely to be less than the costs entailed in delivering care. If suppliers determine the nature and quantity of services, and deliver services for which the costs exceed the benefits, regulation of the supply of services becomes an appropriate mechanism to limit expenditures for medical care.[1]

Recent evidence suggests that there are limits to the creation of demand.[2] Assumptions about the creation of demand are particularly inappropriate to the nursing home market, where demand appears to be largely independent of supply. Nursing homes provide a limited quantity of medically related services, along with a larger array of services to satisfy the residents' basic wants for housing, food, and recreational services. Potential residents or their families can evaluate

[1] This argument assumes that providers will allocate their services in accord with a societal view of need. Such behavior might be motivated by a sense of professionalism. An efficient allocation of the regulated supply might not occur if providers acted on other motives, such as profit maximization, and continued to create demand among potential recipients.

[2] On limits to physicians' ability to create demand, see Hadley, Holahan, and Scanlon (1979). Limits on the hospitals' ability to create demand are suggested by steadily declining occupancy rates.

nursing home care relative to alternative living arrangements, according to their own preferences. The need to defer to providers' judgments about what constitutes appropriate use is absent because of the largely nontechnical nature of the product.

Consumers must make real choices with respect to nursing home care because virtually all users face substantial out-of-pocket costs. Private patients must pay the full cost of their care, and Medicaid patients must sacrifice their entire income, less a small personal-needs allowance, in order to enter a nursing home. Even those with no private income must sacrifice resources on entering a nursing home. These people normally would be eligible for cash-assistance payments and could purchase whatever those payments allowed. Entering a nursing home reduces the payment level to the needs allowance.

Public subsidies, primarily from Medicaid, have drastically lowered the price of nursing home care for many elderly persons, while leaving the prices of alternative systems of care unaffected. Naturally this subsidy influences the choices that people make; many persons undoubtedly can obtain more desirable housing, food, and necessary care in a nursing home than their financial resources would allow outside. Under these circumstances, more people may be seeking nursing home care than objective standards of need would justify, or than the Medicaid program is willing to finance.

Research indicates that the number of persons who demand nursing home care is indeed larger than the number who receive it (Scanlon, 1980). This imbalance is the result of separate policies of state government, designed to achieve conflicting objectives. Eligibility policies, which determine demand, are established with objectives much broader than mere control of the number of persons demanding nursing home care, and may make many more persons eligible than the state is willing to support. The state reveals its financial preferences in other policies—notably reimbursement and CON regulation—that determine the supply of beds in nursing homes. If the objective behind these policies is to control costs, the resulting bed supply is likely to be insufficient to serve the demand encouraged by eligibility policies.

Regulation of the bed supply will not make demand disappear, as it might if suppliers simply created the demand. As long as the current subsidy structure persists, limitations on supply will pose a rationing problem. Only some of the individuals who want nursing home care will receive it, and the decision as to who receives it will be left in the hands of those who operate the nursing homes. For several reasons, operators are likely to discriminate against the persons most in need of care. Unlike hospital care, nursing home care is not a last resort. Hospitals can and do treat patients unable to find nursing home beds. Nursing home operators can readily refuse to admit patients whom they prefer not to serve. To maximize their profits or net revenues, these operators would prefer patients who pay more (private patients) to those who pay less (Medicaid patients), and patients who require a little care to those who need considerable and costly attention. When nursing home beds are insufficient to satisfy demand, the people most in need of the service have the greatest difficulty finding it.

Concern about this problem led us to question the desirability of applying CON rules to nursing homes. To determine whether this assessment of the nursing home market was correct and, if so, how and why states used CON regulations, in the period August through October, 1978, we conducted interviews in eight states: California, Colorado, Georgia, Massachusetts, New Jersey, New York, Tennessee, and Washington.[3] The eight states studied accounted for about 40 percent of Medicaid expenditures on nursing homes in 1977, and were chosen because they represent various levels and rates of increase in nursing home use, and different levels of total Medicaid spending per capita. Table 2 compares nursing home use and expenditures in the eight states with those in the rest of the nation. New York and California enacted CON legislation in the 1960s; the other six states enacted it in the early 1970s. Georgia is the only state in the nation whose CON program applies only to nursing homes, not to hospitals.

Based on interviews with government officials and industry representatives, and on documentary materials from each of those eight states, this paper analyzes the methods and objectives of the states in applying CON policies to nursing homes, the problems faced in achieving the objectives, and the consequences of actions taken, both

[3] Case studies of four—California, Georgia, New York, and Washington—are available (Lennox, 1979).

TABLE 2

Nursing Home Use and Expenditures in Eight States

State	Beds per 1000 Population Aged 65 and over* 1976		Average Annual Growth Rate in Beds per 1000 Population Aged 65 and over* 1969–1976		Average Nursing Home Occupancy Rate* 1976		Total Medicaid Expenditures per Capita† 1976		Medicaid Nursing Home Expenditures per Capita† 1976		Medicaid Nursing Home Expenditures as a Percent of Total Expenditures§ 1976	
	Number	National Rank	Percent	National Rank	Percent	National Rank		National Rank		National Rank	Percent	National Rank
California	65.2	24	3.94	40	90.04	41	$74.40	9	$16.64	35	22.37	48
Colorado	104.3	2	8.87	12	83.90	50	41.43	30	19.97	28	48.20	17
Georgia	66.5	23	10.66	5	95.61	3	51.31	21	22.17	18	43.21	24
Massachusetts	74.7	16	3.57	42	94.44	13	90.53	4	41.79	4	46.16	19
New Jersey	43.2	43	4.11	39	95.04	8	54.93	17	16.69	34	30.38	41
New York	50.5	36	5.91	28	93.09	22	185.35	1	69.29	1	37.38	31
Tennessee	44.4	40	8.83	13	96.02	1	41.53	29	18.68	31	44.97	22
Washington	81.1	11	7.68	17	92.04	28	49.56	22	20.57	25	41.51	26
National mean	64.0		6.49		92.06		53.79		21.64		41.96	
National median	63.2		6.28		92.36		43.71		20.51		41.54	
National range												
Highest	119.1 (Nebr.)		20.06 (Alaska)		96.02 (Tenn.)		185.35 (N. Y.)		62.29 (N. Y.)		68.06 (Wyo.)	
Lowest	23.9 (Fla.)		1.61 (Okla.)		82.57 (Tex.)		15.39 (Wyo.)		5.39 (W. Va.)		16.91 (W. Va.)	

* National Center for Health Statistics, *Master Facilities Inventory*, selected years, unpublished data.
† Data from DHEW, Health Care Financing Administration, Office of Policy, Planning, and Research, *Medicaid State Tables, Fiscal Year 1976*, Table 5. Population figures for all per capita calculations taken from U.S. Department of Commerce, Bureau of the Census, *1977 Statistical Abstract of the United States*, Table 29.
‡ For services in skilled nursing homes and intermediate care facilities in institutions for all, including the mentally retarded. *Medicaid State Tables, Fiscal Year 1976*, Table 5.

in certificate-of-need programs and in other nursing home policies (notably Medicaid reimbursement and utilization review), for the availability and use of nursing home beds. Because eight states cannot be considered representative of the nation, and because the depth of our investigation varied somewhat among the states, we will use the experience of individual states to illustrate the types of policy choices the states face, rather than to make conclusive judgments on nursing home policy as it operates in all states.

CON Methods and Objectives

CON legislation provides a mechanism for review and approval of the growth and replacement of nursing homes. As such, it can be neutral, restrictive, or promotive with respect to a state's total bed stock. In addition, it can be used to influence the types of beds built, e.g., those for skilled nursing facilities (SNFs) or those for intermediate care facilities (ICFs), where in the state the beds are constructed, and which proprietors are allowed to build and own beds. The purpose a CON program actually serves varies with its legislative authorization and the objectives of its administrators.

CON statutes have varied with respect to the level of expenditures and types of actions covered. A law like New York's, which covers any capital expenditure and any change in the number of beds regardless of expenditure, allows greater state control over the nursing home industry than does a law like Washington's, which has limited its review to construction whose cost exceeds $100,000. Exemptions and exceptions for special types of facilities or population groups can also reduce the probable impact of CON legislation, and have varied from state to state.

The importance of statutory variation, however, is declining. Statutes and regulations developed to comply with federal laws now reflect a uniform minimum approach to state regulation of capital expenditures, which allows administrators to influence nursing home growth. Federal influence began in 1972 under Section 1122 of the amendments to the Social Security Act. By this authority, over thirty states established agreements with the Department of Health, Education, and Welfare (HEW) to review all capital expenditures that exceeded $100,000, changed a facility's bed capacity, or involved a "substantial change" in the services provided by health facilities, including nursing homes (Table 3). Any facility acting in spite of a denial under Section 1122 would be refused capital reimbursement under Medicare, Medicaid, and the Maternal and Child Health Program for the expenditures deemed unnecessary. The effectiveness of this sanction has been questioned, because of the facilities' capacity to use private revenues to compensate for reductions in public reimbursement. This argument would seem more relevant to hospital than to nursing home regulation, however, because most nursing homes are more dependent on Medicaid funds. Experience in Georgia suggests

TABLE 3
States with Section 1122 Agreements

Year 1122 Enacted	States
Never	Arizona, California, Connecticut, District of Columbia, Illinois, Kansas, Massachusetts, Rhode Island, South Dakota, Tennessee, Texas
1970 and before	None
1971	None
1972	None
1973	Alabama, Arkansas, Delaware, Indiana, Iowa, Louisiana, Maine, Michigan, Mississippi, Nebraska, New Hampshire, North Carolina, Pennsylvania
1974	Alaska, Colorado, Georgia, Idaho, Kentucky, Minnesota, Montana, Nevada, New Jersey, New York, North Dakota, Oklahoma, South Carolina, Utah, Washington, Wyoming
1975	Vermont
1976	None
1977	West Virginia
1978	None
1979	None

Source: DHEW, Health Resources Administration, Bureau of Health Planning, Division of Regulatory Activity, Certification Programs Branch, July 12, 1979.
Note: Oregon terminated its 1122 programs in 1979; Florida, Maryland, Ohio, Virginia, and Wisconsin, in 1978; Hawaii, in 1977; and Missouri in 1976.

that Section 1122 may have allowed states with relatively narrow CON statutes to extend their influence over the nursing home industry. Georgia officials took advantage of a Section 1122 agreement to get around a CON process designed and influenced by the industry.

A more significant impetus for a consistent minimum standard of state regulation is the National Health Planning and Resources Development Act of 1974. That law requires all states to enact CON laws that meet specified conditions (similar to those required by Section 1122, but with broader sanctions), as a requirement for receipt of funds under Public Health Service programs. States did not rush to comply with the requirements of the Health Planning Act and there has been considerable uncertainty that all states would meet its 1980 deadline. As the deadline approaches, however, more states are seeking and acquiring HEW approval of their programs. As of November 1979, HEW had designated thirty-four states as in compliance with the act. The likelihood is that most states will soon share a common set of minimum standards for the regulation of capital expenditures.

Statutory authority, however, is only a precondition for regulation. Far more critical to a state's influence is the willingness of officials to use their authority, as demonstrated by the criteria they apply in ruling on proposed changes in the bed stock. CON statutes (and regulations implementing the Health Planning Act) typically specify the kinds of factors that regulation of the bed supply must "take into account"— variations on the themes of need, financial feasibility, and the quality or character of nursing home owners. In defining and using these criteria, CON administrators reveal their objectives for the size and composition of the nursing home bed supply. Some states have ignored their CON authority for nursing homes, leaving the determination of the bed supply either to local planning agencies or to the marketplace. In contrast, the states that use CON legislation to control costs tend to impose their review criteria even upon resistant local agencies. The states have employed various criteria to determine bed supply in nursing homes.

Determination of Need

The "certificate-of-need" label implies that need is the primary determinant of decisions on the bed supply in nursing homes. Need, however, is an imprecise term. Used to refer to individuals' need for services, a state's "need" for beds could be interpreted as the number of beds required to accommodate persons in the state who have conditions that experts believe require institutional care. For nursing homes, as with many other health services, there is no consensus on the health status or functional levels that require institutional care. Even if there were consensus, another problem would remain—the relation between objectively defined need and consumer-defined demand. Need for service may have little to do with the number of persons who actually seek nursing home care. Although objectively defined need may influence a person to seek care, the individual's demand will depend on a variety of other factors—personal taste, financial resources, and the price of nursing home care relative to that for other goods and services. Given the generous public subsidy for nursing home care, and the dearth of underwriting of housing and in-home services, limits on bed supply may well mean that more persons will be seeking care than there will be beds available. The result will mean not only a perceived shortage of beds, but also that persons with an objectively determined need for care may not receive it.

The gap between medical need for care and demand for care poses a dilemma for a state government. A bed supply that is adequate to satisfy demand will raise the costs to the state; a bed supply intended to satisfy only need may leave many people inadequately served. The state's choice between these extremes represents its demand for nursing home services, and reflects both its goals for serving the elderly and the disabled population, and the price it is willing to pay to achieve these goals.

Broadly speaking, two methods are used to determine a state's demand for beds. One method projects the number of beds needed in the future on the basis of the number in current use, adjusted for expected changes in the size of the elderly population and for an independently determined standard for nursing home occupancy. The other method establishes a norm or target ratio of beds to population that is independent of current use. The current-use approach, derived from the Hill-Burton program, may reflect neither medical need nor consumer demand. In the last fifteen years, numerous investigations of nursing home use throughout the country have produced estimates of inappropriate placement ranging from 6 to 76 percent (Congressional Budget Office, 1977). Given this range, it is hard to believe that current use of nursing homes reflects any standard of medical need.

There is also reason to question whether the Hill-Burton approach satisfies the demand for care. If other factors affecting nursing home use (in particular, Medicaid policies, the availability of alternative housing and services, and income levels) remain constant, adoption of the Hill-Burton method is a decision to satisfy in future years the same proportion of demand that is satisfied at present. If the bed supply is insufficient to meet demand now, it will continue to be insufficient five years from now.

A state's reliance on the Hill-Burton method suggests indifference, more than a positive decision with respect to need and demand. Unless a state is dissatisfied with the status of its nursing home industry, use of CON legislation to perpetuate existing practices would seem the simplest path to take. Among the states we visited, the Hill-Burton method was commonly used at the outset of a CON program, when hospitals tended to be the primary concern of legislators and administrators and fiscal pressures were not severe. As long as the elderly population is growing, the Hill-Burton method implies little interference with the nursing home industry's ongoing pattern of growth.

The Hill-Burton method, however, can be manipulated to influence and alter growth patterns. Both Georgia and Massachusetts sought to equalize bed distribution within the state by using the state-wide ratio of beds to elderly (instead of locally determined ratios) as a target for beds in all parts of the state. This ratio became a ceiling in high-growth areas, and a goal in relatively underserved areas. Depending upon the existing distribution of beds and the size of the geographic area to which the ratio is applied, this method may allow significant growth. Growth will occur if the geographic area is small (e.g., a county), if bed supply varies considerably across areas, and if beds are not closed in areas with relatively high ratios of beds to population. Growth, as well as redistribution, is encouraged by New Jersey's effort to tie bed projections to the patients' home county, rather than to the county in which they currently receive care. New Jersey compares the number of nursing home users from a county with the number of persons over sixty-five in the county to arrive at a target for beds needed. The objective is to encourage a supply of beds close to home.

In their acceptance of current-use rates, state-wide-ratio and county-of-residence methods resemble the standard Hill-Burton approach. But in their efforts to alter the location of beds to achieve independently determined goals, these methods resemble the normative approach to planning. Some states have departed entirely from current-use rates in establishing targets. Tennessee, for example, projects bed supply to satisfy expected users—the number of the unmarried elderly unable to carry on their major functions. With this approach, Tennessee encourages increases in the bed supply to better accommodate the estimated need for formal care. New York and Massachusetts have attempted to develop more precise estimates of need by surveying samples of the elderly population. Targets for different types of beds (skilled nursing, intermediate care, and domiciliary care facilities) are derived from the survey's identification of the proportion of the elderly who need each level of care. Until recently, New York's assessments of needs justified a considerable expansion of the number of beds in nursing homes. In contrast, Massachusetts' survey projected only a slight increase in beds but a massive change in the types of services available. The surveys and the related methodologies in both states have been criticized—the New York estimate as too heavily weighted toward meeting demand, thereby projecting beds in excess of medical need; the Massachusetts estimate as too heavily weighted toward medical need, and insufficiently sensitive to demand.

Obviously, no method is above criticism; all methods are subject to manipulation to arrive at preconceived objectives. A brief description of experiences in Georgia, Washington, Massachusetts, and New York illustrates the way in which states adapt their methodologies to fiscal concerns.

Georgia began its certificate-of-need program by adopting the state's average ratio of number of beds to number of the elderly (70 beds per 1,000 elderly) as a ceiling on bed increases in individual counties. State officials perceived this method as suitable to a desired redistribution of beds, but as supportive of an overall level higher than was desirable for the state. Although Georgia officials regarded the projection of current-use rates as consistent with the demand for care (90 percent of which was financed by the Medicaid program), they saw it as working at cross-purposes not only with the need to encourage alternatives to institutionalized care, but also with the state's potential future ability to pay. Despite the fact that Georgia's commitment to so-called alternatives was then limited to a demonstration program involving only 400 Georgia residents, the state reduced its target to 55 beds per 1,000 elderly. The target was selected almost arbitrarily, said officials, to accommodate state budgetary objectives.

These officials were under no illusion that their method would ensure service to all persons in need of care. They readily admitted that, at the reimbursement rate they believed necessary to ensure high-quality care, more beds would be supplied and filled with those needing service than the state would be willing or able to finance. Officials justified the reduction in bed projections as perhaps necessary to create a scarcity of long-term inpatient-care service, in order to increase the incentive to find other solutions for those patients who do not need full-time institutionalization. The state's willingness to incur the additional costs of alternative solutions, however, was an open question.

Washington's experience is markedly similar. From 1971 to 1975, the state used the Hill-Burton method to project the need for nursing home beds on a county-by-county basis. By 1975, concern with rising Medicaid costs led to reconsideration of this method. As in Georgia, Washington officials recognized that current use was not determined simply by the availability of beds, but was also a function of the existing pattern of subsidies for institutional care. The task force evaluating the bed-need methodology therefore advised that if the state were prepared to finance noninstitutional alternatives to nursing home care, bed-need projections should assume a 10 percent reduction in the current-use rate and should employ a nursing home occupancy rate of 95 rather than 90 percent. The 10 percent figure was chosen as an estimate (derived from experience outside of Washington) of the number of people placed in nursing homes who had no objectively determined need to be there and could instead be cared for at home. The 95 percent occupancy rate was justified in terms of the relative stability of a nursing home's patient population. The resulting formula would mean a substantial reduction in the state's projected need for beds.

Washington adopted the recommended change in the formula but rejected the condition that had been used to justify it: expanded financing for noninstitutional services. Concern with the cost per service, and the possibility that noninstitutional services would be used by persons not previously served, as well as by those inappropriately placed in nursing homes, led the state to reject a commitment to support noninstitutional services. Washington, then, reduced its bed-supply objectives with the understanding that services were not available to encourage more appropriate use of nursing homes.

Massachusetts demonstrates a similar phenomenon. From 1974 through 1976, the state, like Georgia, used a state-wide-ratio approach to determine bed need. Reconsideration of this approach was initiated not only by concern with the costs of financing the demand for nursing home care, but also by recognition that the formula allowed expansion that exceeded demand. Use of the state-wide ratio of beds to population allowed expansion of the bed supply in areas that already had low occupancy rates. When the formula led the state to reverse a local planning agency's recommendation for denial on these grounds, policy makers demanded a reevaluation of the bed formula. While that reevaluation was in progress, the state declared a moratorium on all nursing home construction.

In Massachusetts, unlike Georgia and Washington, reevaluation involved the use of specified criteria to determine the need for medical care in the elderly population, independent of their current place of residence. After surveys in all types of institutions, and a sampling of high-risk elderly at home, the state arrived at a set of targets that mandated a slight increase in the total number of beds but massive changes in the types of beds then supplied—specifically, a substantial decrease in the number of beds in chronic disease hospitals, ICFs, and rest homes, and an increase in the number in SNFs. When applied to regions, these state-wide targets were to be adjusted for the percent of the elderly who were seventy-five and older, and the percent living alone. The resulting projections were intended, then, to accommodate variations in the need for nursing home care among the elderly population. As in other states, the new method's departure from the projection based on current use was presumably contingent upon a significant commitment of funds for noninstitutional services that no one was certain would be forthcoming. Despite uncertainty about this and other changes in state policy on long-term care, the state adopted the new method, slightly modified. In contrast to Georgia and Washington, however, Massachusetts explicitly declared its method to be an interim approach, and policy makers continued to debate and deliberate an appropriate policy.

Although, until now, New York has explicitly acknowledged a willingness to ignore need estimates when waiting lists or other factors demonstrate a demand for beds, here, too, restrictive pressure is rising. Reacting both to financial concerns and to scandals related to the quality of care, planners have gradually tightened their estimates of need and employed other criteria to restrict nursing home growth. The New York Department of the Budget approves all CON recommendations before final action, and reportedly objects to any departure from the need estimates. Furthermore, official pronouncements increasingly criticize the state's excessive reliance on institutional as opposed to noninstitutional services. Here, as elsewhere, the state is becoming willing to restrict bed-supply growth to levels below the projected demand. Although states may use medical need to justify these restrictions, to date they have been reluctant to establish the noninstitutional services they believe necessary to compensate for unbuilt beds. The actual justification for restriction, then, apparently has less to do with medical need than with limited financial resources and competing demands for funds.

Review of Financial Feasibility

Bed-need restrictions are not the only way the states have used CON statutes to contain costs. CON programs have often been used to enforce restrictions on Medicaid payments or to close loopholes in capital reimbursement policies that lead to higher payments than the state wishes to make. Overall enforcement of Medicaid rates occurs in the CON review of the "financial feasibility" of a proposed project. In this process, analysts assess the applicant's assumptions with respect to the volume and level of payment from Medicaid and from private patients. If the assumptions are inconsistent with Medicaid payment policy, or, in some instances, entail unrealistic projections of the number of private patients, reviewers will find the project infeasible and the certificate of need will be denied.

States differ in the importance they attach to this process. One indication of commitment is reliance on the Medicaid rate-setting agency to perform the CON financial review. This occurs in New Jersey, New York, Washington, and, for some transactions, Georgia. Process alone, however, is not sufficient to ensure consistency between the rates used for CON approval and the rates actually paid. Washington's payment rates have been criticized as different from CON-approved estimates, a result attributed to fluctuations in the rate-setting method and in its administration. In contrast, in New York, CON approval of the costs of a capital expenditure justifies inclusion of those costs in the Medicaid rate. New York's review of capital expenditures is very detailed, involving line-by-line approval of a capital expenditure budget. A finding that capital expenditures will drive the costs of a nursing home above its Medicaid ceiling leads to reduction or denial of the expenditure.

States have also used CON review to close specific loopholes in Medicaid reimbursement policies—in particular, to eliminate reimbursement that allows nursing homes to increase Medicaid revenues by selling or leasing homes. CON review may be used here not simply to enforce Medicaid restrictions in advance, but to impose limits beyond those specified in the payment process. Most often this is achieved by disapproving unacceptable levels of (or methods for calculating) lease or sales costs. But Georgia has gone beyond this to prohibit all sales in areas its need-projections identify as having too many beds. Although the industry objects that need should have nothing to do with sales, Georgia's policy serves the state's primary purpose: to restrict real estate transactions that raise Medicaid rates. Prohibition of sales might force nursing homes to close and thereby reduce the bed supply.

Instead of using CON review to close specific loopholes in reimbursement policy or to enforce reimbursement decisions in advance, some rate-setting agencies operate in complete independence of CON review. This is true in both Massachusetts and California. Massachusetts uses a set of Medicaid-prepared capital-cost estimates to evaluate proposed capital expenditures, and requires a new CON review for expenditures above the approved amount (plus a generous contingency allowance). But those who set Medicaid rates are not bound in any way by the CON approval.

Differences among states in their reliance on CON review reflect variations in payment philosophies and political strategies. In New York, Washington, and Georgia, reimbursement has been sufficiently lucrative to attract a larger supply of beds than the state wants to support. The reasons are too complex to analyze here (Spitz and Weeks, 1978–1979), but they include concern that payment be adequate to support high-quality care, to ensure access for Medicaid patients, and to achieve political peace with the nursing home industry. Whatever the reasons, policy makers regard CON review as a valuable and necessary instrument in payment control. To have the mechanism and not use it, said one New York official, would open the state to charges that "it had missed its chance." Then the state would have to pay the expenses incurred. As long as the state believes this is true, CON review of financial feasibility serves an important function in state policy.

Obviously, other states do not share this belief and need no prior review to enforce their nursing home rates. In Massachusetts, this choice is particularly noteworthy because it differs from the relation between rate setting and CON review that applies to hospitals. For hospitals, rate setters perform and then abide by CON reviews of capital expenditures. A greater willingness to deny nursing home expenditures after the fact may be associated with the lower political risk of disrupting a for-profit as opposed to a nonprofit industry.

Review of Quality
Some states have used CON statutes not only to control the number and cost of beds, but also to control the quality of nursing home care. Like the review of financial feasibility, the review of quality supplements another policy mechanism in the state—licensure. Some states are more willing to prevent the establishment of a new facility, or to deny a facility an opportunity to expand, than they are to revoke the

license of an existing facility. Officials did not try to defend this distinction in terms of quality of patient care, but it makes sense in political terms. Proprietors (and residents) are likely to exercise far more pressure to prevent a loss than to seek a gain. Hence, the state is able to impose different and more restrictive standards by denying a certificate of need than by revoking a license.

Although not unique in its use of the CON program to review quality, New York has carried this review to such an extreme that it has become a significant impediment to nursing home expansion. Like Colorado and Washington, New York reviews an applicant's licensure record, in and out of the state, to determine whether the proprietor has performed acceptably in the past. Unacceptable performance leads to denial of a certificate. In response to scandals about the poor quality of some nursing homes, New York's criteria for acceptability became extraordinarily restrictive. For new facilities, the legislature required the state to review an applicant's licensure record for the preceding ten years, to determine whether the applicant had consistently delivered high-quality care. For chains of nursing homes, the record of each participating home must be reviewed. If an existing facility seeks expansion, the state examines only its current licensure status. In either case, the reviewers make subjective judgments as to the adequacy of performance.

Although New York officials reportedly try to distinguish between "important" (related to patient care) and "unimportant" (paperwork) shortcomings, the state and the industry agree that the criteria are excessively demanding. The fact that cited deficiencies have been rapidly corrected, for example, does not help to clear a record. Furthermore, a state official explained, the documentary evidence of licensure violations makes it easier for reviewers to support a negative than a positive finding. Existing requirements also produce Catch 22 situations. For example, if two partners, one upstanding and the other negligent, own a nursing home, and the negligent partner wishes to leave, the remaining partner would be denied a certificate for change in ownership because of his previous association with an unacceptable operator.

Perhaps even more important than these difficulties is that New York's quality criteria have created a bias in favor of new entrants who have no previous experience in the nursing home industry. Although the state consults better business bureaus and district attorneys' offices to check on these people, the applicants are far less likely than existing operators to have unacceptable characteristics. State officials are dissatisfied with this bias toward inexperience, believing it to be the source of many of the undesirable practices uncovered in recent investigations of the industry. Despite its shortcomings, quality review has become a significant source of CON denials in New York, and has contributed to what state officials increasingly regard as a necessary restriction of the bed supply.

The Effects of CON Policies

Certificate-of-need regulation makes assumptions about or tries to affect almost all aspects of nursing home use and performance. To evaluate CON policy, it is therefore necessary to consider its consequences on several fronts—with respect to the total supply of nursing home beds, the distribution of beds by geographic area and level of care, the availability of beds to different types of users, the quality of care provided, and the costs to the state. Obviously, these aspects of the nursing home market are influenced by other factors as well as by the CON policy. The market is also shaped by the socioeconomic characteristics of the state population and by a combination of policies that include Medicaid reimbursement rates, licensure requirements, and utilization review programs. Detailed examination of these policies was beyond the scope of our study. What follows is therefore a qualitative assessment of the effects of CON policies on the nursing home market, based largely on the perceptions of officials and industry spokesmen in several states.

As long as funds are pouring in, a CON program appears to have some effect on industry behavior, but perhaps not the effect that policy makers intend. Enactment of CON legislation frequently induces substantial increases in the bed supply, as nursing homes seek to shut out competition or avoid future restrictions. Georgia officials estimated that plans for 5,000 beds (roughly a 20 percent increase) were initiated between the date of CON's enactment and its starting date, and Tennessee officials estimate a similar (roughly 25 percent) increase. In California, officials describe the growth spurt associated with its 1969 CON law as so large as to exceed demand for the next several years.

Aside from this initial effect, it is difficult to determine whether CON laws affect the rate of nursing home growth. Application and denial rates have been discredited as indicators, since they are themselves shaped by CON policies. On the one hand, operators may continually submit more applications than they intend to use, to compensate for slow or changing decisions in the state; on the other hand, operators may not bother to submit applications that they feel have little chance of approval. The fact that denial rates for nursing homes appear to have been more common than for hospitals (Lewin and Associates, 1975) may indicate differences in the states' willingness to offend these industries. But it is not possible to use these rates to draw conclusions about the effects of CON policies.

Beyond any impact on the total bed supply in nursing homes, CON programs may serve to encourage bed construction in relatively underserved areas. Tennessee and Georgia officials report that operators respond to bed-need projections by applying to build in areas of identified need. This does not mean, however, that operators do not apply in other areas, or that applications in other areas are disapproved. In states with restrictive policies, state officials, local planning-agency staff, and industry spokesmen claim that the state does indeed adhere to its bed-supply projections in awarding certificates of need. But in Tennessee, where growth was favored, officials appeared willing to depart from their need projections for a variety of reasons, including differences in population characteristics, high rates of occupancy, and political pressure.

Regardless of the state's objectives for total bed supply, reliance on CON regulation to redistribute beds does not always work. If reimbursement policies or private demand make nursing home operation lucrative throughout the state, restrictions on bed supply in some areas may lead to building in other areas. But if nursing homes are not sufficiently lucrative in some areas, building will not occur there, no matter how CON programs are used. Redistribution of beds through use of CON policies is particularly difficult in states where reimbursement does not reflect geographic differences in the costs of care. This is true, for example, in California. But even where reimbursement makes some allowance for geographic differences, payment may be insufficient to attract capital investment in the inner cities, which are high-cost, high-crime areas. California officials reported severe shortages in San Francisco, despite a recognized need for beds. New York reported similar problems in Buffalo, and Massachusetts had a problem in Boston. Without significant alterations in the reimbursement system, building was unlikely to occur in these areas even if they were the only place the state allowed any building at all.

Similar problems arise with respect to CON objectives for redistribution of types of facilities. In Massachusetts, for example, planners proposed to reach bed targets by converting chronic-disease and rehabilitation hospitals to skilled nursing facilities, and by upgrading intermediate care facilities to meet standards for skilled care. Reimbursement policies and certain characteristics of the industry blocked both objectives. Downgrading chronic disease hospitals would have subjected them to nursing-home reimbursement ceilings that did not apply to hospitals. Obviously, institutions prefer the classification that gives them the higher reimbursement, and their interest in downgrading was understandably low. Similarly, operators who made money from ICFs were not inclined to upgrade their institutions to SNF status. The costs of upgrading apparently exceeded the expected returns at SNF rates. An even greater deterrent, the state found, was the fact that 30 percent of existing ICF beds could not meet the standards of SNF Life Safety Code or construction requirements. As a result, the state reported a "disappointing" response to its policies, with only 250–400 beds (of a total 27,000) upgraded in the policy's first year.

Inability to accomplish the objectives behind bed-supply targets has not deterred states from applying restrictive policies. Because states frequently tighten their reimbursement policies for nursing homes at the same time, it is difficult to identify the independent effect of CON restrictions on the bed supply. In some states (e.g., Georgia, Washington, and New York), restrictions on reimbursement were intentionally short-lived. As indicated earlier, these states were unwilling or unable to reduce reimbursement to levels that would sufficiently restrict the bed supply and Medicaid obligations. They therefore perceived CON regulation as a necessary mechanism for controlling Medicaid expenditures for nursing homes. In other states (e.g., California and Massachusetts), reimbursement restrictions have been the primary instrument of controlling cost and supply. Some states have successfully used CON and reimbursement policies, alone or in some combination, to halt growth in their nursing home industries.

As the states themselves predicted, holding bed supply below demand creates serious inequities and inefficiencies. Because nursing home operators control admissions, their decisions become critical determinants of service use. Operators prefer patients who pay more and cost less. When the bed supply is limited, they can—and reportedly do—exercise this preference in their admission policies. The states we visited consistently reported access problems for Medicaid patients, especially for those who needed considerable care. When they cannot find nursing home beds, these patients reportedly stay in hospitals beyond the appropriate time for discharge. Some officials and industry spokesmen argue that bed shortages have effectively eliminated the freedom of Medicaid patients to choose a provider, for, with few beds available, they must take what they can get. As long as they are in the hospital, however, these patients do continue to receive Medicaid benefits. The attempts in Massachusetts and New Jersey to deny hospital payment for patients awaiting placement in nursing homes were blocked by the courts. The state (with perhaps some help from Medicare) therefore bears the costs of these hospital stays. In California, such patients reportedly accounted for Medicaid expenses of $2 million per month. New York estimated that 3,000–4,000 persons per day, financed by Medicaid, Medicare, or other sources, were in hospitals awaiting placement in nursing homes. Massachusetts estimated 1,750 in 1974 and 800 in 1976, and New Jersey 1,300.

Just as very sick patients stay too long in hospitals (or, as some observers argue, go without care), persons needing little care stay too long in nursing homes. Although utilization review could theoretically ensure that available beds are allocated more efficiently, its effectiveness appears to be limited. State officials argued that Medicaid reviewers could not legally or practically demand the discharge of patients whose needs for some form of assistance or housing could not be met in the community. In New York, where an aggressive discharge policy was attempted, it was found unacceptable in court. As the states recognized in advance, failure to provide alternatives to nursing home care in the community makes it difficult to ensure appropriate institutional care.

Restrictions on available beds also interfere with enforcement of quality standards. To paraphrase officials' observations, "You can't close a home when you have nowhere to put its patients." Bed shortages in Massachusetts reportedly led the state to give up on closing a nursing home if it meant finding beds for more than 15 or 20 patients. When hospitals, too, are waiting to place patients, closing a home becomes particularly difficult. "When a new nursing home opened," said one responsible state official, "we had to race the hospital to get hold of the beds."

In sum, the creation of a bed shortage, whether through reimbursement or CON policies, creates what officials in the state of Washington describe as a sellers' market. Not only does a shortage allow operators to pick and choose their patients, reaping the associated financial rewards, but it also improves the operators' negotiating position with respect to quality enforcement and—in some states (e.g., Washington)—reimbursement.

State governments clearly recognize the problems a bed shortage produces, frequently before the problems arise. Once the predicted consequences become fact, the states react in different ways. One response is to expand regulation in order to compensate for undesirable behavior of the industry. Two types of regulation attempt to make existing beds more readily available to Medicaid patients. The first is a requirement that any nursing home licensed or awarded a certificate of need must agree to accept Medicaid patients. This requirement would allow legal recourse in cases of blatant discrimination, and, in Massachusetts, local planners hope to use it to get suburban homes to accept some Medicaid patients from the inner city. But since most homes accept some Medicaid patients, compliance with such laws is possible without major changes in admissions practices. As officials themselves observe, without specification of numbers or percentages, nursing homes are unlikely to substitute Medicaid patients for the more lucrative private patients.

A second type of regulation, used in a few states, is the application of the state's rate-setting authority to private as well as to public payments for nursing home care. Applying a uniform rate to all patients would reduce the existing financial incentive to accept private before public patients.[4] Preferences might still persist, either because of side-payments or because of factors independent of price, such as race, social class, or health or functional status. But uniform rates should make it easier for Medicaid patients to obtain access to care. In addition, control over private rates could delay the time at which private patients will exhaust their assets and become eligible for Medicaid benefits. New York officials cited this route to Medicaid eligibility as a significant impediment to controlling Medicaid costs. If, indeed, the Medicaid program cannot deny coverage to a financially eligible nursing home resident, regardless of health status, concern about the rate at which private patients become public patients is justified.

Regulation of all nursing home beds would improve access for Medicaid patients. But such interference in the private market for nursing home care imposes a cost on private patients who are denied care, for it reduces their ability to use their resources to satisfy their preferences. Restricting the access of private patients may have other and unintended consequences. Private patients may be currently subsidizing Medicaid patients (Scanlon, 1980). A reduction in the number of private patients would either curtail the number of Medicaid patients a home would accept, or would require an increase in the Medicaid reimbursement rate to keep the number constant. In extending their regulation of beds, states should recognize these potential problems with access and costs as well as the inequity of interference in the private market.

Another type of regulatory action, operative in a few states, relates

---

[4] It is interesting to note that rate regulation that allows a differential between private and public rates would probably reduce access to care for public patients. Holding private rates at levels below those set by a free market will make nursing home care attractive to a larger number of private patients. Although rate control will limit the operators' revenues from private patients, they will still be more profitable than public patients. With more private patients in the queue, Medicaid patients will have as much, if not more, difficulty in gaining admission as they would have if private rates went unregulated.

to quality enforcement in shortage conditions. If a home is violating safety or other requirements, statutory provisions for receivership would allow the state to take over the home's operation rather than close it down. Massachusetts is considering such a provision, broadening its current authority to take over nursing homes in public emergencies. Current authority is insufficient, officials say, because it is difficult and time-consuming to establish that a "public emergency" exists. These officials recognized that objections to the state's interference in private industry would pose serious obstacles to legislative support for receivership authority. And, even if the legislature enacted broader authority, such objections are likely to affect the state's willingness to take over a nursing home. State officials may also be reluctant to take on the administrative burden of overseeing nursing home management. Receivership could, however, serve as a useful threat to a recalcitrant operator and, in extreme emergency, would allow the state to protect patients who were without alternative sources of care.

Adding new regulations to compensate for the undesirable effects of existing regulation is not uncommon. But it is widely believed that government cannot gain control over industry in a never-ending process of action and reaction that Christopher Hood (1976) has labeled "reciprocal learning." As a large bureaucracy, constrained by a multitude of legal requirements and fixed procedures, the state lacks the freedom to maneuver—and act arbitrarily—that victory may require. It may therefore be far more effective to reduce than to increase regulation when the original goals cannot be met.

Some of the states we visited were in fact taking this course. Pressure to loosen the restrictions on bed supply comes from legislators whose constituents cannot find beds, from nursing home operators who want to expand, from local planning agencies aware of "unmet need," and—within the bureaucracy—from social workers unable to place Medicaid patients, and from budgetary officials concerned about paying for unnecessary days in hospital. Responses to these pressures may be unsystematic, i.e., on a case-by-case basis, or may involve a systematic reassessment of policy. New Jersey appears to be an example of the first; Massachusetts, of the second.

New Jersey reports that it has abandoned its bed-need projections in order to get more beds for Medicaid patients. If they could control the use of all existing beds, say state officials, the state's current supply would be adequate. But, instead, they find that existing operators limit their admission of Medicaid patients. Although New Jersey has passed a law requiring nursing homes to accept a "reasonable number" of Medicaid patients, regulators believe this law is not sufficiently rigorous to overcome access problems that result from the gap between public and private rates of payment. Instead, they believe it necessary to ignore bed projections (which show too many beds in areas where hospital patients ready for discharge cannot find a nursing home bed), in order to allow entry by investors willing to operate at existing Medicaid rates. Health planners in New Jersey object to this approach so strongly that they have effectively refused to participate in the CON review process. But regulators and rate setters believe that abandonment of CON limits, in combination with some general increases in reimbursement levels and adjustments for existing operators in liberally defined "hardship" cases, will produce more efficient and acceptable nursing home care. A New Jersey official reported that in the past a rate hike ended the problem of placing patients on hospital discharge.

Massachusetts has taken a somewhat different approach. Unlike New Jersey, where rate-setting and CON responsibilities are assigned to the same agency, Massachusetts rate-setting and CON officials have operated independently. At the same time that health planning officials were debating the wisdom of a restrictive CON policy, rate setters altered reimbursement policies in ways that substantially reduced the attractiveness of nursing home investment and, at least temporarily, made it difficult for existing operators to meet outstanding financial obligations. As a result, no matter how the health planners chose to use the CON program, growth in bed supply was significantly slowed. Today, however, rate setters and planners are cooperating in an effort to use payment mechanisms, bed-need criteria, and programs for noninstitutional services to efficiently satisfy the need for all forms of long-term care in Massachusetts.[5]

[5] In addition to the intentional easing of CON restrictions, some nursing homes have obtained legislative exemptions from the Massachusetts CON program. Exemptions will undoubtedly affect the bed supply but, as long as Medicaid rates are restricted, they are likely to affect chiefly the private patients.

To some extent, these adjustments were externally imposed, as CON decisions were appealed and overturned. Appeals resulted from the method the CON program employed to encourage upgrading rather than new construction to meet SNF bed-need projections. In reviewing SNF applications, CON officials did not simply compare the existing number of SNF beds with the target; rather, they summed or "aggregated" the numbers of ICF and SNF beds and compared the sum with the SNF target. They allowed no new construction unless an area showed a net need for beds, counting both types of beds. This aggregation method led to the denial of applications to construct SNF beds. Operators successfully appealed these denials to the Health Facilities Appeals Board, which found the aggregation of ICF and SNF beds inappropriate in the absence of evidence that upgrading did or would occur. The regulators' first response to the board's action was to compromise on their aggregation policy, allowing 50 percent of the projected need to be met through upgrading and 50 percent through new construction. This, too, proved unacceptable to the appeals board, and the CON program abandoned the aggregation method entirely. The change would justify approval of 4,200 new beds, as compared with the 2,800 the aggregation method would have allowed.

The CON program similarly gave way on what officials ultimately decided were unrealistic assumptions about downgrading chronic-disease and rehabilitation hospitals to SNF status. Although the state planned to encourage downgrading, by tying payment to reviews of the appropriateness of care, it was a mistake, said a planning official, to expect large savings from this effort. On grounds that these hospitals were treating patients who required intensive care (patients who could not gain admission to nursing homes), and that the hospitals' fixed costs should be covered to keep them in operation, rate setters and planners agreed to establish a rate specific to these facilities, to reduce it only gradually over time (rather than all at once), and to prevent new construction of this type of facility. As with its decision to eliminate the aggregation method, the state decided to give a higher priority to finding sufficient beds than to redistributing the existing supply to conform to standards of medical need or to saving money.

This general principle also led the state to recognize explicitly that the existing ratio of beds to population (especially for ICFs) could be lowered only if the state made noninstitutional services more widely available. Although the state has not been prepared to raise expenditures on these services to the levels believed necessary to satisfy demand, it has incorporated "slots" for community care in its bed-need projections, which are reportedly to be followed *only* when the assumed slots are actually provided. Funds for noninstitutional services are to be targeted to people identified as probable candidates for nursing home use, and to areas that experience delays in placing hospital patients in nursing homes. The state is also experimenting with placement mechanisms to increase the likelihood that the patients most in need of care will get it.

At the same time, the state is altering its reimbursement policy to provide bonuses to homes that make a specified proportion of beds available to Medicaid patients, as well as to homes that maintain specified quality standards. In contrast to the regulatory approach, which works against the operators' financial interests, bonuses seek to make desirable behavior financially worthwhile. If targets for Medicaid patients are set too high, however, the bonus may be insufficient to change admission practices in nursing homes. Massachusetts is also exploring methods for adjusting reimbursement rates to reflect the degree of the patients' disability, in order to overcome the operators' reluctance to take those who need extra care. But, so far, rate setters have objected to patient-based rates as too complicated to implement.

Overall, it is difficult to tell whether the policy changes in Massachusetts are purely rhetorical or will increase the bed supply to better satisfy need. Nevertheless, the wholesale abandonment of service commitment proved to be politically unacceptable. Hence Massachusetts appears to be engaged in a systematic effort to balance cost with need for service, and to allocate limited resources effectively and efficiently.

Not all states are willing to alter their restrictive policies, even when they recognize the resulting inefficiencies and inequities. Georgia officials gave no indication that they planned to loosen their restrictions, and their noninstitutional services program was still in its infancy. Washington was reevaluating its restrictive policies but, in 1978, conflict between officials anxious to satisfy the demand for service and officials unwilling to pay the price required for satisfaction made the outcome uncertain. In general, it is fair to say that the states perceive both gains and losses from regulating the bed supply in nursing homes. What they decide to do depends upon the weights they attach to each.

Who Wins? Who Loses?

CON restriction is not the only mechanism a state can use to control what it spends on nursing home care. A more direct method, recognized by several states, is to limit the rates Medicaid will pay for nursing home beds. Theoretically, a state can set a rate, independent of the costs of an individual home, that will attract construction of the number of beds the state is willing to support. (An approach that reflects industry costs but not the costs of each individual home is consistent with the federal requirement, under Section 249, that Medicaid nursing home payment be reasonably related to costs.) Unless rates are related to a patient's condition, problems of discrimination against those who need extra care will arise if rate restrictions create a shortage of beds, just as problems arise with CON restrictions. But with free entry into the market (i.e., *without* CON restrictions), nursing homes will compete for patients. The result, some argue, will be both higher quality and greater efficiency in the delivery of care. In such circumstances, CON restrictions would not only be unnecessary but would also actually be destructive, for they would inhibit the competition on which desired performance depends.

Why would a state prefer CON restrictions to reliance on the rate structure to control costs? We believe that the choice has to do with the risks state officials are willing to take. When a state tries to restrict its nursing home payments, the reaction is immediate and vociferous. The operators complain of insufficient funds and imminent bankruptcy. Although state officials may greet these claims with skepticism, standing fast poses a considerable risk. If the new rate is indeed too low, operators may lack the resources to provide adequate care. A new owner or another nursing home may ultimately replace the one that fails. But in the meantime patients may suffer. This risk is not limited to the time when the rates are set, but is a constant element in a competitive market. If patients suffer, or appear likely to suffer, officials will be blamed. The political costs of the market's transition costs may be perceived as too great for state officials to bear. Although they may try to control their rates, they may end up paying more than they want to pay. To avoid uncertainty and political pressure, some states even prefer to pay higher rates, using CON methods both to protect the occupancy rates in nursing homes (assuring them adequate revenues), and to avoid greater utilization than the state is willing to finance.

Awarding monopoly power to nursing home operators at comfortable rates will undoubtedly reduce their threats to reduce the quality of care. But the combined strategy of high rates and restrictive CON policies by no means ensures that high-quality care will be provided. CON restrictions may therefore yield state officials only the control of expenditures. High rates accompanied by CON restrictions will probably cost the state less than high rates in the absence of restrictions on entry, even though these restrictions encourage inappropriate hospital use. These hospital stays may be paid for by Medicare (a federal, not a state program). Or, if paid for by Medicaid, they may fill otherwise-empty hospital beds, for which Medicaid (in most states) would pay a share of fixed costs anyway. Obviously, it is not possible to calculate actual costs without more detailed information. But it is possible that state expenses for hospital patients awaiting nursing home beds are significantly lower than expenses for the new beds that high Medicaid rates would encourage in the absence of entry restrictions.

If expenditure control is the only goal, then the states can be said to win from using CON restrictions. But if, instead, we consider expenditures in relation to services provided, the states appear to lose. By protecting established owners from competition, the states are undoubtedly supporting inefficiencies in production, and spending more for a given supply of beds than is theoretically necessary.

The states' loss in this respect is clearly the nursing home operators' gain. In every state we visited, they recognized the advantages of restricting entry. This was true whether the industry considered Medicaid rates sufficient or grossly inadequate. Where operators found the rates particularly low, they regarded CON restrictions as essential to their survival. Without these restrictions, they feared that new entrants into the industry would rob them of patients; with fewer patients at low rates, they would be forced out of business. In California, for example, a spokesman for the nursing home association described his members as "happy as clams" with entry restrictions, and anxious to ensure that they covered all possible competitive threats, including the reclassification of hospital beds to nursing home status.

Even in the states where Medicaid rates make expansion or new building attractive, nursing home operators do not object to the CON process. In Georgia, which may be an extreme example, the industry was the prime mover behind CON legislation. Their interest was not to prohibit all expansion and new investment, but to establish a mechanism whereby the industry itself could decide who would build where. The state officials' circumvention of the CON program's industry-dominated council did not create opposition to the process. Instead, in Georgia as in other states, the industry tends to oppose specific applications of CON regulation rather than the overall concept of controlling entry. Thus, in Georgia, the industry has opposed CON officials' use of bed-need projections to inhibit sales and, in Massachusetts, the industry opposed highly restrictive estimates of medical need as a basis for bed-supply projections. A spokesman for the Massachusetts nursing home industry emphasized, however, that, despite their opposition to specific CON practices, association members—primarily owner-operators of single homes—were not anxious to expand. Interestingly, he explained their attack on stringent restrictions on bed supply as part of a strategy to get their rates raised for current operations. By demonstrating that more beds were needed, but were unavailable at current rates, the industry believed they could press the state to raise rates for all homes. Even if current operators did not want to expand, they therefore had a stake in convincing the state that more beds were desirable. As long as the state stopped short of allowing expansion that threatened occupancy levels, these operators would be satisfied.

In sum, whatever losses in efficiency CON restrictions impose on the state are gains in revenue and security to nursing home operators. The monopoly power that CON restrictions create is apparently far more valuable to these operators than any new investment they might forego. Their stake in the CON process may explain why the states that are unable to limit their payments to nursing homes are able to use CON restrictions to take actions the industry opposes.

Consideration of winners and losers from CON restrictions is not complete without evaluating their effects on patients. CON restrictions influence price, access, and quality of care. Because patients eligible for Medicaid must pay all their income toward nursing home care, and because their income must be less than the Medicaid rate, price is an issue only for private patients. In the absence of competition, private patients face higher charges than would occur in an open market. Furthermore, although private patients have the advantage in nursing home admissions, CON restrictions will reduce the choices available to them, choices they would have in an open market. CON restrictions unquestionably make access a problem for Medicaid patients, particularly those who need intensive care. The effects of competition on quality are less clear. On the one hand, some states use CON review to prohibit unsatisfactory operators from expanding. Although we have described the problems with this approach, it may give the operators a greater incentive to provide high-quality care. On the other hand, we know that when they cannot find empty beds, the states have difficulty enforcing licensure standards for existing operators. In this respect, CON restrictions clearly detract from the quality of care.

It is difficult not only to determine the combined effect of these factors, but also to compare this effect with the quality of care in an open market. As noted earlier, some officials fear that the "transition costs" of a competitive market—with nursing homes going in and out of business—will cause patients considerable harm. Others believe that the market is not so volatile as to cause serious disruption. Rather, they argue, the threat of competition and some excess of beds over patients will force the operators to maintain good quality in order to stay in business. Implicit in this view is the belief that patients or their agents (families or social workers) can and will evaluate quality in choosing among nursing homes.

Without more evidence, the effects of CON restrictions on quality remain an open question. But the outcome in other areas seems fairly straightforward. Patients lose; nursing home operators win; the state loses in efficiency and gains in budgetary control. It is tempting to conclude, on these grounds, that CON regulation of nursing homes is undesirable. To a state under fiscal and political pressure, however, this conclusion hardly seems helpful. When the political and fiscal environment of a state is taken into account, some broader conclusions are possible.

If fiscal pressure is indeed producing inefficient choices in a state's nursing home policy, it may be appropriate to reconsider the structure of financing for nursing home care. It is questionable whether the availability of nursing home care should depend on economic conditions that vary from state to state and are largely outside the control of any individual state. Shifts in national economic activity mean that some states lose a sizable share of their labor force, so that the elderly constitute a larger share of the state population. The result is a decrease in the state's revenue sources, accompanied by an increase in the number of persons likely to seek publicly financed nursing home care. CON restrictions are one way such states try to cope with inadequate revenues, obviously to the detriment of the needy population. To reduce the pressure for restricting expenditures, the federal government should play a greater role in financing nursing home care.

With or without this change, it is necessary to consider policy measures that can reduce the negative consequences of CON restrictions. If the states cannot satisfy the demand for nursing home beds, they must develop mechanisms for rationing whatever beds they have. There are two strategies for achieving an appropriate bed allocation. The first is a regulatory strategy that relies heavily on utilization review. If the Medicaid provisions allowing recipients free choice of providers were dropped, the state could assert its authority to tell patients where they could go, and to tell nursing homes which patients they could accept. A home could not choose a patient who needed little care over a patient needing considerable care if the Medicaid program would authorize benefits only for the sicker patient. This regulatory approach to rationing assumes far more rigorous restrictions on coverage than have apparently been applied to date. Furthermore, these restrictions would encounter opposition from operators, who would continue to avoid patients whose care required greater expenditures. The regulatory approach to rationing, complicated by the probable opposition of Medicaid recipients and by the difficulties of coordinating and controlling a complex bureaucratic system, hardly seems destined for success.

Altering financial incentives, with reinforcement from utilization review, appears to be a far more promising strategy for allocating beds. To encourage the allocation of beds according to the need for care, a reimbursement system must have several elements. First, rates must vary with the patients' need for care, in order to discourage discrimination against those who need extra care. Second, rates must reward the delivery of appropriate care to all patients. Payments should increase with improvements in patients' health status, and should reward the operators for discharging patients who no longer need nursing home care. Rewards of this sort require utilization review or the planning of patient care in order to work. Using incentives to support a review system should increase its probability of success. But even incentives are unlikely to force discharges unless patients have some other place to go. If the less sick patients are to make room for the very sick, it may be necessary to finance services in the community.

These recommendations are hardly original and are probably difficult to implement. The experience of the states reported here, however, underlines their importance. If policy makers continue to rely on restricting the bed supply to control costs, without confronting questions of bed allocation, government is accepting the inequities and inefficiencies that result.

References

Chulis, G.S. 1977. Medicare: Use of Skilled Nursing Facility Services, 1969–73. *Health Insurance Statistics* HI-75 (February).

Congressional Budget Office, U.S. Congress. 1977. *Long-Term Care for the Elderly and Disabled* (February). Washington, D.C.

Hadley, J., Holahan, J., and Scanlon, W. 1979. Can Fee-For-Service Reimbursement Co-Exist with Demand Creation? *Inquiry* (Fall):247–258.

Hood, C.C. 1976. *The Limits of Administration.* New York: Wiley.

Lennox, K. 1979. Certificate-of-Need and Nursing Homes. Working

Papers 1218–5 to 1218–8. Washington, D.C.: The Urban Institute.

Lewin and Associates, Inc. 1975. *Evaluation of the Efficiency and Effectiveness of the Section 1122 Review Process.* Washington, D.C.

Scanlon, W. 1980. A Theory of the Nursing Home Market. *Inquiry* (in press).

Spitz, B., and Weeks, J. 1978–1979. Medicaid Nursing Home Reimbursement in California, Colorado, Connecticut, Illinois, Louisiana, Minnesota, and New York. Working Papers 1216–0 through 1216–6. Washington, D.C.: The Urban Institute.

The research for this paper was supported by Grant No. 1-RO1-HS 02620–01 from the National Center for Health Services Research. The authors would like to thank Karen Lennox for able research support; and John Holahan, Bruce Spitz, and Pat Butler for valuable comments.

Address correspondence to: Judith Feder, The Urban Institute, 2100 M Street, N.W., Washington, D.C., 20037.

IV The Future

The American

Hospital Association Perspective

JOHN ALEXANDER McMAHON
AND DAVID F. DRAKE

Introduction

Some months ago we were completing a paper for inclusion in the
Milbank Memorial Fund's publication, *Health: A Victim or Cause of
Inflation?* We must respectfully contend that this title provided a
more fruitful point of departure for speculation about the direction
of future public policy than does the title of this volume, *Hospital
Cost Containment: Selected Notes for Future Policy.* One of our
objectives is to demonstrate that hospitals themselves are very much
the victims, rather than the cause, of the current round of inflation in
health care costs.

Regardless of their causal relationship to inflation, hospitals have
participated in a broad variety of voluntary programs designed to
contain costs by emphasizing management solutions. Management
programs to contain costs are partially a response to the deleterious
effects of inflation on access to health care services and, in addition,
contribute to the increased efficiency of an institution's operations.
The American Hospital Association (AHA) has sponsored a variety
of programs intended to improve the management of hospitals. The
AHA has urged the creation of hospital committees on cost containment, cost effectiveness, and productivity. The staff has prepared
materials to aid these efforts, and regional discussions have been

In *Hospital Cost Containment: Selected Notes for Future Policy*, edited by Michael Zubkoff, Ira E. Raskin, and Ruth S. Hanft. New York: PRODIST, 1978.

held on the subject of cost containment. Various publications and packaged programs have been developed to assist hospitals in both cost containment and operations effectiveness. These programs emphasize methodologies that can be tailored to fit the particular needs of individual institutions. Educational institutes have emphasized departmental contributions to cost control, and management data programs have been designed and implemented to aid the evaluation of departmental and institutional performance. Budget and cost allocation programs and management systems have also been established. Research studies not only provide descriptive data, but also lay a foundation for explanation of cost variables.

Devices such as these intended to sharpen management's ability to contain costs can bring about marginal reductions in prices, depending on the situation of the individual institution. Such management-oriented programs will continue, but are likely to have only a limited impact on the rate of cost increases, because the causes of inflation are beyond the control of individual hospital managers. At most, management decisions can take into account the effects of inflation and respond to changes in price levels. The harmful *effects* of inflation can, to some extent, be minimized by good management, but it is not possible that inflation itself can be alleviated because inflation is not generated solely within hospitals. Any program intended to control the rate of inflation will be inadequate if it addresses only the hospital, and ignores the factors which stimulate and sustain the public's demands for and expectations of medical care.

Our second objective is to demonstrate, through an analysis of the nature of long-run hospital inflation, that the problems of inflation can be successfully approached only if the entire health care system or delivery network is examined for its contributions to and encouragement of inflationary tendencies. Cost-containment strategies directed exclusively at hospitals, therefore, not only are likely to fail permanently to reduce the rate of inflation in health care, but will further discredit mechanisms to control costs.

A third objective is to propose national health insurance (NHI) as a method of addressing the problems of systemic or structurally induced inflation. National health insurance represents a means of reorganizing the health care system through the introduction of a mixture of cost-related incentives and disincentives to consumers and providers alike. This paper thus represents a demurrer to the currently popular position that the enactment of NHI must await the discovery and attainment of effective controls on health care and hospital costs. We believe that the nation has postponed for too long the removal of financial barriers to health care for many of its citizens, and that a carefully constructed NHI plan may represent the only real opportunity for finding the elusive handle on health care costs.

Hospitals and Inflation—The Current Problem

In our earlier contribution to a Milbank publication, we discussed the historical development of inflationary tendencies in the hospital industry.[1] We concluded that the prices of hospital services have traditionally been susceptible to "demand-pull inflation," that is, the demand for health care services grows more quickly than the industry's ability to accumulate, without bidding up prices, the resources necessary to produce the quantity and types of services demanded. The most recent inflationary surge in these prices, however, has been of the "cost-push" variety, that is, the inflationary pressure stems from increases in the prices hospitals must pay for the resources needed to produce hospital services, not from an increase in the quantity demanded.

The situation of the hospital industry in regard to inflation can best be depicted by comparing changes in the prices hospitals must pay for nonlabor inputs with changes in the prices paid by consumers and by other industries for articles they regularly purchase. The AHA constructs annually a Nonlabor Input Price Index (NLIP), consisting of changes in the prices of products purchased by hospitals. The Consumer Price Index (CPI) is regularly issued by the Bureau of Labor Statistics and is the most frequently cited measurement of the impact of inflation on consumer purchases. The Whole-

[1] McMahon and Drake (1976); see also Drake and Raske (1974) and Feldstein (1971)

375

TABLE 1   A Comparison of Indices
NLIP, CPI, and WPI
1967-1975

	Index Values			Percent Change		
Year	NLIP	CPI	WPI	NLIP	CPI	WPI
1967	100.0	100.0	100.0	—	—	—
1968	103.6	104.2	102.5	3.6	4.2	2.5
1969	108.1	109.8	106.5	4.3	5.4	3.9
1970	114.0	116.3	110.4	5.5	5.9	3.7
1971	118.8	121.3	113.9	4.2	4.3	3.2
1972	123.5	125.3	119.1	4.0	3.3	4.6
1973	133.8	133.1	134.7	8.3	6.2	12.9
1974	157.1	147.7	160.1	17.4	11.0	18.9
1975	189.7	161.2	174.9	20.8	9.1	9.2

Sources: Bureau of Labor Statistics, Department of Labor; American Hospital Association (1976).

sale Price Index (WPI) is also compiled by the Bureau of Labor Statistics and measures changes in the prices of industrial commodities. Table 1 shows not only that the prices of hospital nonlabor inputs have increased more than consumer and wholesale prices, but also that most of the discrepancy in these rates of growth is of recent origin, specifically arising from the continuing economy-wide inflation. Much of the recent increases in hospital prices can be attributed to increases in the costs incurred by hospitals for nonlabor inputs.

Hospitals have been especially affected recently by increases in the costs of malpractice insurance, fuel, and household and maintenance costs. Almost one-sixth of the 20.8 percent increase in the NLIP in 1975 was due to rising malpractice insurance rates. In 1972, the average premium for basic hospital professional liability insurance was $20,466. By 1974, such a premium had almost doubled in price to $38,583, and during 1975, the cost mushroomed to $118,357.[2] These costs cannot be directly controlled by hospital management, yet they represent inescapable costs of maintaining hospital services.

The experience of hospitals with prices for labor inputs (wages) has been similar, with two-thirds of the inflation of the previous four

[2] Data for 1972 from Survey of Hospital Professional Liability (Malpractice) Insurance; data for 1974 and 1975 from Survey of Selected Hospital Topics. Both surveys were conducted by the Division of Information Services, American Hospital Association.

Table 2   Change in Wage Levels for Hospital and
Total Nonagricultural Workers,
by Dollars and Percent, and Change in CPI, by Percent
1971-1975

| Year | Average Hospital[a] Wage | | Total Private[b] Wage | | CPI |
	$ Amount	% Change	$ Amount	% Change	% Change
1971	2.96	—	3.44	—	4.3
1972	3.08	4.1	3.67	6.7	3.3
1973	3.22	4.5	3.92	6.8	6.2
1974	3.45	7.1	4.22	7.7	11.0
1975	3.83	11.0	4.54	7.6	9.1
Overall increase		29.4		32.0	32.9

[a]Hourly earnings—nonsupervisory workers.
[b]Nonagricultural workers.
Source: Bureau of Labor Statistics, Employment and Earnings.

years occurring in 1974 and 1975. The wage levels for hospital workers traditionally have been somewhat lower than those for workers in other nonagricultural sectors of the economy. Despite recent increases in the rate of growth in hospital workers' wages, this differential has been maintained. Moreover, as Table 2 indicates, from 1971 to 1975, average wages for all nonagricultural workers increased more rapidly than did those for hospital workers. The rates of increase in the wages of hospital workers, in fact, failed to keep pace with the rate of inflation as measured by the CPI. In 1972 and 1973, for example, workers in most other industries had a greater chance of minimizing the effects of inflation on their standards of living because of the wage increases they received. In 1975, this situation changed as the average hourly earnings for nonsupervisory workers in hospitals increased 11 percent. The average hourly earnings of workers in all nonagricultural industries rose 7.6 percent. Over the entire period 1971-1975, the percentage increase in wages received by hospital workers was slightly lower than the overall percentage increase for all nonagricultural workers. Wages for hospital workers increased 29.4 percent during this five-year period, but increased 32.0 percent for all industrial workers. Neither group of workers was able to obtain wage increases commensurate with the 32.9 percent increase in the CPI, however.

The year 1975 was the first full year in which wage and price controls were no longer applied to the hospital industry. It is likely that the wage increases achieved then were at least in part a reaction to the prolonged period of economic controls on hospitals, and in part were a response to the historically lower wages paid to hospital workers. The present continuing round of severe inflation, during which hospital workers made considerable gains in wage levels, began after controls on the hospital industry were lifted in April 1974. Unlike prices in earlier periods of inflation in hospital services, this new set of price increases was fueled by rising prices in the rest of the economy, such as those described earlier. This is cost-push inflation, in contrast to the demand-pull inflation that has prevailed historically.

Figure 1 illustrates the relative impact of these types of inflation in 1969—a period of demand-pull inflation—and in 1975, when inflation in hospital prices was cost-push. In 1969, 65.6 percent of the increases in hospital expenses per adjusted patient day[3] was attributable to increased quantity of goods, services, and labor inputs. In 1975, inflation, or increased prices, was responsible for 73.3 percent of the increase in expenses per adjusted patient day.

Although inflation is a persistent phenomenon affecting all sectors of the economy, over the past few years hospitals have been especially severely affected by inflation because hospital purchases are concentrated in many of the commodity areas where inflation has exceeded the average rate of increase. The prices of hospital services have been increased correspondingly to cover the increased costs of providing services. In 1969, for example, expenses per adjusted patient day were $64.26, and by 1974 they were $113.21 (American Hospital Association, 1975: 4). Hospitals have been victims of inflation, but the damage sustained by them is not irreparable. Of greater concern should be the impact of inflation on access to health care.

Inflation counteracts many developments that have rendered health care more accessible to more people. As the prices of health care services rise, those members of society who are least able to afford health care are the ultimate victims. It is true that access to health care services by the aged and the poor has been improved by

[3]Adjusted patient days are an aggregate figure reflecting the number of days of inpatient care plus an estimate of the volume of outpatient services, expressed in units equivalent to an inpatient day in level of effort.

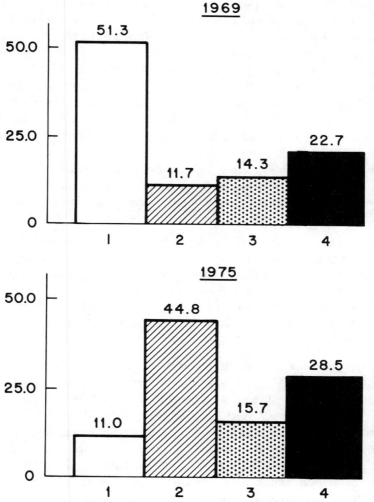

Fig. 1   *Components of Total Hospital Inflation, 1969 and 1975,*
by Percent

Key:

1—Increases in the *quantity* of goods and services purchased
2—Increases in the *cost* of goods and services purchased
3—Increases in the *quantity* of personnel employed
4—Increases in average *wages*

Source: American Hospital Association (1976).

government programs such as Medicare and Medicaid. Inflation has an indirect impact on government funding of these programs, however, because a constant level of expenditures for health care services provides a steadily diminishing amount of care. If public expenditures are increased to maintain a certain level of service, conflicts soon arise with other social programs. One result of such conflicts is that many state Medicaid programs have already been cut back (Taft, 1976). The Ford Administration sought to alter the Medicare program in its budget proposals for FY 1977 by putting a greater share of the cost of illness back onto the very groups the Medicare program was designed to relieve (see Schmeck, 1976, and Taft, 1976). Moreover, even the availability of benefits from such programs has never succeeded in completely eradicating barriers to access. As Karen Davis has written (1975: 480):

> . . . a uniform medical care financing plan has not been sufficient to guarantee equal access to medical care for all elderly persons. Those elderly population groups with the poorest health care are the lowest utilizers of medical care services under the program— the poor, blacks, and residents of the South. Furthermore, differences on the basis of income, race, and location are of sizable magnitude.

Unfortunately, intervention directed at curbing the effects of cost-push inflation cannot be limited to the health care sector alone, because this type of inflation is generated and sustained throughout the entire economy. A decision to combat cost-push inflation necessarily entails government fiscal and monetary intervention. Controls limited to the hospital industry are an inadequate response to inflation of the cost-push variety, as the experience of hospitals with the Economic Stabilization Program illustrates (Ginsburg, 1976). Controls may have postponed price increases, but the retention of controls on hospitals produced the distortions in the marketplace that we experienced in 1974 and 1975. The result was double-digit inflation in the price of hospital services, as the increased costs incurred by hospitals for the purchase of inputs were passed on to consumers and payers. Extensive economy-wide controls, like those of the ESP, distort incentives and lead managers to take a cautious stance because of the uncertainty in the administration of the controls. The development of better fiscal and monetary policies could well have a more important and wider-ranging influence on cost-push inflation than could further experimentation with wage-price controls, either at the health care sector level or at the level of the entire economy. Similarly, political settlement of some of the complex questions about social values involved in the malpractice issue could do a great deal toward reducing the inflationary effects of increasing malpractice insurance premiums.

Hospitals and Inflation—The Long-Run Problem

Even after the momentum of the current cost-push bulge has subsided, most experts agree that the basic inflationary pressures on the hospital will continue to build. Inflation in the prices of hospital and other health care services began in the post-World War II period. Rising incomes, a higher standard of living, and more comprehensive health insurance coverage for a growing proportion of the population all contributed to the growing demand for health care services. Hospitals responded to this increased demand by increasing capacity. Expenditures for hospital care and employment in hospitals became larger. The relatively steady rate of increase in hospital prices was interrupted in the late 1960s after the passage of Medicare and Medicaid (Davis, 1973). The availability of better, more comprehensive, insurance coverage for medical care stimulated demand on the part of two hitherto deprived groups, the poor and the aged. Consequently hospital prices rose sharply in the late 1960s, although the rate of increase abated by the end of the decade (Drake and Raske, 1974).

The unique system of financing health care services through various types of third-party coverage has enabled the industry to provide the sophisticated and expensive types of medical care demanded by the public and their physicians (Feldstein, 1973). Because the *net* costs of hospital care—the single most expensive component of health care costs—have been reduced for consumers through this broad third-party insurance coverage, hospitals have been able to expand their armamentarium of medical technologies.

Without such extensive coverage of otherwise prohibitively expensive care, the demand pressures for increasing health care services would not have distorted supply responses, and rising prices would have served as a rationing device as in other industries. In relation to hospital services, however, rising prices have permitted substantial increases in the intensity, sophistication, and complexity of care.

Demand-pull inflation is partially sustained by this extensive health insurance coverage. In 1950, for example, direct payments were the source of over 68 percent of personal health expenditures. Private insurance benefits covered only 8.5 percent and all forms of public payment about 20 percent of personal health expenditures (Mueller and Gibson, 1976: 17). In 1975, direct payments accounted for only 32.6 percent of personal health care expenditures, while private insurance benefits covered 26.5 percent, and all public sources covered 39.7 percent of such expenditures. Thus, by 1975, private insurers and public sources of payment purchased almost as great a share of personal health care as did direct payments twenty-five years earlier.

Not all health care services are equally covered by third-party payers, however. Hospital care is most heavily covered, with 92 percent of expenditures coming from third-party payments. Physicians' services are also fairly well covered, with 65.5 percent of total expenditures derived from third parties. Only about 15 percent of expenditures for both dentists' services and drugs and drug sundries, however, are derived from third-party payments. About 58 percent of expenditures for other health care services are also covered by third-party payments (Mueller and Gibson, 1976: 15).

Third-party payments directly affect demand because they alter the distribution of resources available for the purchase of health care services. Those types of care that are most extensively covered by insurance or are underwritten by a government program become relatively less expensive to potential consumers as financial obstacles to the receipt of care are lowered. Hospital care is the most expensive single component of health care, and now receives almost 40 percent of all health expenditures. Yet it is also the service most heavily covered by third-party payment, and thus is the service most attractive and financially accessible to consumers. Given a choice between an alternative but less expensive means of receiving care requiring direct payment, and more expensive hospital care covered by some form of third-party payment, the thrifty consumer (and his physician) will choose the latter alternative. At the same time, the availability of funds from these sources of payment and the incentives encouraging greater hospital utilization than might otherwise be required have enabled hospitals to expand the range of facilities and services they offer, including the most up-to-date and advanced technologies.

A second major contributing factor to demand-pull inflation is the unique role of the physician as a primary determiner of demand for health care services (Evans, 1974; Fuchs, 1974). Patients lack information about their illnesses and about alternative modalities of care, and physicians act as their agents in determining the need for and course of care. Physicians are trained to prescribe on the basis of the needs of each individual patient, but they also are trained in the practice of highly technological medicine (Hiatt, 1975). Because of this professional orientation toward the individual case and what Fuchs has called "the technological imperative," physicians have tended to emphasize the results of care without commensurate attention to its cost. This orientation can be seen in the way physicians care for themselves and their families. It has been found that physicians' families have substantially higher rates of surgery than comparable professional groups (Bunker and Brown, 1974).

Medicine is an applied, rather than a pure, science, because of the complexities of diagnosis and the difficulty in controlling all possible factors contributing to an illness. Hiatt (1975: 236) provides a list of once-common procedures which have now been almost abandoned because they were found to be ineffective, not because they were replaced by more adequate therapies. His list includes gastric freezing for peptic ulcer, colectomy for epilepsy, renal-capsule stripping for acute renal failure, lobotomy for mental disorders, and sympathectomy for asthma. Many accepted methods of treatment have never been tested for effectiveness, or compared with alternative forms of treatment (Cochrane, 1972). New technologies and treatments, aisde from drugs, are frequently introduced without testing or evaluation. Not only is effectiveness seldom measured, but the relative cost impact of alternative therapies is similarly ignored. If two procedures were tested and found to produce approximately the same results, that which resulted in lower costs could be encouraged. Few such studies have been undertaken, however. One result is that vast amounts of money can be and have been spent on therapies of questionable value to attain results that, if not dubious, might have been attained at less cost.

A related problem of physician practice is that of variability in the rates at which various procedures are performed. Bunker found that there were twice as many surgeons in relation to population in the United States as compared to England and Wales and that there were twice as many operations (Bunker, 1970; see also Lewis, 1969). A more recent study found that 24 percent of all recommendations for elective surgical procedures were not confirmed when second opinions were solicited (McCarthy and Widmer, 1974). Studies conducted by Wennberg and his colleagues in Vermont and Maine show that the probability of an individual's tonsils being removed ranged from 8 percent to 62 percent among various hospital service areas. Variability existed as well for other surgical procedures, ranging from 24 percent to 52 percent for removal of the uterus, 7 percent to 17 percent for removal of the appendix, and 11 percent to 31 percent for removal of the gall bladder. Hospitalization for bronchitis and upper respiratory infections varied sevenfold (Wennberg, 1976; Wennberg and Gittelsohn, 1973). Thus, in addition to the questions about the value of some types of treatment, considerable discrepancies exist in the rates at which physicians diagnose need and interpret the values of specific modes of treatment. This wide variation indicates considerable professional disagreement about the scope of need for medical and/or surgical intervention. The tendency to recommend elective surgery has implications for health care costs and for patients' health status.

Greater emphasis on peer review, second opinions, and organized group practices may provide one means for creating a professional consensus on appropriate remedies and interventions, with consequences for health care costs and quality of care. To a large extent, such variation in medical practices has been properly viewed as a professional problem. Yet the cost impact of these decisions is on the patient's hospital bill where the facilities for such intervention are housed.

Medical facilities and services reliant upon technology are usually based in hospitals because the general function of hospitals in the health care system is to organize specialized, sophisticated, and complex health care resources for patient care. Modern health care capabilities are best represented by the proliferation of specialists, and as this tendency continues, the integrating function also increases in importance. Services that might otherwise be underutilized or too expensive are affordable in hospitals because of their financial support, because of some of the coverage characteristics outlined earlier, and because of high patient volume.

As new medical technologies increase, the effect is not the more efficient performance of old tasks, but the ability to perform new ones. Innovation is almost always cost-inducing rather than cost-saving in health care because new capabilities are constantly acquired. Some self-proclaimed radical critics of highly technological medicine doubt much of its effectiveness (see Illich, 1976, and Carlson, 1975), but it seems incontestable to us that if technological medical services are to be provided at all, the most appropriate sites for them are hospitals. Not all hospitals should maintain all devices or the ability to perform any type of service, but attempts to apply technologies piecemeal in other locations will only increase inefficiency. Cost increases due to the acquisition of new technologies are likely to be contained only if new technologies are stringently tested and evaluated for their effectiveness before heavy investment is made in them and the technology has proliferated.

With health care expenditures standing at $118.5 billion in 1975 (8.3 percent of GNP), serious questions for public policy have been raised, regarding the need to make social choices among alternative resource deployments. Some have argued that health care expenditures cannot be allowed to continue to increase at their recent rates, or that expensive technologies can be extended to their capacities. Hiatt (1975: 237) cites estimates that the total cost for coronary bypass operations and diagnostic arteriograms could exceed $100 billion per year, an amount almost equivalent to total health expenditures in 1975, if some medical estimates of need were met. Another current example is that of Computerized Axial Tomography (CAT), used to produce head and body scans, a sort of three-dimensional x-ray. At least eleven firms are manufacturing these devices, and over 200 hospitals have already purchased a unit. Body scanners cost between $400,000 and $600,000, plus the costs of maintenance and personnel for staffing the machines (Downey, 1976a; Downey, 1976b; Phillips and Lille, 1976). No consensus has yet been reached on the clinical effectiveness of the body scanner, nor have comparisons been made with other techniques already available to determine the relative diagnostic improvements provided by the more expensive scanners. In short, there has been no determination of the actual benefits to be gained from these sizable investments by hospitals. Physicians collectively must begin to share with hospitals an interest in identifying costly medical procedures which can be reduced without sacrificing the quality of patient care.

As attention shifts from the need to obtain additional resources to the need to make the best use of available resources, not only must new technologies and innovations be carefully evaluated for their cost/benefit effectiveness, but existing technologies and courses of treatments should be similarly evaluated whenever possible. Increasing financial constraints require closer examination of the effectiveness of methods of treatment, but it is not certain that this will actually take place on a systematic basis unless coordinated efforts are made by all segments of the health care system. Greater overall effectiveness of the health care system may then result from efforts to contain health care costs, but a prerequisite for the success of such efforts should be determination of the specific objectives of cost containment.

Demand-pull inflation in the price of hospital services is sustained, then, by the types of choices physicians are trained to make in favoring technological applications of medicine. These decisions are supported by the public despite their cost, because of extensive third-party coverage. Technological medicine is expensive by itself, but costs are increased also by inappropriate or excessive utilization. We feel that many proposals to curb inflation in the price of hospital care are doomed to failure because they fail to address this network of factors that work to maintain a high level of demand for this type of medical care.

Objectives of Hospital Cost Containment

Given the long-run nature of demand-pull inflation in hospital costs, how can a specific policy or policies for containing hospital costs be developed? Frequently, the policy goal is stated in terms of reducing the percentage rate of increases in hospital costs. Should the goal be containment of total hospital costs or expenditures, the costs of units of hospital service, such as per diem or per case costs, or some other measure of relative hospital costs, such as hospitals' share of the Gross National Product or even of total health expenditures? Each of these variables has, at least implicitly, been suggested as the one to minimize in various cost control proposals and there are problems with each as a reasonable goal for public policy.

For example, the goal of minimizing the rate of increase in total hospital costs or expenditures because these are the single costliest component of health care fails to recognize that hospitals provide forms of care other than high-cost, high-technology inpatient acute care. Indeed, the fastest growing hospital service is ambulatory (and presumably, primary) care provided in hospital outpatient clinics and emergency rooms. Between 1965 and 1975, for example, outpatient visits in the nation's community hospitals increased five times more than did inpatient days.[4] Any cost control program directed at total hospital expenditures must recognize that, because ambulatory care is inadequately covered under the current health insurance arrangements, ambulatory care is the first activity that hospitals must curtail when faced with severe financial constraints. The recent New York City financing crisis has vividly illustrated this dilemma.

In addition to the outpatient problem that is ignored in a total expenditure limitation approach, the financial arrangements be-

[4]Calculated from National Hospital Panel Survey Data.

tween the hospital and its medical staff can cause distortions in this overall control approach. Those hospitals that have, or more importantly add, salaried physicians to their medical staffs will report a substantial increase in the level of total hospital expenditures. Cross-national comparisons indicate that there is considerable variation in the share of health expenditures allocated to hospitals in Western industrial nations. Much of this variation stems from the inclusion or exclusion of hospital-based physician services as a component of hospital expenditures. In West Germany, hospital expenditures constituted only 29 percent of total health spending in 1970, as opposed to the nearly 40 percent share in the United States. At the opposite extreme were England and Wales, where the National Health Service allocated 60 percent of its health expenditures for hospitals. France and the Netherlands, on the other hand, each spent about half of their health dollar on hospital services.[5] Until there is greater consensus on the optimum resource allocation and organization of care that defines the appropriate portion and role for the hospital, it would be extremely unwise to set as a goal for hospital cost containment the minimization of the rate of increase in total hospital expenditures or, for that matter, of the relative share of total hospital expenditures in the GNP or in the health care dollar.

In a similar way, the minimization of hospital unit costs as a possible policy goal can be distortive. If we are successful in reducing the use of inpatient hospitalization for dealing with less acute kinds of illness, then we would expect that the remaining patients in hospitals would be acutely ill. Care for these patients would obviously, on a unit basis, be more expensive.

Attempts merely to restrict the amount of money spent on hospital care represent a desire to treat the symptoms of inflation rather than the underlying causes. Limits or caps on the amounts of resources allocated to hospitals simply do not address the problem of providing alternative sources of care to inpatient hospitalization. The appropriate public policy concern is not just to minimize costs or the rate of inflation but to do so without significantly impairing the quality of care available to consumers.

[5] Data from a telephone conversation with Joseph G. Simanis, Office of Research and Statistics, Social Security Administration, July 7, 1976. See also Simanis (1973).

A more appropriate public policy goal than simply limiting the rate of increase in hospital costs is to provide incentives for less costly alternatives to inpatient hospitalization without sacrificing the integrating and coordinating function of the hospital. Such a sacrifice might have to be made if flat and arbitrary limits were imposed on hospital expenditures or unit costs. Recent studies have directed attention to the importance of the organization of medical practice in increasing efficiency and lowering rates of hospitalization (Gaus, et al., 1976; Ellwood, 1976). Physician participation in a group practice, regardless of the type of payment mechanism in effect, and membership on a hospital medical staff are conducive to the development of peer review, coordinated care, better use of resources, and easier access to a broad range of physician services.

If greater organization and rationalization increase the efficiency of physicians' performance, it is quite likely that the efficiency of a health care system in which choices are predominantly made by physicians could also be improved by greater organization. Improved organization should not only include physicians, but also other providers of health care services. The institution best suited by its present role to perform these organizational functions is the hospital. It already deals with similar problems, although on a restricted scale. In order to deal adequately with the inseparable problems of rising costs, especially for inpatient care, and of quality of care, hospitals would have to expand the range of services they provide beyond care for acute illnesses requiring inpatient care. We endorse Freymann's concept (1974) of the "mission-oriented hospital," which not only consists of the traditional facilities and staff, but integrates them with a complex network of interrelated, organized capabilities for providing the whole range of health care services. These include care of the chronically ill, long-term care, home care, nursing home care, outpatient treatment centers, maternity units, and facilities for the terminally ill. Frequently, care of comparable quality can be rendered more efficiently outside the hospital as it is presently constituted. When this is the case, the alternative methods of care should be encouraged. An example is home-based renal dialysis, which can be provided at about one-third the cost of dialysis provided in hospitals (Iglehart, 1976). Alternative means of delivering such services should be welcomed by hospitals because they free resources for other uses. Hospitals themselves should explore the alternatives with regard to both their cost efficiency and their effectiveness and quality.

Experiments and extra-hospital programs will probably operate best when provided in a concentrated and coordinated manner in each community, because each represents a fairly specialized use of resources and manpower that are not readily interchangeable. Isolated or individual units or organizations attempting to provide a similar range and variety of services would be likely to be costly and duplicative. Also, as specialization increases, the need for coordination among specialized units increases. Without it, patients would be unable to receive the appropriate types of care required as their conditions change.

Within a revamped system emphasizing the "mission-oriented hospital," concern would be directed not at hospitals' share of total expenditures or of GNP, but at the ratio of benefits from increased expenditures to their costs. Reorganization of the health care system emphasizing the hospital as an instrument of coordination and integration for a wide variety of services rather than as a site for inpatient care would do away with the issue of the appropriate level of hospital expenditures, because the inflationary inpatient care sector could be reduced in a system making use of complementary methods of care. The problem then becomes one of designing sufficiently attractive incentives to bring about (1) the coordination of services presently provided independently of hospitals; (2) the expansion of hospital responsibilities to encompass a wide range of provider roles beyond inpatient care; (3) the alteration of third-party payment mechanisms to cover sources of care other than inpatient hospital care; and (4) the encouragement of physicians to make use of a variety of coordinated treatment methods rather than to rely so heavily on highly technological diagnostic and therapy regimens.

NHI and Cost Containment

Our analysis of the long-run problem of inflation in the prices of hospital services has emphasized the interrelationship between the preference of physicians for medical treatment dependent on technology and the system of third-party payment which has skewed insurance benefits heavily in the direction of inpatient hospital services. Thus, the most expensive types of health care have been made most accessible to the consumer fortunate enough to be covered by health insurance, while physicians have not been encouraged to explore alternatives to expensive forms of hospital-based care.

We feel that the urgently required changes in the scope of medical insurance benefits and in the delivery system cannot be dealt with in isolation from the issue of equity of access. Policies designed primarily to contain costs are likely to have an unfavorable impact on access, while policies intended to facilitate access alone are likely to be simply more inflationary.

Despite anticipated short-run increases in demand, such as those which followed the inauguration of the Medicare program, we contend that universal, governmentally mandated health insurance provides the only public policy framework sufficiently comprehensive to restructure those components of the health care delivery system that especially support demand-pull inflation. The AHA has long maintained that national health insurance should not simply channel additional funds into a delivery system that remains essentially unchanged. The infusion of these funds should be made conditional on the adoption of structural reforms by providers of health care services. The intentions of these reforms should be specifically mentioned in the NHI statute, although compliance should be initially encouraged through the offering of incentives rather than by the imposition of penalties and sanctions. Providers of health care services should be offered a variety of means to comply with the statutory intent as well, in order to preserve managerial discretion in dealing with particular institutional circumstances.

The salient part of any NHI program will be its schedule of benefits, and the most significant aspect of the benefits will be their contribution to improving access to health care for those currently unable to afford such care. If an NHI plan were to fail to improve access while it successfully contained the rate of inflation, it would ultimately be evaluated as failing to secure its major objectives. Because increased insurance coverage expands utilization and the amounts of resources required to meet greater demand, there is a strong temptation to build into NHI programs devices intended to curb or restrict increased utilization, such as limited benefits or required copayments (McClure, 1975). This curtailment, however, reduces the protection the plan can give, especially to the poor, who are unlikely to be able to afford sufficient care otherwise, and who also may have greater health care needs. Therefore, benefits under NHI must be carefully designed because the potential for conflict between the desire to restrain prices and the desire to improve access is greatest here. It has been proposed that benefits be partially geared to income, to maximize protection for those least able to afford medical care and to minimize the inflationary impact of this protection. Deductibles, copayments, and limits on total out-of-pocket expenditures during a year could all be related to the income of a consumer. Those better able to afford care would be liable for a greater share of their costs, while those with smaller incomes would have a greater proportion of their expenses covered (Donabedian, 1976). A health card mechanism could be established for the collection of these variable copayments.

The determination of the extent of NHI benefits cannot be divorced from consideration of the effect on the system of providers delivering the covered services. Experience with private health insurance plans has driven home this lesson. The present system of benefits provides extensive coverage (and thus incentives) for inpatient hospital care but little coverage for outpatient, long-term, or nursing home care. If NHI benefits are fairly comprehensive and cover a full range of alternate methods of care, one of the artificially imposed causes of inflation in the present health insurance system would be removed, along with the stimulus for overutilization of inpatient hospital care.

Such NHI-mandated financial support for and encouragement of specialized services to supplement traditional inpatient care would be likely to stimulate growth and investment in these services. The primary purpose of such innovations is not simply to shift patients from expensive to less expensive facilities. This would be only one desirable consequence of improved organization within the health care system, intended to maximize the overall amount of care provided in *organized* settings.

We have contended that hospitals, because of their central role in providing health care services to their communities and their historical development, are especially suited to provide this organization. NHI, however, must not go so far as to attempt to mandate centralization of all health care services. Other organizations, such as medical care foundations, health maintenance organizations, and multispecialty group practices, should also be encouraged to participate in integrating and coordinating the health care delivery system. What an NHI plan might encourage through its benefit structure would be growth in the number of group practices of physicians and dentists. This could be done by designing special insurance benefits to cover services provided in these settings, or by covering them more fully than services received from unorganized providers. The provider organization, rather than the delivery site, would then be the requirement for services to be covered by insurance. Hospitals would be only one of several locations at which care covered by insurance would be provided.

Any NHI program should integrate existing regulatory devices intended to contain costs and reduce reliance on uneconomic technology, while monitoring quality. Providing incentives for group practices alone will be insufficient to bring about a reduction in overutilization of expensive sources of care and the full consideration of less expensive alternatives. Health Systems Agencies (HSAs) and Professional Standards Review Organizations (PSROs) have been created across the country for purposes of planning and quality review. These methods of regulation and planning are mandated by federal law, but represent an important departure from previous regulatory policy in the health care sector because they are intended to operate on the local level with guidance from the state and national levels. Dispersal of regulatory authority among a fairly large number of such agencies may be especially important under an NHI plan, but a federal-state regulatory framework should be established to coordinate these decentralized activities. As the federal government becomes increasingly important in creating health insurance benefits, even if it acts through private health insurance carriers, conflicts may develop between government's roles as regulator and as guarantor of benefits for lower income groups, the aged, the disabled, and the unemployed. The separation of government's roles as purchaser and as regulator should be built into the design of an NHI program and the regulatory function decentralized as much as possible.

A deliberate research and development program is an essential feature for NHI. Biomedical research and development may remain relatively unaffected by the transition to NHI because the need for it will continue. General health services research and development should increase markedly in importance, both because there will be a greater need to monitor the costs of care, and because the greater need for coordination in a more unified and tightly organized system will generate a need for feedback information (Wennberg, 1976). Adequate funding for research and development is necessary in order that the new technologies be applied appropriately. The intent should not be to freeze medical technology at its current level or to return to a simpler era, but to apply technology only as it provides positive benefits when compared to alternative therapies at equal or reduced costs. The research and development can be conducted at the level of the individual institution and at the system level, but should be financed as an integral part of the NHI program.

Conclusions

We have contended that the issue of hospital cost containment cannot be successfully approached by means of public policy in isolation from the network of factors that have influenced decisions about the provision of health care over the last thirty years. The system for the delivery of health care is composed of a variety of providers and payment mechanisms, but for policy purposes these institutions are not independent, discrete units. Economic and other incentives have skewed the organization of these components so that sophisticated technologies have been emphasized for treatment of acute illness. Other nonacute health problems have been incompletely recognized by the system because they are less susceptible to these sophisticated medical interventions.

For these reasons we have advocated that public policy responses to the issue of hospital cost containment examine the system of incentives that has made the prices of hospital care prone to inflation. A national health insurance program, we feel, is not only a means for expanding access to care while introducing incentives to redeploy resources for the provision of less costly types of care, but is the only alternative which would not actually imperil the provision of health care services by inappropriate types of controls. Other proposed remedies address only isolated components of the system, such as hospitals, without addressing the reasons for the price increases manifested in those components.

Embarkation on a public policy course of cost containment in the health care field should not be carried to the extreme of repudiating the commitments represented by past national policy— governmental *and* private—to better health care and expanded access. Past health programs, it is now generally conceded, were not designed with cost considerations foremost, but with emphasis primarily on expansion of access, of quality, of manpower, and of facilities. These were program-design flaws, in that the anticipated costs and benefits were not gauged, and in that close monitoring of programs was not often mandated. Yet we believe that lessons can be absorbed by policy makers from these experiences and that trade-offs are not demanded between cost consciousness intended to hold down inflation and the desire to provide good quality health care to all citizens. A national health insurance program should include from the outset a range of services broader than those covered by current health insurance plans to ensure the efficient utilization of health care facilities based on medical suitability rather than on financial accessibility. Contributions by individuals toward the cost of care in proportion to their ability to pay will serve as an inducement for proper utilization of health care services and help defray the cost of care to the public.

Public policy attention to inflation should properly be a concern in all social welfare programs and in all phases of governmental operation. It should never be allowed to become the sole or predominant policy goal of any program, nor should concern about the impact of inflation be made the excuse for postponing badly needed reforms of the health care delivery system. A focus on inflation and the distortions it produces in the economy cannot justify the politically popular step of initiating anti-inflation programs that satisfy political demands but do little either to remove the causes of inflation or to improve the delivery of services.

References and Acknowledgment

The authors wish to thank David M. Kozak, Policy Analyst, Office of Program and Policy Development, for his assistance in the preparation of this chapter.

American Hospital Association
  1975   Hospital Statistics. 1975 Edition. Chicago: American Hospital Association.
  1976   The Hospital Economy. Division of Information Services.
Bunker, J.P.
  1970   "Surgical manpower: A comparison of operations and surgeons in the United States and in England and Wales." The New England Journal of Medicine 282 (January): 135–143.
Bunker, J.P., and B.W. Brown, Jr.
  1974   "The physician-patient as an informed consumer of surgical services." The New England Journal of Medicine 290 (May): 1051–1055.
Carlson, R.J.
  1975   The End of Medicine. New York: John Wiley & Sons.
Cochrane, A.L.
  1972   Effectiveness and Efficiency: Random Reflections on Health Services. London: The Nuffield Provincial Hospitals Trust.
Davis, K.
  1973   "Hospital costs and the Medicare program." Social Security Bulletin 36 (August): 18–36.

1975   "Equal treatment and unequal benefits: The Medicare program."
            Milbank Memorial Fund Quarterly/Health and Society (Fall):
            449–488.

Donabedian, A.
1976   "Issues in national health insurance." American Journal of Public
            Health 66 (April): 345–350.

Downey, G.W.
1976a   "A scanner for every hospital?" Modern Healthcare (February):
            16S–16X.
1976b   "Cat fever." The New England Journal of Medicine (April 22):
            954–956.

Drake, D.F., and K.E. Raske
1974   "The changing hospital economy." Hospitals, Journal of the
            American Hospital Association 48 (November 16): 34–40.

Ellwood, P.M., Jr.
1976   "Health delivery in transition: from group practice to HMO to
            multigroups." Statement before Congress of the United States,
            House of Representatives, Subcommittee on Health and Envi-
            ronment (February 10).

Evans, R.G.
1974   "Supplier-induced demand: Some empirical evidence and impli-
            cations." Pp. 162–173 in Mark Perlman, ed., The Economics of
            Health and Medical Care. New York: John Wiley & Sons, Inc.

Feldstein, M.S.
1971   The Rising Cost of Hospital Care. Washington, D.C.: Informa-
            tion Resources Press.
1973   "The medical economy." Scientific American 229 (September):
            151.

Freymann, J.G.
1974   The American Health Care System: Its Genesis and Trajectory.
            New York: Medcom Press.

Fuchs, V.
1974   Who Shall Live? Health, Economics and Social Choice. New
            York: Basic Books, Inc.

Gaus, C.R., B.S. Cooper, and C.G. Hirschman
1976   "Contrasts in HMO and fee-for-service performance." Social
            Security Bulletin 39 (May): 3–14.

Ginsburg, P.B.
1976   "Inflation and the economic stabilization program." Pp. 31–51 in

Michael Zubkoff, ed., Health: A Victim or Cause of Inflation? New York: Prodist for Milbank Memorial Fund.

Hiatt, H.A.
1975   "Protecting the medical commons: Who is responsible?" The New England Journal of Medicine 293 (July 31): 235–241.

Iglehart, J.K.
1976   "Kidney treatment problem readies HEW for national health insurance." National Journal 8 (June 26): 895–900.

Illich, I.
1976   Medical Nemesis: The Expropriation of Health. New York: Random House.

Lewis, C.E.
1969   "Variations in the incidence of surgery." The New England Journal of Medicine 281 (October 16): 880–884.

McCarthy, E.G., and G.W. Widmer
1974   "Effects of screening by consultants on recommended elective surgical procedures." The New England Journal of Medicine 291 (December 19): 1331–1335.

McClure, W.
1975   "The medical care system under national health insurance: Four models that might work and their prospects." Paper presented to the American Political Science Association, Panel on National Health Insurance, September 2. San Francisco, California.

McMahon, J.A., and D.F. Drake
1976   "Inflation and the hospital." Pp. 130–148 in Michael Zubkoff, ed., Health: A Victim or Cause of Inflation? New York: Prodist for Milbank Memorial Fund.

Mueller, M.S., and R.M. Gibson
1976   "National health expenditures, fiscal year 1975." Social Security Bulletin 39 (February): 3–21.

Phillips, D.F., and K. Lille
1976   "Putting the leash on 'CAT'." Hospitals, Journal of the American Hospital Association 50 (July 1): 45–49.

Schmeck, H.M., Jr.
1976   "Limiting the cost of major illness would benefit three million patients." The New York Times (January 22).

Simanis, J.G.
1973   "Medical care expenditures in seven countries." Social Security Bulletin (March): 39–42.

Taft, J.
    1976   "States put scalpel to Medicaid in budget-cutting operation."
            National Journal 8 (May 1): 581–586.
Wennberg, J.E.
    1976   "National health planning goals." Unpublished manuscript
            (March).
Wennberg, J.E., and A. Gittelsohn
    1973   "Small area variations in health care delivery." Science 182
            (December 14): 1102–1108.

Research Needs for Future Policy

RALPH E. BERRY, JR.

Introduction

As has been noted countless times, the cost of hospital care has been rising rapidly over an extended period of time. The average cost per patient day in nonfederal short-term general hospitals, for example, is approximately six times as high as it was twenty years ago. Moreover, the rate of increase of hospital costs has generally been accelerating. In fact, hospital cost inflation is not a problem of recent vintage, but represents a phenomenon with a rather long history that has displayed a marked tendency to intensify in recent years.

As hospital costs have risen, and particularly as these costs have been translated into a public burden through governmental budgets, more and more pressure has been brought to bear to control these costs. A variety of proposals designed to effect a control on hospital costs have appeared or reappeared in recent years. Incentive reimbursement mechanisms, prospective budgeting, rate regulation, areawide planning, certificates of need, and even structural reform of the medical care sector have been suggested as potential solutions to the cost problem—some have even been tried.

There has been some experience with cost containment in recent years as various mechanisms have been tried in several jurisdictions. There was even the brief period from 1971 to 1974 when price and wage controls were in effect nationally under the Economic Stabilization Program. A review of the experience to date, however, as

In *Hospital Cost Containment: Selected Notes for Future Policy,* edited by Michael Zubkoff, Ira E. Raskin, and Ruth S. Hanft. New York: PRODIST, 1978.

reflected in the several papers in Part III, does not inspire particular confidence in the current capacity to contain hospital costs. It seems not unreasonable to conclude that evidence from evaluation studies of specific cost-containment efforts is not overwhelming and does not indicate a significant degree of success. This book is indicative of the general concern with hospital cost inflation. Or perhaps it represents more the growing frustration with the propensity for hospital costs to rise in spite of a general awareness of the problem, specific public policy concern, and actual efforts to contain hospital costs.

What are the prospects for hospital cost containment? Do such mechanisms as rate regulation, prospective budgeting and reimbursement, planning and certificate of need, utilization review, and the like, have the potential to control or contain cost inflation in the hospital sector? As several of the earlier papers in this volume imply, the answers to these questions derive from the answers to several more fundamental questions. What is the structure of the hospital industry? What behavioral patterns are associated with varying market conditions? What are the dimensions of the problem of hospital cost inflation? What impact will various cost-containment mechanisms have on structure, behavior, costs, and productivity? In effect, several of the papers imply that the lack of success to date may be a function of a lack of knowledge and, hence, that successful cost containment may be enhanced by future research. There is also the implication that actual policies have often been designed without taking full account of even the limited available knowledge and, hence, that more successful cost containment may be enhanced by a better application of previous research.

The purpose of this paper is to outline some thoughts about the research needs for future policy. The intent is not to provide answers, but rather to ask questions. There is no presumption to offer any specific research agenda. Rather, it seems more appropriate and useful to reflect on a research strategy; to delineate the set of questions that should be asked in any research context and to consider the answers to those questions in the context of hospital cost containment.

Ralph E. Berry, Jr.

A General Research Strategy

Whenever one sets out to research a problem, especially when the eventual objective is to define a policy solution to that problem, success usually necessitates first specifically answering several fundamental questions. In effect, in policy-related research or policy analysis, the degree of success is often related to the extent to which the approach to the research or the analysis has been systematic.

First, and perhaps foremost, it is necessary specifically to ask and to answer the question "What is the real problem of concern?" Although this may seem obvious and perhaps perfunctory, there is no shortage of unsuccessful research that can be traced essentially to a failure to formulate the right research question. Obviously, the more specifically the research questions can be formulated, the easier it is to seek answers, and the more likely it is that answers, when found, will have operational significance and provide the basis for enlightened policy. Similarly, one could cite a litany of unsuccessful policy or policy with unintended results that derives from a failure to ask the right question.

Once the question is specifically formulated, the researcher should answer a second fundamental question: "What is the ideal set of data necessary to answer the question?" Of course the ideal set of data is rarely available, but one needs to know what it is in order to specify an appropriate research design and to delineate specific data requirements. It is also useful to reflect on the ideal set of data in order to interpret and to qualify any findings generated from a less than ideal data set.

Next, the researcher must ascertain what part of the necessary data set is known or can be approximated by available surrogates. In essence, this simply requires that a systematic review of available data and relevant research literature must be undertaken.

Finally, the researcher can identify the gap between what is known and what needs to be known in order to answer the question. Closing this gap is what research is really about.

Different questions can be answered with different sets of data or information. One does, however, need a specific question to begin the process. Moreover, the appropriate degree of specificity can serve to limit the research effort and enhance the potential for success. Thus, for example, one might consider the question "What will happen if Congress enacts a national health insurance program?" But what is the real question? What will happen to what— prices? patterns of utilization? supply responses? Moreover, there is quite a difference between questions such as "Is utilization likely to increase under national health insurance?" and "Is utilization likely to increase by as much as 10 percent under national health insurance?"

The question whether utilization is likely to increase can be answered with a minimal data set. In fact, if we simply know whether there is any elasticity to the demand and supply curves we can provide an answer by reference to a simple comparative statics supply and demand analysis. Although this represents an oversimplification, and is only an approximation, it does provide an answer— and a reliable one at that. But if the question is whether utilization is likely to increase by as much as 10 percent, the data set necessary for an answer is considerably more complex. At the very least, we now need reasonably accurate estimates of specific elasticities. Questions of supply response, especially in the health sector, are exceedingly complex, and the necessary data set is more complex by an order of magnitude. It should be remembered that although we often use simple supply and demand curves to deal with questions of direction of change, with some confidence; and even use them to deal with questions of relative magnitude of change on occasion—albeit with somewhat less confidence; in fact, since we are rarely if ever concerned with competitive industries, there is really no such thing as a supply curve.

Some simple-sounding questions are often quite complex. Fortunately, some complex problems often involve relatively simple questions. But the first principle of successful research is to ask the right question. When the right research question has been formulated, there is some possibility that it can be answered. If we know the question and the ideal set of data necessary to answer it, then we can identify the gap between what is known and what we need to know. We can, in other words, identify the research needs.

Ralph E. Berry, Jr.

Hospital Cost Containment—
What Is the Problem?

Although the phenomenon of hospital cost inflation has been around for a long time, and the problem of cost containment has received the considered attention of analysts and policy makers for much of that time, it does not seem unreasonable to argue that cost containment has rarely been defined in a clear concise way. In fact, even a casual reading of several of the papers in Part I of this volume suggests that we actually have a choice of cost-containment problems. Some view the problem in terms of the price inflation of hospital services. Others concentrate on the rate of increase of total expenditures for hospital care. A related concern would derive from the relative proportion of health expenditures, especially for hospital services, in the Gross National Product. Still others would view the problem in terms of the growing government budget for hospital services. It is not at all clear just what it is that is to be contained. Is policy to be designed to contain the rate of price inflation; the rate of increase of total expenditures; the share of GNP; or the size of the government budget?

Indeed, we might press the issue back one step to some heuristic advantage. Do price increases, total expenditure increases, shifts in GNP shares, or increases in government expenditures necessarily imply a problem at all? One could cite several hypotheses consistent with the observed increases, and not all of them would be cause for concern.

Total expenditures would be expected to increase if population increased; undoubtedly, some part of the increase in total expenditures for health services results from population growth. Moreover, changes in the mix of the population might explain part of the increase. The proportion of certain subgroups in the population, such as the aged, that tend to utilize more health services has increased over time. If policy is to be designed to contain the increase in total expenditures, what account must be taken of that part of the overall increase consistent with population growth and a changing composition of the population?

One might, as an alternative, look rather at the rate of increase of per capita expenditures. Per capita expenditures, by definition, abstract from increases induced by population growth. Are increases in per capita expenditures indicative of some problem and an unambiguous candidate for containment? Again one could postulate reasonable hypotheses that would suggest a degree of caution. Certainly some part of the increase in per capita expenditures can be traced to increased income, or put another way, hospital services are a normal good—that is, the income elasticity of demand for hospital services is positive. Now one does not usually consider constraining the consumption of normal goods when income rises, except in very special sets of circumstances. Or perhaps a relevant hypothesis would be that tastes have changed—a more difficult hypothesis to test, but a reasonable one and not necessarily indicative of a problem to be dealt with through cost containment policy.

What of relative shifts in the shares of Gross National Product for hospital services and other things? To the extent that the increasing proportion of hospital services in GNP represents an increase in the share of the nation's scarce resources used in this sector, does it not warrant containment? Perhaps, but again one could postulate certain hypotheses that would at least bear testing. The observed increases in the proportion of hospital services, given increases in income, are consistent with a hypothesis that hospital services have an income elasticity greater than one, for example. Perhaps hospital services are luxury goods. Indeed, the question whether hospital services are luxury goods or necessities is a research question that seems well worth answering. Income elasticity estimates from cross-section data imply that they are necessities—the elasticities tend to be well below one. On the other hand, time-series data imply that they may be luxuries—the income elasticity tends to be greater than one.

This particular example may be worth some elaboration in the context of our current concern. Suppose we take as given that cross-section and time-series data imply quite different income elasticities of demand for hospital services, and ask what relevance this might have to future research needs for cost-containment policy. Now the shortcomings of empirical demand estimates are well-known, and considerable care must be exercised in interpreting either cross-section or time-series estimates. One drawback to the cross-section estimate, of course, is the need to assume tastes are constant over persons and/or over space. But a similar problem arises in the time-series context—it is necessary to assume that tastes are constant over time. Our current concern is not with whether the same household at different points in time is more or less likely to have similar tastes than different households would at the same point in time, but rather with whether a given cost-containment policy would have the same effect regardless of whether the income elasticity was greater or less than one. Clearly it would not. Co-insurance rates, for example, could perhaps be applied with some success as a mechanism for constraining the quantity demanded and thus containing total cost. But if hospital services are a luxury good, then over time, as income increases, the co-insurance rate would have to be raised more than proportionately to effect the same proportionate constraint.

Perhaps more significant to future policy than the differential impact of a given policy instrument is the issue of whether different policy instruments entirely are suggested by the answers to certain research questions such as "Are hospital services a luxury or a necessity?" Suppose, for example, that we assume for present purposes that at a point in time consumers behave as though hospital services were a necessity, but that over time they behave as though they were luxury goods. Indeed, such may well be the case. It is not inconceivable that over time consumer preferences shift toward hospital services for a variety of reasons. Let me cite one plausible explanation. Suppose that consumers in general have elastic expectations relative to real or perceived technological advances and medical research. Then over time, as consumers become aware of changes in medical technology—or even anticipate that they have occurred—their preferences may shift toward medical services, and any estimate of the income elasticity over time will be greater than a corresponding cross-section estimate. Now quite apart from the issue of whether or not cost-containment policy is appropriate, given this phenomenon, if it were determined by some process that cost containment should be implemented, then an instrument that reflected this phenomenon would clearly have a greater chance of success than one that did not. Thus, a constraint on new equipment that embodied technological progress, for example, would work better than a general constraint on new equipment—particularly if the consumer were made aware of the implication of the constraint.

Of course, all that is really being argued is that we simply reflect on the demand for hospital services and recognize that the quantity demanded is a function of own price, the price of substitutes, the price of complements, income, insurance, and tastes. In this context we could cite any number of hypotheses consistent with shifts in the demand curve as well as movements along the demand curve. Moreover, to this point we have avoided those arguments in the demand function that are most likely to represent potential problems that are more obvious candidates for cost containment—prices and insurance. We might also note the obvious, that demand side considerations are only half the story.

Indeed, this line of argument was prompted by the question of just what is the problem that occasions such concern for cost containment. We have observed, in the case of hospital services, relative price inflation, increased total expenditures, a growing share of GNP, and higher government budgets. These phenomena are simply data; they represent the outcome of the interaction of such supply and demand factors as prevail in the market for hospital services. Taken alone, such data would not connote anything negative. In a market system prices are signals—rising prices signal sellers that buyers now value the good more highly and serve as an incentive for increased production. If we told someone sensitive to the issues and problems of economic development that the relative share in GNP of a particular service industry had grown consistently over the past few decades, he might think, "how fortunate." In fact, the reason that these specific data are viewed as symptomatic of a problem is because we think the market for hospital services is characterized by significant market imperfections. In effect, there is a problem precisely because we don't like the outcome—we don't think the market is working.

In a fundamental sense, the function of a market is to balance value in consumption with opportunity cost. If a market is working reasonably well, market prices tend to reflect scarcity values of both resources and consumer goods. The problem with the market for hospital services, of course, is that we can't trust prices to reflect scarcity values, especially of the consumer good in question. If we observed a particular consumer paying $100 to purchase a wool coat, we might take that price as a reasonable approximation of the value of the coat in consumption. But if we observed the same person consuming a day of hospital care that cost some third-party payer $100, we would be less inclined to accept the cost as indicative of the value in consumption. And therein lies the fundamental problem. Relative price inflation, increased expenditures, higher government budgets, and especially the increased proportion of GNP are considered indicative of the wrong rate of output.

Hospital cost containment, in any sense except that of constraining relative price increases for a given output, involves constraining the rate of output. Whether the policy instrument employed involves demand constraints or supply constraints, the implicit intended effect is the same.

It would seem that the most fundamental research question in the context of hospital cost containment is "What is the right rate of output of hospital services?" If that is the right question, is it any wonder that we are so far from an answer?

But, in fact, cost-containment efforts have been employed in the past and will undoubtedly continue to be employed. It should be clear, however, that the actual policy intent of cost containment is based on either of two implicit assumptions: (1) whatever the right rate of output is, it is less than the actual rate of output; or, (2) the actual rate of output is acceptable, but the only increases that will be tolerated are those generated by real productivity increases. Of course, given the relative success of cost-containment efforts to date, it would appear that neither constraint has been particularly binding.

Thus, we can formulate a small number of fundamental research questions in the context of hospital cost containment that involve the rate of output. First, what is the right rate of output of hospital services? Second, quite apart from the right rate of output, how can the actual rate of output, or more particularly the rate of increase of that output, be constrained? Third, given the actual output, how can we constrain relative price increases for that output?

The full implication of the first question is presumably obvious. The implications of the second and third may not be, however. In fact, if cost-containment policy is implemented and succeeds in constraining the rate of increase of actual output over time—in effect constraining increases that might have derived from income increases, population changes, or shifts in consumer preferences, for example—that will be equivalent to the normative assumption that whatever the right rate of output is, it is less than the actual rate of output. In effect, cost-containment policy would serve to reduce the gap between some unspecified desired rate of output and the actual rate of output.

If cost-containment policy is implemented and succeeds in constraining relative price increases for a given level of output, that will be equivalent to the normative assumption that the actual rate of output is acceptable, but increases in output must be limited to those generated by real productivity increases. This constraint is somewhat less binding, in principle, but increases that might have derived from income increases, population changes, or shifts in consumer preferences, for example, may well be constrained. In essence, if such increases would have exceeded real productivity increases, then this constraint is only a modification of the more binding one and implicitly involves the same normative assumption that whatever the right rate of output is, it is less than the actual rate of output.

When the implications of the second and third questions are spelled out, the relative importance of the first question is the more clear. Undoubtedly the general support for cost-containment efforts derives from the widespread acceptance of the implicit assumption that the actual rate of output exceeds the right rate of output. There is no doubt that the output of the hospital sector includes necessary services, quality, and necessary complexity, but is also includes unnecessary services, inappropriate complexity, and undoubtedly some waste. To the extent that cost-containment policy is implemented successfully, one might expect that it will serve to eliminate unnecessary services, inappropriate complexity, and waste. In effect, cost-containment mechanisms should serve to eliminate the gap between the actual rate of output and the right rate of output. But how will we know when the gap has been eliminated? The more successful any set of cost-containment instruments, the more likely we will go too far. Hence, the more research contributes to answering the second and third questions, the more critical it is to answer the first question.

Policy makers who sit in the catbird seat and must cope more immediately with the implications of accelerating hospital cost inflation and the burden of growing budgets are undoubtedly not particularly placated by such a point, no matter how correct it might be in a strict conceptual sense. They undoubtedly view the actual outcome to be sufficiently off mark as to warrant cost-containment efforts without specific knowledge or delineation of the desired outcome. Most researchers who have studied the hospital sector would probably agree. The known market imperfections are such that the relative inefficiency is considered to be of a significant order of magnitude albeit not specifically measured. Most knowledgeable persons would agree that successful cost containment would have to go quite far indeed before one had to worry much about going too far. Certainly it would have to go farther than efforts to date have succeeded in going. Thus, it would seem that research has something to offer, even research that stops short of answering the fundamental question. And on that encouraging note we might move on to the kinds of questions with operational significance that might be asked, and more specifically to a consideration of where some of the answers might be found.

Where Do the Answers Lie?

In the most fundamental sense, the relevant questions can only be answered when we have a more complete understanding of the market for hospital services, the imperfections that prevail in that market, and the implications of those imperfections. If one could will into being any set of data one wanted, the ideal set for assessing the market for hospital services would include three principal components. First, one would need consumer preferences and such data as are necessary to derive the market demand for hospital services. Second, one would need the technological and factor market data necessary to derive the production function or the relevant cost curves for hospital services. Finally, one would need the several parameters that define the relevant industry structure. Indeed, if one had such a set of data, one could even answer the question of what is the right rate of output—at least the right rate of output given the prevailing income distribution. (In fact, if one had the foresight to will into being sufficiently robust consumer preference data, one could even approximate the right rate of output for alternative income distributions.) Moreover, given the parameters that define the structure of the market for hospital services, one could assess both the causes and the extent of such allocative inefficiency as might prevail. Intervention such as cost-containment efforts to improve the performance of the hospital services industry would be rather straightforward.

Unfortunately, we can't will ideal data sets into being. Even economists are afforded such luxury only when they are either fantasizing or teaching introductory principles courses. Rather, we must make do with the less than ideal data that are available or can be generated from systematic research efforts. But a consideration of the ideal data set does serve to outline the practical data requirements and to guide the search for answers in the right general direction. In order to answer the relevant questions in the context of cost-containment policy we need at least some reasonable approximation of both the demand for hospital services and the cost of production over the relevant range of output, and some knowledge of the characteristics of the market for hospital services that might serve significantly to affect the outcome. Most especially, we need knowledge of the peculiar characteristics of supply response in the hospital services market.

Of course, the available data set is not a null set. The body of knowledge is not insignificant and research efforts over a number of years have provided useful estimates and insight. There have been several empirical studies of the demand for hospital services, for example. Thus, although not immune to specific empirical criticism, the relevant literature contains estimates of the elasticity of the demand for hospital services with respect to such as own price, price of substitutes, income, and insurance. Moreover, the influence on demand of such surrogates for taste parameters as race, sex, age, education, marital status, and the like have been estimated. Within a tolerable margin of error, available estimates of the relevant demand elasticities are probably sufficient to approximate the effect of such demand constraints as co-insurance and deductibles. This is not to say that these estimates cannot be refined and improved, or that the margin of error cannot be reduced significantly—indeed, one of the major research efforts of recent years, the Rand National Health Insurance Experiment (Newhouse, 1974), was designed for just that purpose—but rather to note the availability of specific surrogates for necessary demand data. Whether or not the available surrogates are sufficient for any specific future cost-containment policy, of course, can only be determined on an ad hoc, as-needed basis. They are probably sufficient for policy efforts that do not depend on a high degree of specificity for success. But if cost-containment policy is to become more effective and demand constraints are to have a significant role in such policy, as might be the case under certain national health insurance programs, for example, there will be a need for more refined estimates of demand elasticities. More and better demand analysis is a research need for future policy.

Much the same can be said for hospital cost analysis. Although there has been considerable research effort devoted to estimating hospital cost functions—and in fairness it should be noted that much of this research has provided useful knowledge and insight—it is still the case that much more needs to be known about hospital cost functions if they are to provide the basis for more refined or sophisticated hospital cost-containment policy. The empirical cost functions estimated to date have only limited usefulness in the context of cost containment.

The paper in this volume by Lipscomb, Raskin, and Eichenholz indicates the potential of empirical cost estimates, but it is also illustrative of the limited usefulness of currently available estimates. The authors addressed themselves particularly to the incentive under rate regulation for hospitals to adjust their volume of output because short-run marginal cost is below average cost. Their analysis of more than a dozen different hospital cost studies tended to support the modifications employed by the Cost of Living Council under Phase IV. Still, it seems fair to conclude that their analysis only supports the contention that the modification represented a move in the right direction. The range of marginal cost estimates in the several studies was rather broad and the authors were able to cite problems in model specification, sampling, and estimation techniques worthy of further research.

Of course, it could be argued that earlier cost studies were not designed to provide a basis for cost-containment policy and it is not fair to judge them by how specifically they might serve that purpose. And such is not the current purpose. Rather, the intent is only to note the nature of the available data set and indicate the extent to which it will meet the needs of future cost-containment policy. It would seem that hospital cost analysis is a prime research need.

The paper by Lave and Lave represents the potential of cost analysis designed specifically to address questions in the context of cost-containment policy. Their estimates suggest that there is a stable hospital cost structure that is relatively insensitive to certain output specifications. They were able to estimate marginal costs and isolate the effect of certain hospital characteristics. The availability of specific empirical estimates such as those generated by the Laves provide the basis for more specific rules and constraints and hence enhance the potential of cost-containment policy. In essence, they are akin to more specific demand elasticity estimates in the context of demand constraints.

The analysis completed by the Laves provides other insights with potential for future cost-containment policy. Thus, for example, they found the cost structure constant across regions, but not across hospital size. Moreover, they found that the cost effects of increasing and decreasing occupancy rates were not symmetrical. On balance, their research is exceedingly useful in its own right, and it does augur well for cost analysis designed specifically to address questions in the context of cost-containment policy. Still, the authors consider their work preliminary rather than definitive and argue for further research with more than the traditional polite caveat. In the spirit of our concern they offer several specific suggestions including the use of better estimating techniques, the use of data bases with more information, and more precise modeling of hospital supply responses.

Undoubtedly the weakest part of the available data set is that which involves the peculiar characteristics of supply response in the hospital services market. In attempting to assess the parameters that define the structure of the hospital industry one must cope with several typical problems such as differentiated products, lack of knowledge, geographical markets, and the like. But one must in addition cope with several rather unusual problems such as the dominance of nonprofit enterprises on the supply side of the market, the possibility that supply-side actors have influence on demand, and the fact that buyers and sellers are not alone in the market but are both significantly affected by the actions of third-party financiers. Some of the papers in this volume dealt with certain aspects of these problems, but perhaps not enough emphasis has been given to the fact that the real constraint on cost-containment policy may be the sheer magnitude of the gap between what is known and what needs to be known about the structure of the hospital industry and especially the behavioral patterns within the industry.

Effective public policy critically depends on the ability to predict the supply response to varying market conditions and specific public policy instruments. One can only expect cost containment to be as effective as the policy makers' ability to take specific account of the impact of varying mechanisms and instruments on hospital behavior and hence to predict supply response. The traditional theory of the firm that postulates a producer attempting to maximize profits (or a specific utility function with profit as a dominant argument) subject to technological and market constraints is useful because it allows prediction of supply response. But as noted before, the conceptual framework alone is sufficient only for predicting the direction of supply response. Specific empirical testing of the model in actual markets is a necessary condition for predicting the relative magnitudes of supply response because actual behavior depends not only on the utility function being maximized, but on the nature of the constraints imposed as well. Thus, for example, if one is willing to assume behavior consistent with profit maximization, one can predict the likely impact of an oil embargo or general energy shortage. In the short run prices can be expected to rise, profits will increase, and efforts to increase supply will be made as prevailing market conditions allow for the processing and refining of a supply characterized by higher marginal cost. Moreover, if the relative shortage persists, one would predict an increase in investment in a variety of contexts in the long run. But without specific empirical data concerning the structure of the oil industry and behavioral patterns among firms in the industry, there would be no way to predict precisely how much prices would rise, how much profits would increase, or how much investment would take place. In essence, neither the short-run nor long-run supply response could be approximated with any degree of precision without some specific empirical knowledge.

The economic behavior of nonprofit enterprises has drawn considerably attention in the past decade, especially from economists interested in the market for hospital services. But studies to date have been essentially conceptual and somewhat speculative in nature. Those who have attempted to model hospital behavior have concentrated on specifying utility functions for nonprofit hospitals. Hospital utility functions have been postulated in terms of such arguments as quantity, quality, prestige, net income, and the income of the medical staff. These conceptual efforts are important, but little has been done to test these models empirically. Without specific empirical testing of hospital behavior models in actual markets, they cannot provide the basis for predicting the relative magnitudes of supply response either to varying market conditions or to specific cost-containment mechanisms.

The problem, of course, is analogous to the simple supply and demand analysis of any market. One need only know that supply and demand have some elasticity in order to predict the direction of change likely with any given change in market conditions. But, in order to predict the relative magnitude of the change, one needs specific empirical estimates of the elasticities. Similarly, knowing that quality and the complexity of services are in the objective function of hospital decision makers is sufficient to predict that any demand increase induced by increased income, increased insurance, or new government programs will result in a supply response that includes a higher quality, more complex service. But one would need specific empirical data in order to predict the precise nature of the supply response. Therein lies the dilemma for cost-containment policy. Containment implies constraining the extent and the nature of the supply response. Just as the policy maker would need specific elasticity estimates in order to determine how much of a deductible or co-insurance to apply to generate a given demand constraint, he would need specific empirical estimates in order to constrain the supply response to effect a given supply constraint.

It would seem that the general lack of success of prior cost-containment efforts can be viewed in the context of the lack of specific knowledge concerning the characteristics of supply response in the market for hospital services. Certainly several of the papers in Part III of this volume would tend to support this contention either directly or indirectly. Hellinger, for example, has summarized the findings of evaluation studies of several prospective reimbursement schemes. In general, the studies did not find hospital costs to have been lowered significantly. Although one might suggest several viable explanations for the specific findings, including the confounding effect of national wage and price controls in certain instances, the voluntary nature of several of the reimbursement experiments, and even the methodological shortcomings of certain evaluations, there is reason to suspect that significant cost containment might not have been expected. A systematic review of the several mechanisms employed, for example, suggests that the instruments implemented to contain costs were formulated in the absence of sufficient empirical knowledge of their likely impact on hospital behavior, and more especially of hospital reaction to that impact. Rate regulation by formula in New York is among the strictest forms of cost containment implemented to date, for example. Still, the net effect of cost containment even in that context is modified considerably by induced adjustments in hospital behavior. It may be, as Bauer concluded, that "rate setting . . . is just a highly complicated tinkering operation, plugging up leaks in one small section. . . ." In any event, it seems not unreasonable to conclude that the failure to contain costs is related to the failure to understand or more fully account for likely hospital reaction to specific market constraints.

Salkever and Bice have provided more direct evidence of the influence of unintended supply response in frustrating actual cost-containment efforts. They have analyzed the effect of certificate-of-need regulation by examining its effect on investment patterns and costs while controlling statistically for other factors that influence investment. In essence, they found that certificate-of-need constraints have no significant impact on total investment but rather serve to encourage a redirection of investment from bed expansion to the addition of new services and facilities. They conclude that the net effect of certificate of need not only was not cost containment, but might actually have exacerbated hospital cost inflation.

Effective cost containment will depend critically on the ability to predict the supply response to varying market conditions and specific cost-containment instruments. Undoubtedly the weakest part of the available data set is that which involves the characteristics of supply response in the market for hospital services. Conceptual models of hospital behavior have been formulated and help us understand the cause of past failures. But since specific empirical testing of such behavioral models in actual markets is a necessary condition for predicting the relative magnitudes of supply response, it would seem that such efforts are a prime research need for future cost-containment policy.

What Are Some of the Gaps?

In assessing future research needs, whatever the aspect of the problem, it is probably safe to conclude that efforts could be productively directed at generating better data, applying improved estimating techniques, and empirically testing conceptual models.

Although the emphasis on each might and probably should vary, the same general conclusion is valid for demand analysis, cost analysis, and analysis of supply response in the market for hospital services. Moreover, there are undoubtedly external economies that will derive from even incremental advances in any case, since there is a clear interdependence among data, estimation, and theory as well as across demand, cost, and supply response.

There is, of course, a considerable body of existing research that can be reviewed to some advantage both to serve policy in the near term and to guide future research for policy in the long term. The state of knowledge has expanded rather dramatically in the past fifteen years as researchers have responded to the significant public policy relevance and the intellectual challenge of this rapidly growing sector of the economy dominated by nonprofit enterprises and often characterized by atypical economic behavior.

Since most of this research has been systematically reviewed and summarized periodically, the task of assessing what is known and identifying specific gaps in knowledge is considerably eased. Most of the research published before 1965 has been summarized by Klarman (1965), and his extensive survey represents a basic reference for earlier research not only on hospitals, but on health economics in general. Research relevant to hospitals has been reviewed rather extensively by Berki (1972). The essay in this volume by Lipscomb, Raskin, and Eichenholz sets out many of the findings of hospital cost analysis as they relate to the concept of marginal cost. Finally, most of the econometric studies of health economics have been reviewed recently in a particularly systematic and useful way by M. Feldstein (1974).

The purpose of this section is not to undertake a systematic and extensive review of existing research, but rather to reflect on some of the gaps that remain and represent research needs for future policy. Although it will often prove useful to refer to representative previous research in order to facilitate the flow of the discussion, there will be no attempt to be either complete or critical in what follows.

Albeit the demand side of the problem has received little attention in this volume, it has been well researched in general. As noted above, there have been a considerable number of empirical studies of the demand for hospital services. Moreover, it seems fair to conclude that in relative terms demand analysis has progressed somewhat further than either cost analysis or analysis of supply response in the market for hospital services—such is certainly the case in an empirical sense.

In general, demand studies have employed econometric techniques to estimate a traditional demand equation with the quantity of hospital services dependent on own price, prices of substitutes and complements, income, insurance, and such surrogates for taste parameters as race, sex, age, education, marital status, and the like. While most researchers have specified rather complete demand equations, the state of knowledge has been advanced by varying the emphasis on the several factors likely to influence demand as well as the preciseness with which the several independent variables were approximated.

Thus, for example, earlier demand studies, such as that by Rosenthal (1970), tended to concentrate on own price elasticity. Given the widespread contention that hospital utilization was not responsive to price, but was determined exclusively by technical medical considerations, the early demand studies that demonstrated a negative price elasticity were of some significance. Of course, given the importance of insurance, considerable care must be taken in interpreting price elasticity estimates. Later demand studies that specifically accounted for the fact that the net price paid by the patient depends on both the gross price of hospital services and the extent of insurance coverage, such as that by M. Feldstein (1971), facilitated the interpretation of price elasticity estimates. Additional demand studies that have concentrated on the role of insurance in the demand for hospital services, such as those by Phelps and Newhouse (1972) and Rosett and Huang (1973), have served to clarify still further the interrelated influences of price and insurance. Finally, several recent studies, including those by Acton (1972) and Grossman (1972), have introduced the patient's time as an integral part of the total price.

Although most demand studies have tended to emphasize own

price elasticity, some research has begun to analyze cross-elasticities and the influence of substitutes and complements on the demand for hospital services. Davis and Russell (1972), for example, estimated the cross-elasticity of inpatient care with respect to the price of outpatient services and found the expected direct relationship. Martin Feldstein (1971) included the numbers of general practitioners and medical and surgical specialists per capita in his demand equation. His findings suggest that general practitioners represent substitutes for inpatient care and that specialists represent complements.

As noted above, most demand studies have found the income elasticity to be rather low. The work of Anderson and Benham (1970) and P. Feldstein and Carr (1964) are representative and their results, as those of most cross-section studies, imply that hospital care is a necessity.

Even this somewhat brief and incomplete review of demand studies is indicative of the volume of research that has been completed. What is perhaps not indicated is the extent to which future policy and research can benefit from the economies of scale implicit in that volume. Thus, for example, the sheer number of estimates provides a useful range and a basis for approximating relevant elasticities. Moreover, a systematic analysis of comparable and related elasticity estimates can provide a basis for assessing the relative magnitudes of bias that derive from several sources, most notably general data problems, specification and estimation problems, and the interaction of insurance and price elasticity. Last, but not least, they serve collectively to point the way for future research.

Any future research that serves to refine the several elasticity estimates or to reduce the bias in such estimates will enhance future policy. In a general sense better data and better estimation would serve to close a research gap. One gap that exists in this context is especially significant—the inability to date adequately to capture product heterogeneity in the dependent variable. Very little has been done to account for product differences—quality and complexity of hospital services—in the demand function.

One gap on the demand side, however, would seem to be of

primary significance—not enough is known about the role of the physician in determining the demand for hospital services. Are hospital services final goods, or intermediate goods? Estimating a demand equation that has the quantity of hospital services dependent on own price, other prices, and such consumer characteristics as income, insurance coverage, race, age, sex, education, and the like, is equivalent to assuming that hospital services are a final good. Virtually all empirical demand studies have followed this route. An alternative perspective would view the consumer's demand to be for "medical care." Physicians would be viewed as entrepreneurs who combine several inputs, including their own time and hospital services, to produce medical care. The demand for hospital services, in effect, would be a derived demand. Such a perspective was outlined in some detail by P. Feldstein (1966), and has been alluded to by others rather often, but little if any empirical demand research has been based on such a conceptual model.

Suppose in fact that consumers do enter the market to demand medical care from physician entrepreneurs who in turn demand hospital services to combine with other inputs to produce that product. The demand for hospital services, as any factor of production, would depend on the marginal revenue product and the marginal cost of hospital services.

As an aside, it is interesting to notice how this formulation of the problem provides a simple and logical explanation of Roemer's Law that the supply of hospital beds creates a demand for their use. If hospital services are an input to the physician's production of medical care, one would expect the physician to demand more or less as the price was lowered or raised—that is, a movement along the relevant demand curve. But what is the "price" that physicians pay for hospital services? It is certainly not a money price (except in the sense that out of the total price of medical care the physician receives less as the patient pays more on a separate bill to the hospital—in which case the money aspect of price is likely to be reflected in the marginal revenue product). Rather, the price is expressed in terms of such as peer pressure and pressure from hospital administrators and perhaps trustees as the individual physician's demand for beds varies. Thus, for example, for a given number of beds it is likely that any physician who seems to be using more than his fair share would feel the pressure, however subtle. What effect does the supply of beds have? Clearly as the supply of beds varies the relevant price of beds varies to the individual physician. An increase in the supply of beds will lower the pressure (there may even be a different form of pressure to use the beds), and at the lower "price" the physician will demand more beds.

Is the demand for hospital services to be considered in the context of consumers maximizing their utility as would be the case if they are treated as a pure final good? Or is it to be considered in the context of physician entrepreneurs maximizing their utility as would be the case if they are treated as a pure intermediate good? It seems likely that neither extreme represents the state of the real world. An alternative that is intermediate and has considerable intuitive appeal would treat the physician as an agent for the patient in the market for hospital services. This is a relatively new idea and holds much promise for learning more about the role of the physician in determining the demand for hospital services.

Ross (1973) has done some preliminary theoretical modeling of agency in a general equilibrium context; and M. Feldstein (1974) has speculated in a general way on the potential of the agency relationship for understanding behavior in the health sector; but no specific conceptual models of the physician as agent have been formulated; and of course no empirical testing of the agency model in actual markets has been done. It would seem that future research directed at analyzing the extent to which the physician is an agent might be fruitful.

A crucial question, of course, is the extent to which the agency relationship holds. At one extreme, if the physician is a perfect agent, then the existing demand estimates are quite appropriate—in principle there is no difference between a consumer maximizing his own utility and an agent maximizing it for him. At the other extreme if the physician is not an agent (a perfect nonagent?), then the existing demand estimates are quite inappropriate—the correct model would involve the physician as an entrepreneur maximizing utility, and the demand for hospital services should be treated strictly as a derived demand. More likely, the agency relationship is relevant but it holds in a more or less imperfect form. Several alternative forms could be postulated and tested. Closer to the perfect agent form, for example, one might treat the physician as a utility maximizer, but include the patient's utility as an argument in the relevant maximand. Closer to the nonagent form, one might consider the case where the physician seeks to maximize utility subject to the constraint that the patient's utility (health care) is maintained at some minimum level (standard).

Indeed, this formulation of the problem serves to put the role of the physician and its potential impact on the cost of hospital care into proper perspective. Few would argue with the contention that a physician, entrusted with the care of the patient, should seek to maximize the patient's well-being. In fact, even those who are most concerned with cost containment in their public roles would at least secretly hope that if the need arose in their own cases, their physicians would seek to maximize their well-being, and perhaps even "spare no cost" in so doing. But the present structure of the market for hospital services puts the physician in an untenable position. If he is to act as an agent for the individual patient, he cannot simultaneously act as an agent for society. Future cost-containment policy would be well served by any research that contributes to the development of mechanisms that keep the physician on one side or the other.

There has also been considerable research effort devoted to hospital cost analysis. Most of the earlier cost studies tended to concentrate on the question of whether or not hospital services were produced subject to economies of scale. On balance, the weight of evidence is that economies of scale, however significant statistically, are not of a significant order of magnitude in real terms. Whatever hospitals may be, they do not have the long-run cost curves of a natural monopoly. Approximately constant returns to scale can be inferred from the long-run data analyzed in this book by Lipscomb, Raskin, and Eichenholz. This is consistent with the findings of M. Feldstein (1968) for British hospitals and Evans (1971) for Canadian hospitals. These latter two studies are significant in this regard since the availability of case-mix data in England and Canada allows product-mix differences to be taken into account and hence avoids a source of bias that prevails in most cross-section studies of U.S. hospitals.

In the short run, marginal costs tend to be significantly below average costs. This result is rather consistent among all cost studies and has some relevance for cost-containment policy as outlined in Lipscomb, Raskin, and Eichenholz's paper.

Hospital cost analysis has been hindered by the lack of available data to account adequately for the known heterogeneity of hospital output. Most researchers have tried to cope with the problem with varying degrees of success, but none has succeeded in overcoming it. Hospitals are multiproduct firms both in terms of their products—patient care–teaching–research—and the quality and complexity of these products. Even abstracting from the problems of isolating the influence of teaching and research—which is feasible for a large subset of hospitals—the problems inherent in patient care output measures remain and represent a research need of primary significance.

Recent cost studies and related efforts have approached the problem of product heterogeneity from several directions. Extensions of certain of these approaches would seem to have sufficient promise to warrant further research. One such approach is to use explicit measures of hospital case mix in estimating cost functions as was done for a subset of U.S. hospitals by Lave, Lave, and Silverman (1972) and Lee and Wallace (1973). A related approach would involve the development of an index of output based on case-mix variations building on the work of Rafferty (1972). Unfortunately, such efforts are currently constrained by a lack of data. There is very little case-mix data generally available for U.S. hospitals—there is no case-mix data available on a national basis. The gap in this context is a data gap.

An alternative approach would be to attempt to group hospitals to minimize the degree of heterogeneity in the output measure. Berry (1973) has grouped hospitals according to facilities and services. In fact his groupings are based on inputs rather than outputs, but the technique has some merit, and the implications for certain cost-containment mechanisms seem obvious.

However limited the knowledge of hospital cost functions, even less is known about the production function for hospital services. There are no engineering production functions, and a lack of relevant data constrains attempts to generate empirical estimates. Moreover, the restrictive assumptions required to apply available estimating techniques are hardly met by the conditions that prevail in the market for hospital services.

Production function information is not generally available for most products, but it is of special concern in the case of hospital services and in the context of cost containment. In general, it is expected that market incentives will suffice to stimulate firms to select reasonably efficient factor combinations and output levels. But in a sector dominated by nonprofit enterprises, with supply-side actors influencing demand, and reimbursement by third parties serving to scramble the signal of scarcity values to both sides, it is quite unlikely that the market serves this function reasonably well, if at all. If cost-containment policy is to be brought to bear to improve the performance of the hospital sector, then policy instruments have to be designed to stimulate the selection of more appropriate factor combinations and/or output levels. The irony of intervention is exposed in its classic form in this context. How can you fine-tune what you cannot see? This is a gap of considerable magnitude, but even partial closing of it would enhance future cost-containment policy by a comparable order of magnitude.

The production function is obviously related directly to supply response. In the previous section it was noted that the weakest part of the available data set is that which includes the characteristics of supply response in the market for hospital services. Although that is the case, even that set is not empty. Some important conceptual work has been done and several models of hospital behavior based on the maximization of specific utility functions have been developed.

Newhouse (1970), for example, has postulated that hospitals seek to maximize prestige, which is a function of quantity and quality. Lee (1971) suggested prestige maximization as well, but defined it more in terms of the conspicuous production of complex quality services. Evans (1970) postulated that hospitals seek to maximize surplus. Pauly and Redisch (1973) have modeled the hospital as a physicians' cooperative that seeks to maximize the income of the medical staff.

These conceptual efforts are important, and can be used to predict hospital behavior. The gap in this context is that the theories have not been tested empirically in any rigorous way in actual markets. Hence, they cannot provide the basis for predicting with any degree of certainty or confidence the relative magnitudes of supply response to varying market conditions or to specific cost-containment mechanisms.

On balance, it would seem that there is a major gap in the context of supply response. The real constraint on cost-containment policy may well be the sheer magnitude of the gap between what is known and what needs to be known about hospital behavior and supply response.

On the other hand, however limited, there is a minimal data set. It can be used to some advantage in predicting input and output behavior of hospitals in response to certain cost-containment policy instruments, albeit in a gross directional sense. In fact, several of the papers in Part III of this volume imply that in part the lack of success of cost-containment efforts to date reflect an apparent gap between what is known and what is applied.

A Final Note on Cost Containment

As hospital costs have risen, and particularly as these costs have been translated into a public burden through governmental budgets, pressure has increasingly been brought to bear to control these costs. The exuberance for cost containment reflects the growing dissatisfaction with the performance of the hospital sector. The widespread support for some form of cost-containment policy is indicative of the general acceptance of the notion that the hospital sector is not producing the right rate of output in some sense. Policy makers and most others have come to the conclusion that the extreme market imperfections preclude an acceptable performance in this sector without some form of external intervention.

But what form should the intervention take? There is a range of choice. Given the failings of the existing sector, should it be replaced, regulated, or repaired?

There are those who believe the choice is clear-cut. Interestingly enough, those would include supporters of each of the three alternatives. Perhaps the choice is not so clear-cut.

The basic presumption of this volume is that the general level of performance in the hospital sector is unacceptable and some policy effort is in order to affect the outcome. On balance, whether intended or unintended, taken as a whole this volume would seem to come out closer to the regulation alternative. Perhaps this derives from the selection of papers. Perhaps it reflects the nature of prior cost-containment efforts. Perhaps it is simply indicative of the likelihood that regulation will prevail over the foreseeable future. Many would hold that such emphasis is appropriate. They would argue that the relevant question is not should the hospital sector be regulated, but rather how should it be regulated. But others would undoubtedly hold that such emphasis is not appropriate. Some would argue that the failings of the existing sector are not such as to be amenable to regulation. They would cite the failures of regulation efforts as well as the failures of the sector and conclude that only a new planned health system was capable of performance consonant with social objectives. Still others would argue that the system could and should be repaired. They would also cite the failures of regulation—not only in health—and conclude that the baby ought not to be thrown out with the bath water. They would note with some concern that it is not that improving the market has been tried and found wanting—rather, it has not been tried.

In the last analysis, whether the policy choice is to replace, regulate, or repair the existing market for hospital services, such efforts will depend critically on what is known and what needs to be known in order to effect the desired outcome. Ironically, if one could will the ideal data set into being, there would be little to choose among the three alternatives. But since the policy maker will have to make do with something less than an ideal data set, in making his choice, he would do well to consider the practical implications and limitations of what is known and what might be generated by feasible research. As policy moves from certain interventions to improve the market to more sophisticated changes, through regulation designed to affect supply constraints by modifying supply response, or eventually to replacing the market for hospital services, the necessary data and knowledge base becomes increasingly more complex. The gap between what is known and what needs to be known in order to affect the outcome in the desired way increases by a significant order of magnitude.

The available data set would seem to be most likely to serve the needs of policy designed to unscramble the signals of scarcity values in the market for hospital services. One possibility in this context would provide incentives for the consumer to become more cost-conscious through reform of the current insurance system. The use of co-insurance and deductibles could effect a demand constraint by limiting moral hazard. In fact, by the straightforward mechanism of eliminating all but catastrophic health insurance, the consumer would be in a position to reflect directly on scarcity values in all but extreme cases. The available data set does lend some credence to this argument, and in any event, the research needs to effect policy along such lines seem quite tractable.

The available data set is somewhat less likely to serve immediately the needs of policy designed to modify the influence on demand of supply-side actors. An interesting possibility in this context would involve the encouragement of a system of competitive HMOs. Now variations of this policy instrument have in fact been implemented with rather less success than might have been expected by some. One way to view the HMO is as an agent for the patient. If HMOs are competitive, presumably the ones that perform the agency role better will be more successful. An alternative way to view the HMO is as a producer of medical care that must face the real cost of the hospital services input. Presumably the introduction of cost consciousness will mean that those that use the input more efficiently will be more successful. Perhaps the lack of success in previous HMO policy might be in part due to asking the wrong question, or at least clouding the right question by mixing it up with several other questions. In fact, it would seem that the critical question is whether or not it is possible to devise a mechanism for putting the physician on the demand side of the market for hospital services. The potential improvements in performance likely in this context would seem to warrant research efforts, and the research needs would seem to be feasible.

The available data set would seem least likely to serve the immediate needs of policy designed to effect specific containment objectives through modifying the supply response in a sector dominated by nonprofit enterprises. Such regulatory efforts as rate regulation and certificate of need are hampered by a lack of knowledge specific to behavior patterns and have been frustrated by unintended or perhaps unanticipated supply responses. The research needs in this context are significant, but certain of them seem feasible.

It was not my intention to develop a treatise on policy choices, or to present a balanced assessment of the arguments pro and con for any alternative. Nor did I intend to analyze any of them in terms of political feasibility, or even to predict the likely choice. Rather, I intended only to reflect on each briefly from the perspective of the research needs that must be met if success is to be expected from the pursuit of any particular policy choice.

The fundamental question in the context of cost containment is "What is the right rate of output of hospital services?" The answer to this question must be phrased in several dimensions. First, what is the appropriate level of output in the aggregate; how much of the nation's scarce pool of resources is to be devoted to the production of hospital services? Second, given the level of aggregate output, what particular mix of services is to be produced? Third, what is the appropriate way to produce any desired output; what combination of inputs represents a reasonably efficient production choice? Fourth, what is the appropriate pattern of distribution of hospital services among the population; who gets what part of the total output? The first three questions refer to the relative efficiency of the allocation of resources. The fourth question refers to the equity of the distribution of the produce of those resources.[1]

[1] Some would argue that the equity question is more properly treated in the context of income distribution, and that the issue of the right rate of output should be resolved

In assessing the potential for any policy choice it is necessary to reflect on how it will serve to answer these questions. In determining the research needs for any policy choice it is necessary to reflect on the gap between what is known and what needs to be known in order to answer these questions.

A planned system and a regulated system would answer the question of the aggregate level of output by means of setting a specific supply constraint. But even abstracting from the ultimate supply constraint, several critical questions remain to be answered, and the available data set does not augur well for answering them in the near term.

What particular mix of hospital services is to be produced, for example? How much coronary care, cancer therapy, renal dialysis, and so forth, will be included among hospital output? What will be the proportions of inpatient care and outpatient services? However one views the mechanisms that serve to answer those questions in the current system, or the answers that obtain, one should not lose sight of the fact that the questions will have to be answered in any event and under any alternative system. More important, one should be aware of the kinds of data needed to answer them and the likelihood that they will be sufficient to render the answers less rather than more arbitrary.

Given the level of aggregate output and mix of services, what factor combinations are to be employed in producing them? In the absence of production function information, it is not clear how questions concerning input mix are to be answered.

What will be the pattern of distribution among the population of the given output? Now some might think that removing health care from the market would negate such a question. Not so. It is not quite clear what making health care a right would imply in this context, but it is not likely that any aggregate supply constraint chosen would ever allow for consumption by all to the point where the marginal utility in consumption was zero, for example. Rather more reason-

for the given income distribution. Others hold the view that health care is a right and that the distribution of health care among the population should not depend on the prevailing distribution of income. Since our current purpose is limited and would not be particularly served by resolving this issue one way or the other, it seems reasonable to leave the question.

able conceptual alternatives would be consumption to the point where the value in consumption was equal to marginal cost, or consumption up to some point necessary to provide a given minimal health standard for all. There would seem to have to be a more practical alternative, given any likely total supply constraint for the system, but what data would provide for even an approximation to such a solution? Clearly no such data set currently exists. Still some answer must be found to the distribution question. If the system does not provide enough renal dialysis for all who might benefit from it, for example, who will get it and who will be left out?

There is no question about the relatively poor performance of the hospital sector. Similarly there is no doubt but that some form of cost-containment policy will be in place in the years to come. In a world of perfect information and perfect policy instruments, rational cost-containment policy could be implemented to bring about the right rate of output in the hospital sector—to eliminate unnecessary complexity and waste while retaining necessary complexity and quality. Unfortunately, this is a world of poor information and less than perfect policy instruments. At present, there are no data sufficiently robust to discriminate among quality, necessary complexity, unnecessary complexity, and waste. We do not have sufficient production function information. Not enough is known about the role of physicians and how to modify their influence on the demand for hospital services. And too little is known about the peculiar characteristics of supply response in this sector. Research is needed to close the several gaps. But judicious selection of policy alternatives is needed as well to take advantage of what is known and to move in those directions that can be aided by feasible research.

References

Acton, J.P.
1972 "Demand for health care among the urban poor, with special emphasis on the role of time." Santa Monica, Calif.: RAND Publication R-1151-OEO/NYC. October.

Anderson, R., and L. Benham
   1970   "Factors affecting the relationship between family income and
            medical care consumption." Pp. 73-95 in H. Klarman, ed.,
            Empirical Studies in Health Economics. Baltimore: The Johns
            Hopkins Press.
Berki, S.E.
   1972   Hospital Economics. Lexington, Mass.: Lexington Books, D.C.
            Heath & Co.
Berry, R.E., Jr.
   1973   "On grouping hospitals for economic analysis." Inquiry 10
            (December): 5-12.
Davis, K., and L. Russell
   1972   "The substitution of hospital outpatient care for inpatient care."
            Review of Economics and Statistics 54 (May): 109-120.
Evans, R.G.
   1970   "Efficiency incentives in hospital reimbursement." Unpublished
            doctoral dissertation, Harvard University.
   1971   "'Behavioral' cost functions for hospitals." Canadian Journal of
            Economics 4 (May): 198-215.
Feldstein, M.S.
   1968   Economic Analysis for Health Service Efficiency. Amsterdam:
            North-Holland Publishing Co.
   1971   "Hospital cost inflation: A study of nonprofit price dynamics."
            American Economic Review 61 (December): 853-872.
   1974   "Econometric studies of health economics." In M. Intriligator
            and D. Kendrick, eds. Frontiers of Quantitative Economics II.
            Amsterdam: North-Holland Publishing Co.
Feldstein, P.J.
   1966   "Research on the demand for health services." Milbank Memo-
            rial Fund Quarterly 44 (July): 128-165.
Feldstein, P.J., and W.J. Carr
   1964   "The effect of income on medical care spending." Proceedings
            of the Social Statistics Section, American Statistical Association:
            93-105.
Grossman, M.
   1972   "On the concept of health capital and the demand for health."
            Journal of Political Economy 80 (March-April): 223-256.
Klarman, H.E.
   1965   The Economics of Health. New York: Columbia University
            Press.

Lave, J.R., L.B. Lave, and L.P. Silverman
  1972   "Hospital cost estimation controlling for case mix." Applied Economics 4 (September): 165–180.
Lee, M.L.
  1971   "A conspicuous production theory of hospital behavior." Southern Economic Journal 28 (July): 48–58.
Lee, M.L., and R.L. Wallace
  1973   "Problems in estimating multi-product cost functions: An application to hospitals." Western Economic Journal (September): 350–363.
Newhouse, J.P.
  1970   "Toward a theory of nonprofit institutions: An economic model of a hospital." American Economic Review 60 (March): 64–74.
  1974   "A design for a health insurance experiment." Inquiry 11 (March): 5–27.
Pauly, M., and M. Redisch
  1973   "The not-for-profit hospital as a physicians' cooperative." American Economic Review 63 (March): 87–99.
Phelps, C., and J. Newhouse
  1972   "Coinsurance and the demand for medical services." Santa Monica, Calif.: RAND Publications R-964-OEO. May.
Rafferty, J.A.
  1972   "Hospital output indices." Economic and Business Bulletin (Winter): 21–27.
Rosenthal, G.
  1970   "Price elasticity of demand for short-term general hospital services." Pp. 101–117 in H. Klarman, ed. Empirical Studies in Health Economics. Baltimore: The Johns Hopkins Press.
Rosett, R., and L. Huang
  1973   "The effect of health insurance on the demand for medical care." Journal of Political Economy 81 (March–April): 281–305.
Ross, S.
  1973   "The economic theory of agency: The principal's problem." American Economic Review 63 (May): 134–139.

Inflation and Hospital Capital Investment
PAUL B. GINSBURG

Cochrane, A.L.
    1972   Effectiveness and Efficiency. London: Nuffield Provincial Hospital Trust.

Davis, K., and R. Foster
    1973   Community Hospitals: Inflation in the Pre-Medicare Period. Social Security Administration, Research Report No. 41. Washington, D.C.: Government Printing Office.

Dowling, W.L.
    1974   "Prospective reimbursement of hospitals." Inquiry 11 (September): 163–180.

Feldstein, M.
    1971   "A new approach to national health insurance." The Public Interest 23 (Spring): 93–105.
    1973   "The welfare loss of excess health insurance." Journal of Political Economy 81 (March/April, part 1): 251–280.

Ginsburg, P.B.
    1972   "Resource allocation in the hospital industry: The role of capital financing." Social Security Bulletin (October): 20–30.

Havighurst, C., ed.
    1974   Regulating Health Facilities Construction. Washington, D.C.: American Enterprise Institute.

Lave, L., and J. Lave
    1974   The Hospital Construction Act: An Evaluation of the Hill-Burton Program, 1948–1973. Washington, D.C.: American Enterprise Institute, Evaluative Studies 16.

Marine, D. and J. Henderson
    1974   "Trends in the financing of hospital construction." Hospitals, Journal of the American Hospital Association 48 (July 1): 56.

Newhouse, J., and V. Taylor
    1970   "The subsidy problem in hospital insurance." Journal of Business 43 (October): 452–456.

Index

443